MEDICINE
AND THE
ETHICS OF CARE

MEDICINE
AND THE
ETHICS OF CARE

Diana Fritz Cates and Paul Lauritzen
Editors

Georgetown University Press / Washington, D.C.

Georgetown University Press, Washington, D.C.
© 2001 by Georgetown University Press. All rights reserved.
Printed in the United States of America

10 9 8 7 6 5 4 3 2 1   2001

This volume is printed on acid-free offset book paper.

Library of Congress Cataloging-in-Publication Data

Cates, Diana Fritz.
    Medicine and the ethics of care / edited by Diana Fritz Cates and Paul
    Lauritzen.
        p. cm.
    Includes index.
    ISBN 0-87840-824-X (cloth : alk. paper)
    1. Medical ethics.   2. Feminism—Health aspects.   I. Lauritzen, Paul.
    II. Title.
    R725.3.C38   2001
    174′.2—dc21   00-061026

For
Julia Coffey Lauritzen

And in Memory of
Edward H. Fritz
(1927–1998)

CONTENTS

CONTRIBUTORS

Barbara Hilkert Andolsen is Helen Bennett McMurray Professor of Social Ethics at Monmouth University in West Long Branch, New Jersey.

Sidney Callahan, Ph.D., is an author and psychologist in Ardsley-on-Hudson, New York.

Paul F. Camenisch is Professor of Religious Studies, DePaul University, Chicago, Illinois.

Diana Fritz Cates is Associate Professor of Ethics in the School of Religion at the University of Iowa in Iowa City, Iowa.

Russell B. Connors, Jr., is Associate Professor of Theology at the College of St. Catherine in St. Paul, Minnesota.

Chris A. Franke is Professor of Theology at the College of St. Catherine in St. Paul, Minnesota.

Christine E. Gudorf is Professor of Religious Studies at Florida International University in Miami, Florida.

Paul Lauritzen is Chairperson, Department of Religious Studies, and Director, Program in Applied Ethics at John Carroll University in University Heights, Ohio.

John P. Reeder, Jr., is Professor of Religious Studies at Brown University in Providence, Rhode Island.

Ruth L. Smith is Associate Professor of Religion in the Humanities and Arts Department at Worcester Polytechnic Institute in Worcester, Massachusetts.

Edward Collins Vacek, S.J., is Professor of Christian Ethics at Weston Jesuit School of Theology in Cambridge, Massachusetts.

Laurie Zoloth is Associate Professor of Social Ethics and Chair of the Jewish Studies Program in the College of Humanities at San Francisco State University in San Francisco, California.

ACKNOWLEDGMENTS

The production of this volume was supported by a University of Iowa Arts and Humanities Initiative grant and a College of Liberal Arts Semester Assignment award. Much of my work was completed at the University of Iowa Obermann Center for Advanced Studies, which is directed by Jay Semel. I am grateful for the support of its staff. (Diana Fritz Cates)

Work on this volume was supported also by a George E. Grauel Faculty Fellowship from John Carroll University. I am grateful to the university for this award, and to Frederick Travis, Nick Baumgartner, and Sally Wertheim for their strong administrative support for my research over the years. Special thanks to Mary Jane Ponyik for her help in preparing the volume for publication. (Paul Lauritzen)

Introduction

Diana Fritz Cates and Paul Lauritzen

As recently as 1992, Hilde Lindemann Nelson could accurately report that "bioethics has largely bypassed feminist insight" and that "the standard works [of bioethics] have neither corrected for medicine's male bias, nor adopted feminist methodologies" (Nelson 1992, 8). Since that time, however, feminist approaches have made their way into mainstream biomedical ethics. For example, the fourth edition of the classic text *Principles of Biomedical Ethics* (Beauchamp and Childress 1994) was expanded to include a discussion of the ethics of care, and the chapters on justice and virtue are clearly informed by feminist reflection.[1] This may be the best known text in biomedical ethics to exhibit the transformative effects of feminist thought, but it is not the only one. There are a growing number of books that focus specifically on feminist biomedical ethics (Holmes and Purdy 1992; Mahowald 1993, 1998; Sherwin 1992; Tong 1997; Wolf 1996; and others). The journal literature reflects the same growing interest (Carse and Nelson 1996; Little 1998; Tong 1998; Walker 1993; and others).

Medicine and the Ethics of Care is intended to be a further contribution to this literature. Although it engages less explicitly in feminist criticism than some of the work just mentioned, this collection of essays is motivated and shaped by feminist ethical concerns. It is designed to clarify and extend the influence that feminist ethics in general and the ethics of care in particular exert on biomedical ethics. This volume is intended also to demonstrate some of what religious ethics can contribute to the ethics of medicine and of care. Few of the religious ethicists gathered here develop explicit theological interests in their essays, but most of them consider the meanings and requirements of care and justice in light of religious texts and traditions.

SITUATING THE ESSAYS

In order to introduce the following essays, it is necessary to locate them not only in relation to recent work in feminist biomedical ethics, but also more broadly in relation to some other conversations that have given shape to contemporary ethics. To begin with, the essays in this volume are informed by several decades of debate about standard modern Western philosophical accounts of moral agency and decision making. Taking aim primarily at Kantianism and utilitarianism, a variety of critics have questioned such features as the individualism, the universalism, the rationalism, and the act-centeredness of these ethical models. Some critics have questioned the way that these models represent persons as separate and independent centers of moral agency who ought to be unconstrained in their decision making by everything but their own rational powers (Keller 1986; Taylor 1989). Some have questioned the way that Kantianism and utilitarianism require persons to reason about moral matters from an objective and disinterested point of view, abstracting from the particulars of their identities and the requirements of their personal and communal relationships in order to judge what "anyone" ought to do in a given moral predicament (Benhabib 1992; Blum 1980, 1990; Sandel 1982). Others have also questioned the way that these models encourage persons who make moral assessments to focus on acts, and the rightness of acts, rather than on the persons who commit the acts and the stories within which their acts make sense (Hauerwas, Bondi, and Burrell 1977; MacIntyre 1981).

It is in the context of these and other debates about the modern moral self that the ethics of care first came into view, with the publication of Carol Gilligan's *In a Different Voice* (1982). Gilligan offers a critique of Lawrence Kohlberg's six-stage theory of moral development (Kohlberg 1981). According to Gilligan, there are two main problems with Kohlberg's theory. The first is that the theory is intended to be universally applicable; it is intended to help identify the stage of moral development reached by any given child. Yet it has its empirical basis in a study of 84 boys and no girls (Gilligan 1982, 18). When Kohlberg's theory is used to measure girls' development, girls appear as a group to be morally less mature than boys. Gilligan argues that it is unfair to measure girls according to a male-defined standard. Girls tend to have their own patterns of moral development, which Gilligan seeks to elucidate.

A second and deeper problem is that Kohlberg's psychological theory has philosophical roots in a modern Western conception of the self and morality. This has become increasingly clear to Kohlberg's critics (Blum 1993; Crysdale 1994; Friedman 1987; Flanagan and Jackson 1993; Gilligan 1987; Kohlberg 1984; Larrabee 1993). Kohlberg thinks of moral development as a process of separation and individuation by which one becomes capable of thinking impersonally, impartially, and universally about moral dilemmas, in terms of rights, duties, and the "primacy of justice" (Flanagan and Jackson 1993, 79, 81). He has observed in many male subjects a tendency to subordinate personal relationships to rules (his stage four) and rules to universal principles of justice (his stages five and six) (Gilligan 1982, 18). However, it is the moral theory that he brings to his investigations that allows him to conclude that children who exhibit these tendencies are more advanced morally than those who focus in their decision making on, say, information provided by emotions or the requirements of particular relationships.

When one studies girls with the awareness that "the moral point of view" need not be defined ahead of time as an impartial perspective focused on the fair adjudication of competing rights, then something interesting occurs. As Gilligan observes,

> the outline of a moral conception different from that described by Freud, Piaget, or Kohlberg begins to emerge and informs a different description of development. In this conception, the moral problem arises from conflicting responsibilities rather than from competing rights and requires for its resolution a mode of thinking that is contextual and narrative rather than formal and abstract. This conception of morality as concerned with the activity of care centers moral development around the understanding of responsibility and relationships, just as the conception of morality as fairness ties moral development to the understanding of rights and rules. (Gilligan 1982, 19)

The idea of an ethic of care was thus originally used by Gilligan to characterize the distinctive voice that she heard in her research on the moral development of girls and women.

As a research psychologist, Gilligan has left most of the psychological work of developing an ethic of care to others. One writer who made an early attempt is Nel Noddings. Noddings' book, *Caring*, opens with a passage that Gilligan easily could have written. "One might say," Noddings begins, "that ethics has been discussed largely in the language of the father: in principles and propositions, in terms such as justification, fairness, justice. The mother's voice has been silent" (Noddings 1984, 1). Like Gilligan, Noddings wishes to identify and make more audible the voice of care, which gives expression to the moral insights of many girls and women.

For Noddings, an ethic of care is distinct from an ethic of justice or principles in several significant respects. We can mention only some of these.

An ethic of principles is ordinarily associated with individualistic conceptions of the self. Persons who adhere to an ethic of principles imagine that they stand alone before the court of their own impartial reason, and that this is the best position from which to survey their moral obligations toward others. An ethic of care, on the other hand, is rooted in a conception of the self as fundamentally relational. Persons who adhere to an ethic of care imagine that they become who they are in and through processes of caring and being cared for, and that it is within contexts of mutual care that they are best suited to reflect on their moral responsibilities toward others (Noddings 1984, 49–51). An ethic of principles is motivated by reverence for the universal moral law, whereas an ethic of care is motivated by an emotion-laden longing to "remain in the caring relation and to enhance the ideal of ourselves as one-caring" (5). An ethic of principles tends to regard emotions as distorting influences that constrain the ability to determine what any rational being ought to do in a given situation. An ethic of care regards emotional engrossment in the lives of others as basic to discerning what we ought to do on their behalf (19). An ethic of principles is primarily concerned with the form of moral reasoning, and it tends to construe moral reasoning as a kind of mathematical problem solving (1). An ethic of care is concerned with discerning what is needed by particular persons in particular contexts. "We do not begin by formulating or solving a problem," says Noddings, "but by sharing a feeling. Even when we move into the problem identification stage, we try to retain alternative phases of receptivity" (31). There are other ways that Noddings distinguishes an ethic of care from an ethic of principles, but this is enough to indicate the significance of the shift.

Several feminists and other moral theorists have responded critically, on several different fronts, to Noddings' "feminine" construction of an ethic of care (Cates 1997; Gudorf 1994; Hoagland 1991; Lauritzen 1989; Tronto 1993). Many have sought independently to develop more feminist critical ethics of care and justice (Held 1993; Jaggar 1989; Kittay and Meyers 1987; Mullet 1988; Okin 1989; Tronto 1993). Related movements in moral philosophy and religious ethics have contributed to these developments. Most notable is the recent resurgence in Aristotelian and other classical approaches to ethics. This resurgence is significant for many reasons; we can mention only some that are particularly relevant to this volume. An Aristotelian approach takes moral selves to be constituted in and through ongoing relationships with other selves, especially friends; hence, a critical retrieval of Aristotle can provide a way past individualistic conceptions of the self (Blum 1980; Groenhout 1998; MacIntyre 1981; Sherman 1989). In addition, Aristotle's ethic provides a well-developed theoretical framework within which to analyze care as a virtue or as an emotion that can and ought to be ordered by virtue: it provides a theory of virtue, a theory of emotion, and a theory of the cultivation of virtuous emotion (Rorty 1980a; Sherman 1989). Aristotle's ethic also provides a framework within which to understand care and justice as related virtues, so that we are not compelled to associate care with virtue or emotion and justice with an affect-less obedience to abstract moral principles (Nussbaum 1993). An Aristotelian approach has a place for moral principles, but it de-emphasizes their use and places greater importance on context-sensitive discernment of what is at issue morally in a given situation (Blum 1994). An Aristotelian approach construes practical reason as a power that functions partly through the work of perception and emotion, so it can help us overcome reason-emotion dichotomies (Nussbaum 1986, 1994). Although feminist reconstructions of Aristotle may provide the most promise for the ethics of care, feminist reconstructions of Hume and Kant are also notable (Baier 1987, 1993; Lind 1990; O'Neill 1996; Sherman 1990).

Within religious ethics, there has been a parallel resurgence in the ethics of St. Thomas Aquinas. Like Aristotle, Thomas conceives of persons as being fundamentally relational creatures. As a Christian, however, Thomas holds that humans function best when they enjoy a certain kind of relationship with God, as well as with other human beings. Thomas conceives of rightly ordered relationships with God and with others in terms of love and friendship, which suggests strong analogies to relationships of care. There is an immense and diverse literature within Christian ethics that addresses love as a power that calls humans into being, heals their brokenness, and transforms their moral characters and communities. Not all of this is written in a Thomistic vein, but all of it is influenced by Thomistic studies (Harak 1993; Hauerwas and Pinches 1997; Heyward 1982, 1989; Johann 1966; Wadell 1991; and others). Several of the authors in this volume situate their accounts of care, implicitly if not explicitly, in relation to an account of Christian love. This involves them in many overlapping debates, including debates about the relationship between love and justice—between love for persons near and dear and love for persons as such, and between both of these forms of love and the requirements of social justice (Andolsen 1994; Judish 1998; Meilander 1981; Outka 1972; Reeder 1998; Santurri and Werpehowski 1992). It involves them in debates about the relationship between love and justice as virtues and love and justice as moral principles, and more broadly, debates about the role of principles in the moral life (DuBose, Hamel, and O'Connell 1994).

Like Aristotle, Thomas also provides his readers with full-blown accounts of human action, emotion, and the virtues that order both action and emotion (Harak 1993; McInerny 1992; Porter 1990, 1992; Westberg 1994). A feminist critical retrieval of Thomas can thus provide theoretical grounding for contemporary accounts of friendship, love, compassion, or care (Cates 1997; Vacek 1994; Wadell 1989). Because Thomas conceives of the person who loves as a soul-body composite, a Thomistic approach can also account for the embodiment of care. It can account, for example, for the way that care disposes us to experience certain bodily changes at the perception of persons in pain; for the way that bodily care sustains us as caring persons; and for the way that care moves us to tend to the bodies of others (Harak 1993, 1996). It can also expose the need to order virtuously the distribution of the burdens and benefits of bodily care (Andolsen 1985; Reeder 1998). Scholars are only beginning to unpack the significance that these and other developments in the ethics of virtue may have for the ethics of medicine and biomedical research (Cahill and Farley 1995; Drane 1994; Kilner, Orr, and Shelly 1998; McKenny and Sande 1994; Pellegrino 1985; Pellegrino and Thomasma 1996; Phillips and Benner 1994).

Other related movements that provide some of the context for the work in this volume include those in the philosophy of mind, specifically the philosophy of emotion, and in moral psychology, which straddles the fields of normative ethics and empirical psychology (Flanagan and Rorty 1990, 1). Theorists of emotion seek to elucidate the sorts of things that emotions are compared to other psychological states (Calhoun and Solomon 1984; de Sousa 1987; Oakley 1992; Rorty 1980b). In this way, they help to define what care is—whether an emotion, an attitude, a disposition, an action, or something else—so that we know what we mean when we use the term. Theorists of emotion also help clarify the relation between emotion and knowledge, which is particularly important for an ethic of care, given the tendency in adherents like Noddings to characterize care as both "feminine" and "essentially nonrational" (Jaggar 1989; Lauritzen 1998; Noddings 1984, 25; Stocker and Hegeman 1996). They also help to clarify the role that emotions play in moral decision making (Callahan 1995). Because these theorists have one foot in the field of psychology, they are able to articulate moral ideals that reflect "knowledge of the basic architecture of the mind, core emotions, patterns of development, social psychology, and the limits on our capacities for rational deliberation" (Flanagan and Rorty 1990, 1).

In this way, they help ethicists to conceive realistic ideals of caring and being cared for (Flanagan 1991).

The focus within the ethics of virtue on understanding and shaping the many dimensions of moral character is connected to a conception of persons as characters who are embedded within personal and communal narratives. There has been a recent explosion of interdisciplinary inquiries that explore the relationship between ethics and literature. These inquiries range from investigations into narrative as the necessary form of our understanding of human beings and their actions (Charon 1994; Crites 1971; Hauerwas 1977; Lauritzen 1996; MacIntyre 1981; Walker 1989), to studies of literature as means for moral education (Booth 1988; Cates 1998; Eldridge 1989; Lauritzen 1994; Nussbaum 1990). These inquires also range from personal story-telling offered as a mode of moral reasoning and persuasion, particularly within the arena of medical ethics (Charon et al. 1996; Hawkins 1999; Kilner, Orr, and Shelly 1998; Montello 1995; Phillips and Benner 1994; Reich 1991), to studies of the literary structure of medical knowledge (Chambers 1996; Hunter 1991, 1996).[2] The ethics of medical care will likely be enhanced by further investigations into the ways that "textual analysis, literary theory, and the reading and writing of literature can contribute . . . to an understanding of how we recognize and deal with ethical issues in medicine" (Clouser and Hawkins 1996, 239).

Finally, nearly all of the inquiries that we have mentioned take place in both feminist and more traditional philosophical and theological modes. A feminist ethic of care emerges within the context of several decades of debate in feminist philosophy, theology, religious studies, and ethics. Ethicists who are committed to the liberation of all women from sexism and other related forms of oppression continue to critique various traditional teachings and practices. More than ever, they are extending their critiques into the medical arena and exposing ways that relationships among medical professionals and other care providers, relationships between providers and patients, modes of providing patient care and performing medical research, and so on, ignore or misunderstand women, and as a consequence diminish women's well-being, injuring different women in different ways (Andolsen 1993; Farley 1985, 1995; Gudorf 1994; Lebacqz 1991; Sanders 1994; Sherwin 1996; Wheeler 1998). In addition to offering critique, liberation ethicists offer constructive arguments that are presently redefining biomedical ethics to reflect the interests and experiences of diverse women (Lauritzen 1995; Lebacqz 1995; O'Connor 1995; Roberts 1996; Sanders 1995; Tong 1996; Townes 1998).

It is exciting and perhaps daunting to realize that the ethics of care, particularly as it pertains to the ethics of medicine, is not only situated within these and many other converging conversations, but also has all of these resources at its disposal. The most helpful scholarship in medical ethics will draw upon and contribute to these resources. The essays in this volume are distinguished by the way that they reveal the powerful insights into the ethics of care and medicine that can be reached through concerted work in philosophy, empirical psychology, religious studies, literary studies, women's studies, education, and other fields once considered disparate.

INTRODUCING THE ESSAYS

Given the variety of conversations that inform the chapters in this volume, it would be possible to order the chapters in any number of ways. We have chosen to highlight three of the themes that recur repeatedly in discussions of the ethics of care, namely, those of community, emotion, and narrative. Ongoing critical reflection upon these themes is essential to the development of an ethic of medical care. Our volume is, accordingly, divided into three parts, which track these themes in overlapping and intersecting ways.

Part one is titled "Care, Justice, and Community." The chapters in this section attend to the problem of framing the relationship between care and justice. It is not enough to say that care highlights community, emotion, and narrative, whereas justice emphasizes individualism, rational argumentation, and abstract cases. The relationship between care and justice is much subtler. We begin, therefore, with an essay by John P. Reeder, Jr. that reflects critically on justice and care as moral concepts or virtues. Reeder notes that justice and care are commonly thought to address different problems and involve distinct moral considerations. Justice, some say, addresses the problem of the distribution of resources and is associated with the language of fairness, consistency, and rights. By contrast, care addresses the importance of being properly attached to the good of self and other and speaks the language of need and responsibility. According to Reeder, although it is true that justice and care are distinct virtues, to say that justice and care address different problems and do so in fundamentally different vocabularies is mistaken. Reeder analyzes several possible positions in the justice/care debate, and he indicates how construing justice and care as distinct but overlapping virtues can help us articulate the complexity of the moral considerations that enter into good medical ethical decision making.

The complexity of the relationship between care and justice is further elaborated by Barbara Hilkert Andolsen in the second chapter of part one.

Writing about the appropriation of an ethic of care within the nursing profession, Andolsen explains both why an ethic of care is attractive to nurses seeking to articulate their professional moral responsibilities, and why an ethic of care takes us beyond most discussions of nursing ethics. An ethic of care is attractive because its vocabulary allows nurses to capture the sense of obligation that they feel toward many of the persons in their charge. It is not surprising that most discussions of the relevance of care ethics to nursing have focused on the nurse-patient relationship.

At the same time, however, attending to the needs of patients and how those needs are met necessarily takes us beyond the merely personal interaction between nurses and patients. As Andolsen demonstrates, care, justice, and community are all inextricably connected. Although it is true that individual nurses care for individual patients, the nurses provide that care within an institutional context that shapes in decisive ways how care is delivered. Thus, attending to the needs of particular others leads us beyond the personal interaction between nurse and patient to the social or communal context in which that interaction is located. Care leads us to concerns about social justice. We must consider whether certain institutional structures support unjust relationships between health care providers and persons in need, but also whether these structures support unjust relationships among providers themselves. When we ask about the relationships among providers, we run up against the decidedly social and communal questions of class and racial discrimination.

The first two chapters of part one begin to delineate theoretically the web of relationships that exist between care, justice, and community. The third chapter in this first group of essays, written by Christine Gudorf, examines these relationships in more detail and with reference to a particular case. Like Reeder and Andolsen, Gudorf wants to articulate the separate but interdependent status that care has relative to justice. Her chapter thus completes part one because it attends to the similarities and differences in the virtues of justice and care. At the same time, Gudorf's chapter points to parts two and three of the volume because her analysis unfolds through the story of her son's battle with Guillain-Barre Syndrome. Her decision to instruct through narrative, as well as her willingness to allow her emotional engagement with her son's story to inform the lessons that she draws, foreshadow the themes explored later in the volume.

Gudorf narrates the story of her son's treatment, and she reflects on how the different ethical approaches that were exhibited by his medical care providers affected that treatment. She describes, for example, how "principlist" physicians initially refused to give pain medication to her son through an IV or intramuscularly because the general rule is that, in long-term care, pain medication should be delivered through feeding tubes. The fact that this treatment complicated the management of her son's nutritional needs was obscured by a commitment to the general rule. As Gudorf notes, the doctors relented in their rule-bound treatment only after a crisis. Gudorf's reflections show the need for integrating care ethics into the principled provision of competent medical care.

Part two, "Care and Emotion," begins with a chapter by Edward Vacek that explores the centrality of emotion to the moral life generally and to medical care in particular. Vacek argues that emotions are cognitions that involve an openness to value and to the perception of particular values. For example, a parent's immediate experience of joy and wonder at his or her newborn child is a recognition of the preciousness of human life and of *this* human life. As intentional acts, emotions open persons up to objective values. Regrettably, emotions are frequently not treated as intentional, and they are mistakenly reduced to subjective psychological states. Sometimes the values apprehended by emotions are reduced to subjective choices, as if, for instance, the newborn child is precious because the parent values the child, and not because the child has objective value that is apprehended in the parent's emotional response. If we understand emotions properly, however, we see that they are modes of registering what is important in human life. Emotions are thus integral to determining what we ought to do to protect or enhance what is important.

Our habits of feeling emotion are learned. Sometimes these habits are mis-learned and must be re-learned. Vacek examines what is involved in the deliberate formation of persons' emotions. Taking the Christian community as an example, he argues that to the degree that Christians share a common ethos, it is because they read scriptural stories that elicit similar emotions and thereby sustain similar valuations. Vacek suggests that a similar strategy could be pursued among health care workers who might, for example, create a common ethos by sharing "their own set of horror and hero stories."

Vacek's defense of the importance of emotion to the provision of adequate health care is echoed in the second chapter of part two written by Sidney Callahan. Callahan draws extensively on the literature of psychology to explain the nature and function of emotions like care. This allows her to clarify the relationship between the emotion of care and the principles of bioethics. Far from supplanting the traditional principles of bioethics, Callahan shows caring to be an integral part of the project of understanding and adhering to these principles. According to Callahan, each midlevel principle of bioethics—beneficence, nonmaleficence, autonomy, and justice—embodies an "emotional prototype" of care. Thus, although we can distinguish these midlevel principles from care, "the emotion of care motivates, infuses, and informs" them.

Callahan also explores the implications that construing care as an emotion has for our thinking about the relationship between care and justice. For Callahan, care and justice are neither polar opposites nor complementary. Both involve reason and emotion; both involve a "reflexive, mutually interacting round of continuing thought and emotional response." Care and justice thus mutually interpenetrate, and each necessarily implies the other.

The last chapter of part two, by Diana Fritz Cates, moves from the theoretical considerations about the nature and role of the emotions found in the chapters by Vacek and Callahan to an exploration of the practical implications of taking emotions seriously in medical decision making. Her example is the decision to have an abortion. As with other medical decisions, informed consent is an important part of the decision to abort a fetus. But what precisely does informed consent involve? Asking that question in light of the work of writers like Vacek and Callahan leads us to see that providing an informed consent to an abortion may require reaching an embodied, emotional awareness of the seriousness of one's act. Careful attention to the stories of women who have had abortions reveals that emotions like grief and guilt can sometimes enhance women's understanding of what they are consenting to, and can therefore help them to consent in a more autonomous way.

Reflecting further on the meaning of informed consent, Cates considers the kind of autonomy that persons are generally expected to exhibit in providing consent. She compares the views of autonomy that appear in standard discussions of informed consent to a view that emerges from stories told by women who have made abortion decisions. By explaining the way in which many women are autonomous, yet at the same time relationally constituted and embedded, Cates seeks to move beyond an individualistic conception of autonomy toward a conception of "relational autonomy."

Part three, "Care and Narrative," begins with a chapter by Russell Connors and Chris Franke. They model the importance of narrative to an ethic of care by exploring several narratives of care, putting these narratives in conversation with each other, and considering the implications of their conversation for our thinking about good medical care. Connors and Franke explore the stories of God's interactions with persons in pain, in Psalm 23 and the Book of Job from the Hebrew Bible, and in the story of Lazarus from the New Testament. According to Connors and Franke, these narratives help us distinguish two approaches to medical care: one that emphasizes the centrality of curing illness, and one that emphasizes providing comfort in the face of possibly incurable illness. What all three Biblical narratives share is a view of God as Immanuel, God-with-us. To hear, and to share with others, stories about a god whose presence can comfort even in the darkest valley makes manifest that caring is not equivalent to curing, a point made more clear with Franke's discussion of her treatment for breast cancer.

Consider Connors' and Franke's reading of Job. Resisting the standard interpretation that Job is silenced into submission in the face of God's overwhelming power, Connors and Franke instead suggest that Job ceases to mourn for his losses because of the comforting way that God finally responds to his cries for help. Whether or not theirs is an adequate interpretation of the text, we see the fruitfulness of the effort to wrestle with a powerful and beautifully written story. As Connors and Franke struggle to understand the behavior of Job's friends, we come to see ourselves in them. We may, for example, come to see the ways we fail properly to care for those in need by seeing how Job's friends failed properly to care for him. What we see is that the most significant failure of care is when a person's suffering goes unrecognized and unresponded to.

Connors' and Franke's essay dovetails nicely with the next chapter, written by Paul Camenisch. Just as Chris Franke narrates the story of her treatment for breast cancer in order to gain insight into the nature of medical care, Camenisch tells the story of his emergency coronary by-pass surgery as a way of reflecting on the important concepts of healing, care, community, and trust. What both chapters demonstrate is that the careful sorting out of personal experience, partly through the construction of a narrative of that experience, is a means to better understanding the moral dimensions of medical care. Camenisch's call to understand healing in holistic terms is strikingly similar to Connors' and Franke's insistence that care not be reduced to cure. For all three, narratives of personal illness and recovery reveal the need to understand how illness may be a comprehensive threat to the very core of the self. In the face of such a threat, one needs more than good technical care, one needs what Camenisch describes as "communal presence." Although such support typically comes from friends and families, that is, from our personal communities, it can also come from medical professionals who, like Chris Franke's caregivers, deliver flowers to lift a flagging spirit.

If attending to narratives of illness and recovery demonstrate that caring must not be reduced to curing, then the story narrated by Laurie Zoloth in the third chapter of part three shows that even death does not put an end to the demands of care. Drawing on her experience as a member of a *chevra ḳadisha,* a group responsible for the ritual preparation of Jews for burial, Zoloth shows that the embodied work of preparing a lifeless body for burial is an act of profound care. In narrating the concrete details of this ritual, from the cleaning of fingernails to the brushing of hair, and in mining these details for ethical insight, Zoloth follows in a tradition of feminist ethics that makes the mundane the center of moral attention. In a sense, her focus on a ritual of death is the logical extension of work like that of Sara Ruddick (1989) and Caroline Whitbeck (1984), who explore the moral significance of childbirth and mothering. Zoloth's chapter reveals the important insights that can be gained by reflecting on the ordinary business of caring for humans. It also reveals the way that religious ritual can help participants embody these insights.

In addition, Zoloth's work illustrates a point that Martha Nussbaum has long insisted on, namely, that form and content are closely related. In Nussbaum's words, "Certain thoughts and ideas, a certain sense of life, reach toward expression in writing that has a certain shape and form, that uses certain structures, certain terms (Nussbaum 1990, 4). Although it is true that much of the substantive content that Zoloth conveys about the importance of embodied caring and equality in the face of death could perhaps be communicated in traditional philosophical prose, there is a power and a vividness to Zoloth's narrative that helps us not only to see but to feel the truth of what she says. Moreover, according to Zoloth, the very telling of the story in this particular form is potentially transformative; in her case, telling the story of the *chevra ḳadisha* was crucial to her understanding of Jewish bioethics. Thus, according to Zoloth, "narrative ethics is in part about how to pass on the truthful, and in part about how telling the truthful is a transformative act."

The book concludes with a chapter by Ruth Smith that expresses the significance of rhetorical-spatial transactions for the conduct of biomedical ethics. Smith notes that discussions of care frequently ignore the power relations that occur in the rhetorical spaces of care. Most work in ethics appears to occur in geometric space, a world apart from the tactile, auditory, and visual world in which ethics is actually transacted. Fortunately, there are narratives that force us out of the geometric space of conventional biomedical ethics and into the rhetorical landscape of sensate life. One such narrative is Abraham Verghese's account of his work as an infectious disease physician treating HIV/AIDS patients in rural Tennessee. Smith uses Verghese's book, *My Own Country*, to display the importance of place for medical ethics. As Smith notes, Verghese's medical practice confounds the geometric space of traditional bioethics because it is not confined to the usual institutional location of bioethics. Verghese visits his patients in their trailers; he goes to the local gay bar; he travels the country roads of rural Tennessee, all the while reflecting on his own sense of place. *My Own Country* is not easily recognizable as a work of bioethics, but Smith makes the case that it is one nonetheless.

Smith's point is "not only that spaces considered outside medical institutions are morally significant for medicine and ethics, but that spaces participate in behaviors and events." Ethics thus may have an improvisational quality that defies neat summation. When locating, responding, and listening are understood to be key to bioethics, ethics itself is reconstituted as an activity that is always located, always rhetorically structured in particular ways, and always in flux.

Taken together, the following essays extend or open up the boundaries of conventional biomedical ethics. Informed by many of the conversations highlighted in the first part of the introduction, these essays evoke significant changes in (or at least additions to) the way that biomedical ethics is conceived and done. These changes have the potential to make bioethics even more interesting than it already is. These changes also have the potential to improve the lives and work of medical professionals and their patients. The essays go beyond talking about the need to overcome individualistic, overly rationalistic, and act-centered constructions of moral selves. They exhibit what medical ethics becomes when medical professionals and their patients are seen as relational moral agents with complex emotional lives, who are informed by the stories of their professional, social, and personal communities, and are in need of help in extending these stories or constructing new ones that are true to their experiences of illness, helping, feeling helpless, recovering, and dying.

Endnotes

1. John Arras has commented that Beauchamp and Childress have revised the fourth edition so extensively in response to their critics that they could be considered the "Borg of bioethics," after the Star Trek characters, the Borg, who conquer by assimilating their enemies. See Arras (1997).

2. For discussion of various uses of narrative in bioethics, see Nelson (1997).

References

Andolsen, Barbara Hilkert. 1985. A Woman's Work is Never Done: Unpaid Household Labor as a Social Justice Issue. In *Women's Consciousness, Women's Conscience: A Reader in Feminist Ethics,* ed. Barbara Hilkert Andolsen, Christine E. Gudorf, and Mary D. Pellauer, 3–18. San Francisco: Harper and Row.

———. 1993. Justice, Gender, and the Frail Elderly: Reexamining the Ethic of Care. *Journal of Feminist Studies of Religion* 9 (spring/fall): 127–45.

———. 1994. Agape in Feminist Ethics. In *Feminist Theological Ethics: A Reader,* ed. Lois K. Daly, 146–59. Louisville, Ky.: Westminster John Knox Press.

Arras, John. 1997. Nice Story, But So What? Narrative and Justification in Ethics. In *Stories and Their Limits,* ed. Hilde Lindemann Nelson, 65–91. New York: Routledge.

Baier, Annette C. 1987. Hume, the Women's Moral Theorist? In *Women and Moral Theory,* ed. Eva Feder Kittay and Diana T. Meyers, 37–55. Totowa, N.J.: Rowman and Littlefield.

———. 1993. What Do Women Want in a Moral Theory? In *An Ethic of Care: Feminist and Interdisciplinary Perspectives,* ed. Mary Jeanne Larrabee, 19–31. New York and London: Routledge.

Beauchamp, Tom L., and James F. Childress. 1994. *Principles of Biomedical Ethics,* 4th ed. Oxford: Oxford University Press.

Benhabib, Seyla. 1992. *Situating the Self: Gender, Community and Postmodernism in Contemporary Ethics.* New York: Routledge.

Blum, Lawrence A. 1980. *Friendship, Altruism, and Morality.* London: Routledge and Kegan Paul.

———. 1990. Vocation, Friendship, and Community. In *Identity, Character, and Morality: Essays in Moral Psychology,* ed. Owen Flanagan and Amelie Oksenberg Rorty, 173–97. Cambridge, Mass.: MIT Press.

———. 1993. Gilligan and Kohlberg: Implications for Moral Theory. In *An Ethic of Care: Feminist and Interdisciplinary Perspectives,* ed. Mary Jeanne Larrabee, 49–68. New York: Routledge.

———. 1994. *Moral Perception and Particularity.* New York: Cambridge University Press.

Booth, Wayne. 1988. *The Company We Keep.* Berkeley: University of California Press.

Cahill, Lisa Sowle. 1995. "Embodiment" and Moral Critique: A Christian Social Perspective. In *Embodiment, Morality, and Medicine,* ed. Lisa Sowle Cahill and Margaret A. Farley, 199–215. Dordrecht, The Netherlands: Kluwer Academic Publishers.

Cahill, Lisa Sowle, and Margaret A. Farley, eds. 1995. *Embodiment, Morality, and Medicine*. Dordrecht, The Netherlands: Kluwer Academic Publishers.

Calhoun, Cheshire, and Robert Solomon, eds. 1984: *What is an Emotion? Classical Readings in Philosophical Psychology*. New York: Oxford University Press.

Callahan, Sidney. 1988. The Role of Emotion in Ethical Decisionmaking. *Hastings Center Report* (June/July): 9–14.

Carse, Alisa L. 1991. The "Voice of Care": Implications for Bioethical Education. *The Journal of Medicine and Philosophy* 16: 5–28.

Carse, Alisa L., and Hilde Lindemann Nelson. 1996. Rehabilitating Care. *Kennedy Institute of Ethics Journal* 6/1: 19–35.

Cates, Diana Fritz. 1997. *Choosing to Feel: Virtue, Friendship, and Compassion for Friends*. Notre Dame, Ind.: University of Notre Dame Press.

———. 1998. Ethics, Literature, and the Emotional Dimension of Moral Understanding. *Journal of Religious Ethics* 26/2 (fall): 409–31.

Chambers, Tod. 1996. From the Ethicist's Point of View: The Literary Nature of Ethical Inquiry. *Hastings Center Report* 26/1 (January-February): 25–32.

Charon, Rita. 1994. Narrative Contributions to Medical Ethics: Recognition, Formulation, Interpretation, and Validation in the Practice of the Ethicist. In *A Matter of Principles? Ferment in U.S. Bioethics*, ed. Edwin R. DuBose, Ronald P. Hamel, and Laurence J. O'Connell, 260–83. Valley Forge, Penn.: Trinity Press International.

Charon, Rita, Howard Brody, Mary Williams Clark, Dwight Davis, Richard Martinez, and Robert M. Nelson. 1996. Literature and Ethical Medicine: Five Cases from Common Practice. *The Journal of Medicine and Philosophy* 21 (June): 243–65.

Clouser, K. Danner, and Anne Hunsaker Hawkins. 1996. Literature and Medical Ethics. *The Journal of Medicine and Philosophy* 21 (June): 237–41.

Crites, Stephen. 1971. The Narrative Quality of Experience. *Journal of the American Academy of Religion* 39/3 (September): 291–311.

Crysdale, Cynthia. 1994. Gilligan and the Ethics of Care: An Update. *Religious Studies Review* 20/1 (January): 21–28.

de Sousa, Ronald. 1987. *The Rationality of Emotion*. Cambridge, Mass.: MIT Press.

Drane, James F. 1994. Character and the Moral Life: A Virtue Approach to Biomedical Ethics. In *A Matter of Principles? Ferment in U.S. Bioethics*, ed. Edwin R. DuBose, Ronald P. Hamel, and Laurence J. O'Connell, 284–309. Valley Forge, Penn.: Trinity Press International.

DuBose, Edwin R., Ronald P. Hamel, and Laurence J. O'Connell, eds. 1994. *A Matter of Principles? Ferment in U.S. Bioethics*. Valley Forge, Penn.: Trinity Press International.

Eldridge, Richard. 1989. *On Moral Personhood: Philosophy, Literature, Criticism, and Self-Understanding*. Chicago: University of Chicago Press.

Farley, Margaret. 1985. Feminist Theology and Bioethics. In *Women's Consciousness, Women's Conscience: A Reader in Feminist Ethics*, ed. Barbara Hilkert Andolsen, Christine E. Gudorf, and Mary D. Pellauer, 285–305. San Francisco: Harper and Row.

————. 1995. North American Bioethics: The Feminist Critique. In *Meta Medical Ethics: The Philosophical Foundations of Bioethics*, ed. Michael A. Grodin, 131–45. Dordrecht, The Netherlands: Kluwer Academic Publishers.

Flanagan, Owen. 1991. *Varieties of Moral Personality: Ethics and Psychological Realism*. Cambridge, Mass.: Harvard University Press.

Flanagan, Owen, and Amelie Oksenberg Rorty. 1990. Introduction. In *Identity, Character, and Morality: Essays in Moral Psychology*, ed. Owen Flanagan and Amelie Oksenberg Rorty, 1–15. Cambridge, Mass: MIT Press.

Flanagan, Owen, and Kathryn Jackson. 1993. Justice, Care, and Gender: The Kohlberg-Gilligan Debate Revisited. In *An Ethic of Care: Feminist and Interdisciplinary Perspectives*, ed. Mary Jeanne Larrabee, 69–83. New York: Routledge.

Friedman, Marilyn. 1987. Care and Context in Moral Reasoning. In *Women and Moral Theory*, ed. Eva Feder Kittay and Diana T. Meyers, 190–204. Totowa, N.J.: Rowman and Littlefield.

Gilligan, Carol. 1982. *In a Different Voice: Psychological Theory and Women's Development*. Cambridge, Mass.: Harvard University Press.

————. 1987. Moral Orientation and Moral Development. In *Women and Moral Theory*, ed. Eva Feder Kittay and Diana T. Meyers, 19–33. Totowa, N.J.: Rowman and Littlefield.

Groenhout, Ruth. 1998. The Virtue of Care: Aristotelian Ethics and Contemporary Ethics of Care. In *Feminist Interpretations of Aristotle*, ed. Cynthia Freeland, 171–200. University Park: Pennsylvania State University Press.

Gudorf, Christine E. 1994. A Feminist Critique of Biomedical Principlism. In *A Matter of Principles? Ferment in U.S. Bioethics*, ed. Edwin R. DuBose, Ronald P. Hamel, and Laurence J. O'Connell, 164–81. Valley Forge, Penn.: Trinity Press International.

Harak, G. Simon, S.J., ed. 1996. *Aquinas and Empowerment: Classical Ethics for Ordinary Lives*. Washington, D.C.: Georgetown University Press.

————. 1993. *Virtuous Passions: The Formation of Christian Character*. New York: Paulist Press.

Hauerwas, Stanley, and Charles Pinches. 1997. *Christians among the Virtues: Theological Conversations with Ancient and Modern Ethics*. Notre Dame, Ind.: University of Notre Dame Press.

Hauerwas, Stanley, with Richard Bondi, and David B. Burrell. 1977. *Truthfulness and Tragedy: Further Investigations in Christian Ethics*. Notre Dame, Ind.: University of Notre Dame Press.

Hawkins, Anne Hunsaker. 1999. *Reconstructing Illness: Studies in Pathography*. 2d ed. West Lafayette, Ind.: Purdue University Press.

Held, Virginia. 1993. *Feminist Morality: Transforming Culture, Society, and Politics*. Chicago: University of Chicago Press.

Heyward, Carter. 1982. *The Redemption of God: A Theology of Mutual Relation*. Lanham, Md.: University Press of America.

———. 1989. *Touching Our Strength: The Erotic as Power and the Love of God*. San Francisco: Harper and Row.

Hoagland, Sarah Lucia. 1991. Some Thoughts about "Caring." In *Feminist Ethics*, ed. Claudia Card, 246–63. Lawrence, Kans.: University Press of Kansas.

Holmes, Helen Bequaert, and Laura M. Purdy, eds. 1992. *Feminist Perspectives in Medical Ethics*. Bloomington: Indiana University Press.

Hunter, Kathryn Montgomery. 1991. *Doctors' Stories: The Narrative Structure of Medical Knowledge*. Princeton, N.J.: Princeton University Press.

———. 1996. Narrative, Literature, and the Clinical Exercise of Practical Reason. *The Journal of Medicine and Philosophy* 21 (June): 303–20.

Jaggar, Alison M. 1989. Love and Knowledge: Emotion in Feminist Epistemology. *Inquiry: An Interdisciplinary Journal of Philosophy* 32/2 (June): 151–76.

Johann, Robert O. 1966. *The Meaning of Love: An Essay Towards a Metaphysics of Intersubjectivity*. Glen Rock, N.J.: Paulist Press.

Judish, Julia E. 1998. Balancing Special Obligations with the Ideal of Agape. *Journal of Religious Ethics* 26/1 (spring): 17–46.

Keller, Catherine. 1986. *From a Broken Web: Separation, Sexism, and Self*. Boston: Beacon Press.

Kilner, John F., Robert D. Orr, and Judith Allen Shelly, eds. 1998. *The Changing Face of Health Care: A Christian Appraisal of Managed Care, Resource Allocation, and Patient-Caregiver Relationships*. Grand Rapids, Mich.: William B. Eerdmans.

Kittay, Eva Feder, and Diana T. Meyers, eds. 1987. *Women and Moral Theory*. Totowa, N.J.: Rowman & Littlefield.

Kohlberg, Lawrence. 1981. *The Philosophy of Moral Development*. San Francisco: Harper and Row.

———. 1984. *Essays on Moral Development. Volume II: The Psychology of Moral Development*. New York: Harper and Row.

Larrabee, Mary Jeanne, ed. 1993. *An Ethic of Care: Feminist and Interdisciplinary Perspectives*. New York: Routledge.

Lauritzen, Paul. 1989. A Feminist Ethic and the New Romanticism—Mothering as a Model of Moral Relations. *Hypatia* 4/2 (summer): 29–43.

———. 1994. Listening to the Different Voices: Toward a More Poetic Bioethics. In *Theological Analyses of the Clinical Encounter*, ed. Gerald P. McKenny and Jonathan R. Sande, 151–70. Dordrecht, The Netherlands: Kluwer Academic Publishers.

———. 1995. Whose Bodies? Which Selves? Appeals to Embodiment in Assessments of Reproductive Technology. In *Embodiment, Morality, and Medicine*, ed. Lisa Sowle Cahill and Margaret A. Farley, 113–26. Dordrecht, The Netherlands: Kluwer Academic Publishers.

———. 1996. Ethics and Experience: The Case of the Curious Response. *Hastings Center Report* 26/1 (January-February): 6–15.

———. 1998. The Knowing Heart: Moral Argument and the Appeal to Experience. *Soundings* 81/1–2: 213–34.

Lebacqz, Karen. 1991. Feminism and Bioethics: An Overview. *Second Opinion* 17/2 (October): 11–25.

———. 1995. The "Fridge": Health Care and the Disembodiment of Women. In *Embodiment, Morality, and Medicine*, ed. Lisa Sowle Cahill and Margaret A. Farley, 155–67. Dordrecht, The Netherlands: Kluwer Academic Publishers.

Lind, Marcia. 1990. Hume and Moral Emotions. In *Identity, Character, and Morality: Essays in Moral Psychology*, ed. Owen Flanagan and Amelie Oksenberg Rorty, 133–47. Cambridge, Mass.: MIT Press.

Little, Margaret. 1998. Care: From Theory to Orientation and Back. *Journal of Medicine and Philosophy* 23/2 (April): 190–209.

McInerny, Ralph M. 1992. *Aquinas on Human Action: A Theory of Practice*. Washington, D.C.: Catholic University of America Press.

MacIntyre, Alasdair. 1981. *After Virtue: A Study in Moral Theory*. Notre Dame, Ind.: University of Notre Dame Press.

Mahowald, Mary. 1993. *Women and Children in Health Care: An Unequal Majority*. New York: Oxford University Press.

———. 1998. *Disability, Difference, Discrimination: Perspectives on Justice in Bioethics and Public Policy*. Lanham, Md.: Rowman and Littlefield.

Meilander, Gilbert C. 1981. *Friendship: A Study in Theological Ethics*. Notre Dame, Ind.: University of Notre Dame Press.

McKenny, Gerald P., and Jonathan R. Sande, eds. 1994. *Theological Analysis of the Clinical Encounter*. Dordrecht, The Netherlands: Kluwer Academic Publishers.

Montello, Martha. 1995. Medical Stories: Narrative and Phenomenological Approaches. In *Meta Medical Ethics: The Philosophical Foundations of Bioethics*, ed. Michael A. Grodin, 109–23. Dordrecht, The Netherlands: Kluwer Academic Publishers.

Mullett, Sheila. 1988. Shifting Perspective: A New Approach to Ethics. In *Feminist Perspectives: Philosophical Essays on Method and Morals,* ed. Lorraine Code, Sheila Mullett, and Christine Overall, 109–26. Toronto: University of Toronto Press.

Nelson, Hilde Lindemann. 1992. Against Caring. *Journal of Clinical Ethics* 3/1 (spring): 8–15.

————. 1995. *The Patient in the Family: An Ethics of Medicine and Families*. New York: Routledge.

————. 1997. *Stories and Their Limits: Narrative Approaches to Bioethics*. New York: Routledge.

Noddings, Nel. 1984. *Caring: A Feminine Approach to Ethics and Moral Education*. Berkeley: University of California Press.

Nussbaum, Martha C. 1986. *The Fragility of Goodness: Luck and Ethics in Greek Tragedy and Philosophy*. New York: Cambridge University Press.

————. 1990. *Love's Knowledge: Essays on Philosophy and Literature*. Oxford, U.K.: Oxford University Press.

————. 1993. Equity and Mercy. *Philosophy and Public Affairs* 22 (spring): 83–125.

————. 1994. *The Therapy of Desire: Theory and Practice in Hellenistic Ethics*. Princeton, N.J.: Princeton University Press.

Oakley, Justin. 1992. *Morality and the Emotions*. London: Routledge.

O'Connor, June. 1995. Ritual Recognition of Abortion: Japanese Buddhist Practices and U.S. Jewish and Christian Proposals. In *Embodiment, Morality, and Medicine*, ed. Lisa Sowle Cahill and Margaret A. Farley, 93–111. Dordrecht, The Netherlands: Kluwer Academic Publishers.

Okin, Susan Moller. 1989. *Justice, Gender, and the Family*. New York: Basic Books.

O'Neill, Onora. 1996. Kant's Virtues. In *How Should One Live? Essays on the Virtues*, ed. Roger Crisp, 77–97. Oxford, U.K.: Clarendon Press.

Outka, Gene. 1972. *Agape: An Ethical Analysis*. New Haven, Conn.: Yale University Press.

Pellegrino, Edmund D. 1985. The Caring Ethic: The Relation of Physician to Patient. In *Caring, Curing, Coping: Nurse, Physician, Patient Relationships*, ed. Anne Bishop and John Scudder, Jr., 8–30. University: University of Alabama Press.

Pellegrino, Edmund D., and David C. Thomasma. 1996. *The Christian Virtues in Medical Practice*. Washington, D.C.: Georgetown University Press.

Phillips, Susan S., and Patricia Benner, eds. 1994, *The Crisis of Care: Affirming and Restoring Caring Practices in the Helping Professions*. Washington, D.C.: Georgetown University Press.

Porter, Jean. 1990. *The Recovery of Virtue: The Relevance of Aquinas for Christian Ethics*. Louisville, Ky.: Westminster/John Knox Press.

————. 1992. The Subversion of Virtue: Acquired and Infused Virtues in the *Summa Theologiae*. In *The Annual of the Society of Christian Ethics*, ed. Harlan Beckley, 19–41. Washington, D.C.: Georgetown University Press.

Reeder, John P., Jr. 1998. Extensive Benevolence. *Journal of Religious Ethics* 26/1 (spring): 47–70.

Reich, Warren Thomas. 1991. The Case: Denny's Story. Commentary: Caring as Extraordinary Means. *Second Opinion* 17/1 (July): 41–56.

Roberts, Dorothy E. 1996. Reconstructing the Patient: Starting with Women of Color. In *Feminism and Bioethics: Beyond Reproduction*, ed. Susan M. Wolf, 116–43. New York: Oxford University Press.

Rorty, Amelie Oksenberg, ed. 1980a. *Essays on Aristotle's Ethics*. Berkeley: University of California Press.

———, ed. 1980b. *Explaining Emotions*. Berkeley: University of California Press.

Ruddick, Sara. 1989. *Maternal thinking: Toward a Politics of Peace*. Boston: Beacon Press.

Sandel, Michael J. 1982. *Liberalism and the Limits of Justice*. Cambridge, U.K.: Cambridge University Press.

Sanders, Cheryl J. 1994. European-American Ethos and Principlism: An African-American Challenge. In *A Matter of Principles? Ferment in U.S. Bioethics*, ed. Edwin R. DuBose, Ronald P. Hamel, and Laurence J. O'Connell, 148–63. Valley Forge, Penn.: Trinity Press International.

———. 1995. African Americans and Organ Donation: Reflections on Religion, Ethics and Embodiment. In *Embodiment, Morality, and Medicine*, ed. Lisa Sowle Cahill and Margaret A. Farley, 141–54. Dordrecht, The Netherlands: Kluwer Academic Publishers.

Santurri, Edmund, and William Werpehowski, eds. 1992. *The Love Commandments: Essays in Christian Ethics and Moral Philosophy*. Washington, D.C.: Georgetown University Press.

Sherman, Nancy. 1989. *The Fabric of Character: Aristotle's Theory of Virtue*. Oxford, U.K.: Clarendon Press.

———. 1990. The Place of Emotions in Kantian Morality. In *Identity, Character, and Morality: Essays in Moral Psychology*, ed. Owen Flanagan and Amelie Oksenberg Rorty, 149–70. Cambridge, Mass: MIT Press.

Sherwin, Susan. 1992. *No Longer Patient: Feminist Ethics and Health Care*. Philadelphia, Penn.: Temple University Press.

———. 1996. Feminism and Bioethics. In *Feminism and Bioethics: Beyond Reproduction*, ed. Susan M. Wolf, 47–66. New York: Oxford University Press.

Stocker, Michael, with Elizabeth Hegeman. 1996. *Valuing Emotions*. Cambridge, U.K.: Cambridge University Press.

Taylor, Charles. 1989. *Sources of the Self: The Making of the Modern Identity*. Cambridge, Mass.: Harvard University Press.

Tong, Rosemarie. 1996. Feminist Approaches to Bioethics. In *Feminism and Bioethics: Beyond Reproduction,* ed. Susan M. Wolf, 67–94. New York: Oxford University Press.

———. 1997. *Feminist Approaches to Bioethics: Theoretical Reflections and Practical Applications*. Boulder, Colo.: Westview Press.

————. 1998. The Ethics of Care: A Feminist Virtue Ethics of Care for Healthcare Practitioners. *Journal of Medicine and Philosophy* 23/2 (April): 131–52.

Townes, Emilie. 1998. *Breaking the Fine Rain of Death: African American Health Issues and a Womanist Ethic of Care*. New York: Continuum.

Tronto, Joan C. 1993. *Moral Boundaries: A Political Argument for an Ethic of Care*. New York: Routledge.

Vacek, Edward Collings, S.J. 1994. *Love, Human and Divine: The Heart of Christian Ethics*. Washington, D.C.: Georgetown University Press.

Wadell, Paul. 1989. *Friendship and the Moral Life*. Notre Dame, Ind.: University of Notre Dame Press.

————. 1991. *Friends of God: Virtues and Gifts in Aquinas*. New York: Peter Lang.

Walker, Margaret Urban. 1989. Moral Understandings: Alternative "Epistemology" for a Feminist Ethics. *Hypatia* 4/2 (summer): 15–28.

————. 1993. Keeping Moral Space Open: New Images of Ethics Consulting. *Hastings Center Report* 23:33–40.

Westberg, Daniel. 1994. *Right Practical Reason: Aristotle, Action, and Prudence in Aquinas*. Oxford: Clarendon Press.

Wheeler, Sondra Ely. 1998. Broadening Our View of Justice in Health Care. In *The Changing Face of Health Care: A Christian Appraisal of Managed Care, Resource Allocation, and Patient-Caregiver Relationships*, ed. John F. Kilner, Robert D. Orr, and Judith Allen Shelly, 63–73. Grand Rapids, Mich.: William B. Eerdmans.

Whitbeck, Carolyn. 1984. The Maternal Instinct. In *Mothering: Essays in Feminist Theory*, ed. Joyce Trebilcot. Totowa, N.J.: Rowman and Allanheld.

Wolf, Susan M., ed. *Feminism and Bioethics: Beyond Reproduction*. New York: Oxford University Press.

PART I

CARE, JUSTICE, AND COMMUNITY

1

Are Care and Justice Distinct Virtues?

John P. Reeder, Jr.

The relation of justice and love is one of the enduring questions in Western thought, especially in Christian traditions. One thinks immediately of Reinhold Niebuhr, for example, who argued that justice pertains to conflicts of interest within "history," whereas love as the ultimate moral ideal can only be realized in the Kingdom of God "beyond history." One thinks also of Carol Gilligan's more recent thesis that the moral "domain" is not only comprised of justice and rights, but also of the voice of "care." Care, construed as an affective attachment to the good of self and other, is a dimension of moral experience that is not reducible to considerations of justice; we simply bring both nonintegratable perspectives to bear on moral questions.

Much has been written on Niebuhr and other figures in the Christian tradition (see Outka 1972); Gilligan's thesis (1982) has also generated an impressive literature. But what is the relation of these two pivotal figures and the interpretations and debates that they have generated? One answer might be that they have little in common. Their concerns are very different, one might say, although the terminology they use is in some respects similar. Niebuhr (1956 [1935]) inherited a certain picture of the sacrificial love (*agape*) of the founding figure of his religious tradition; his problem was how to relate heedless, self-giving devotion to others to the historical struggles of self-interested individuals and groups. Thus he develops a vertical model of the relation of love and justice: love is the ultimate moral ideal, of which justice is an "approximation" within the conditions of history. Love both grounds and transcends justice. Gilligan's problematic seems very different. Her research on the psychology of moral development reveals that males tend to use the justice perspective, whereas females tend to think and speak in the voice of care. Although the two perspectives are available to and appear in both sexes, Gilligan argues that due to certain forms of early child care and social conditioning the two moral perspectives seem to be correlated with gender roles. Gilligan, in order to retrieve care from its place as a marginalized expression of women's experience, posits a horizontal model of the two categories: justice and care are independent and irreducible dimensions of the moral life.

Thus one might argue that despite some superficial terminological resemblances, the underlying concerns in debates around Niebuhr and Gilligan are simply different. Although traditions may overlap to some extent about justice, agapistic "love" is not really similar to "care." For Gilligan, self-sacrificing care for others is only a stage that reflects the social ideal of the nurturing mother; care in its full development extends to love of self. Moreover, Christian theological accounts have a source—the imitation of Christ—that is absent from Gilligan's view that morality is a natural expression of two primordial features of human experience, namely, the struggle for equality and autonomy (justice) and the vulnerability to loss of attachment (care). We should not conflate debates in two very different traditions.

I am sympathetic to the thesis that Niebuhr and Gilligan (and those who follow them) had very different concerns. I also agree that terms such as "justice" and "love" can be given various senses in order to debate certain issues within particular traditions. I will assume, however, that there is more in common between these debates than meets the eye. Although I readily acknowledge that conceptions of love and care can be formulated so that they differ from one another (and from other categories such as benevolence), and that diverse meanings of justice abound, I presently hold the view that these represent two families of moral considerations: one takes shape in conceptions such as justice, rights, autonomy, and equality; the other is expressed in notions such as care, love, benevolence, and compassion. These families are interpreted and related in various traditions in various ways, given broader assumptions about human nature and moral experience. I want to stand against the thesis that the worlds of theological ethics and Gilligan are constructions of moral experience that have very little if anything in common. I want to uphold a view that asserts that there are surprising unities in human experience, without denying that they are shaped in decisive ways in different traditions. I want to shape a view of the relation of love or care and justice that moves away from Niebuhr's model toward Gilligan's, but which leaves open the possibility of a theological interpretation.

For some years now, there has been a lively discussion of the significance of Gilligan's views with regard to morality in general and biomedical ethics in particular (see, e.g., Carse 1991; Kuhse 1997). More generally, there has been an interest in bringing concepts other than justice and rights to bear in biomedical ethics (see, e.g., Ladd 1978). In what follows I set out my view of justice and care as distinct virtues in light of some questions that arise in biomedical ethics.[1] I argue that William Frankena (1964, 1973a, b) was wrong to suggest that justice alone, not benevolence, judges the proper distribution of benefits and burdens, and that Gilligan was wrong to suggest that considerations of care are entirely distinct from justice. Instead I argue for a partial truth in each of these views: care needs distributive guidelines, and, despite some overlap, justice and care often do express differing considerations. I maintain that concepts of justice and care (and related concepts) pertain both to relations to persons as such and to relations between particular persons. Although considerations of justice and care can conflict in special relations, a compound of justice and care at the level of persons as such can be the framework for more determinate notions of social justice.

GILLIGAN

One can read Gilligan (1982, 1987) as a critic of liberal individualism, understood as a closely related family of moral traditions and theories.[2] Liberal individualism images morality as a type of requirement that is independent of a vision of the good or emotional ties of sympathy or allegiance,[3] binding on all persons qua persons, and demanded by reason and certain basic features of human experience (Reeder 1994). Gilligan's basic move, to rehearse the familiar, is to say that what liberal individualism pictures as the whole of morality is only one of its dimensions, namely, "justice." This is the dimension of morality principally allocated to men in a patriarchal division of labor; men have often taken their experience of morality for the whole. There is another dimension of morality, however, which is "care," principally allocated to women. Gilligan takes the care that is often regarded as optional or supererogatory from the point of view of justice to be a constitutive element of morality.[4] Care encompasses not only positive responsibilities, but negative ones as well; it enjoins not only helping, but also not hurting.[5] Unlike some, therefore, who want to reject liberal individualism altogether, who want to supplant it with another vision of morality as a whole, Gilligan seems (at least early on) to accept liberal individualism as justice, but to supplement it with care.[6] There are then two irreducible and nonintegratable dimensions of the moral domain (Gilligan 1987).

Thus Gilligan develops the well-known set of contrasts (to summarize briefly): (1) justice specifies a set of duties or obligations correlated with individual rights, whereas care speaks of how one should respond to the other in relationships; (2) justice rests on a demand of reason, whereas care rests on emotional attachment;[7] (3) justice applies to persons as such, whereas care pertains in the first instance to particular persons (although it can expand to anyone in need)[8]; (4) the duties and rights of justice are formulated in general principles or rules, whereas care responds directly to each situation.[9] These four contrasts correspond to four major sorts of issues: (1′) the difference between justice and care as moral concepts or virtues; (2′) the role of emotion in the moral life, for example, the nature of sympathy and compassion; (3′) the moral role of special relations, as well as respect for persons as such (this issue involves but is not the same as two other questions, namely, the difference between personal and impersonal relations, and the tension between partiality and impartiality); (4′) the role of general principles or rules in moral judgments, in contrast to the function of narrative or emotional responses to particular situations.

I focus on (1′) here, and only touch on (2′), (3′), and (4′). I argue for the view that justice and care are related, but distinct virtues.[10] What I set aside are two other views: care or love is more fundamental than justice and in some sense is its basis; and justice or at least some independent sense of moral demand is more fundamental and in some sense the basis of facets of care such as compassion.[11]

THE NEO-ARISTOTELIAN OBJECTION

If the sketch above is a good reading of Gilligan, or at least some of her work, consider the following objection to her account: what Gilligan calls justice, what she takes as a general feature of morality—which liberal individualism wrongly identified with morality as a whole—is in fact a liberal individualistic view of justice. The problem is not, a neo-Aristotelian could say, that liberal individualism has taken the justice dimension of morality for the whole; the problem lies with liberal individualism's view of morality itself, including justice.

Moreover, the critic could continue, a neo-Aristotelian view of justice has the basic features that Gilligan assigns exclusively to care:[12] For the neo-Aristotelian, the moral self exists in a web of social roles and relationships. Justice is not independent of our vision of the good and our ties of emotion, as if it rested on some independent demand of reason; it is an ingredient in our vision of the best human life within a community, and it finds expression in character. Further, justice pertains first to persons in specific roles and only secondarily to strangers. Finally, from a neo-Aristotelian perspective, rules or principles are subordinate to narratives, which depict the details of relationships.

A GILLIGAN RESPONSE

Your sense of the distinctiveness of care, the neo-Aristotelian in effect, says Gilligan, depends on taking one view of justice as justice per se. If you adopted a neo-Aristotelian view of justice, you could accommodate within it the basic features you associate with care. Gilligan (or *a* Gilligan) could respond as follows: Even if I amended my view of justice, I would still insist that there is a distinct virtue of care. Although I now grant that there is a view of justice that connects it to a "thick" view of the good and to a web of relationships, which are both ingredient in and instrumental to that good, I still think there is a distinct virtue of care, a type of affective attachment not subsumable under any conception of justice.[13] Justice and care could both be understood as virtues in that they are dispositions to feel, desire, and act in certain ways (Yearley 1990). But they are distinctly different features, so the argument would go, of moral experience.[14]

TWO VIRTUES

In putting these words into Gilligan's mouth, I am putting forward an interpretive hypothesis: Gilligan's concern was to criticize the ethos of liberal individualism from a perspective concerned about gender and the marginalization of women.[15] But at the same time—by naming liberal individualism *justice* and contrasting it with *care*—she employed, and took a view of, an ancient contrast.[16] Gilligan accepted a liberal individualist view of justice, but tried to augment its view of kindness or affective concern.[17]

Compare Gilligan's picture to the view that Judith Jarvis Thomson espouses in her famous abortion essay: There is a sphere of justice consisting of negative rights of noninterference with life and liberty and positive rights generated by specific commitments (1997). There is no general positive right of aid parallel to negative rights, but Minimally Decent Samaritanism (MDS)—a sort of kindness or positive concern for others—occupies the place of a general positive duty. MDS seems to have the independence from justice that Gilligan ascribes to care.

Does Thomson mean that MDS is optional, or is it required? Is it something one ought to have, and therefore not merely optional, but not something one must have? My sense is that for Thomson, MDS is not optional, whereas Good or Splendid Samaritanism is optional and hence supererogatory. MDS, as I read Thomson, is a disposition to desire and to act, which one ought to have, and it may be something one must have.[18] But it is not the sort of requirement of duty or obligation that falls under justice. If care or love is seen as something not required, as a gift, then it will be sharply distinguished from justice as something owed or due, something one can claim or demand. Thomson's MDS seems to be required, although its exercise, like the exercise of justice, requires judgment.[19]

Moreover, MDS can even trump justice in some situations: A woman has a right to determine what happens in and to her body, and thus a fetus (considered hypothetically as a full moral person) has a right to life support only if a woman confers that right through her voluntary commitment, which presumably can be withdrawn. The special relation is constituted by a conditional commitment. But if a very short time of pregnancy remains, and the cost of bearing is minimal, MDS intervenes to say that it would be wrong to abort; MDS in some circumstances limits the *right* to determine what happens in and to one's body.

What Gilligan does then can be interpreted as a move beyond Thomson's virtue of kindness to others at minimal cost to a more fully developed picture of attachments to others (and self).[20] Gilligan might even say that Thomson's MDS is care seen from the perspective of justice; such care is imaged from "within the justice construction," and is akin to mercy, forgiveness, supererogation, or a "choice to sacrifice the claims of the self" (Gilligan 1987, 24). Gilligan thus argues that each of the *perspectives* construes the other perspective in its own way. I would put the point differently: there are various *interpretations* of justice, care, and their relation, of which Thomson's and Gilligan's are instances.[21]

Therefore, I argue that the basic structure of Gilligan's and Thomson's views is similar: a sphere of justice, paralleled by an independent form of moral consideration variously construed in different traditions as charity, kindness, benevolence, love, or care.[22] Gilligan's construction is similar to Thomson's on the justice side, but the care dimension is changed. Justice is still connected to individual rights and notions of autonomy and equality; but care is elucidated more broadly in terms of the notion of affective attachment and a disposition to further the good of self and others. One has a disposition to be averse to people's suffering and to like their flourishing, a set of emotional attachments, as well as a disposition to desire and act to further their good.

DISTINCTIVENESS

My claim then is that Gilligan argues on two fronts: She wants to criticize liberal individualism, and she wants to distinguish the virtues of justice and care. Even if she were persuaded to change her early view of justice, and hence fully extend her critique of liberal individualism, she could presumably still insist that justice and care are distinct virtues.[23]

To support the distinctiveness of justice and care, Gilligan, or anyone else who takes up the torch at this point, could try to point to features that seem to belong to each virtue. I will begin to develop such an account, and then amend it. First, justice and care speak to different problems or issues. Care is the virtue, one might argue, that provides for a certain sort of attachment and devotion to the good of others and self. Justice is the virtue that addresses the question of a rightful or fair distribution of benefits and burdens.[24] One thus would adopt the sort of division of labor between "beneficence" and "justice" suggested by Frankena.[25] Frankena argues that beneficence (do good and prevent harm) and justice are the twin principles of morality (Frankena 1973a, 34, 45, 47–48). Interestingly, Frankena treats non-injury and noninterference with liberty, as well as "the principle of utility" (seek the greatest balance of good over evil), as prima facie rules derived from beneficence, not from justice, which seems to have to do solely with distribution (48–52). Justice answers the question, whose good? (45–53). Frankena argues for a mixed theory—justice and beneficence are irreducible parts of morality that must be combined in moral decisions (see also 1964, 217, 220–21).[26]

Justice would speak, therefore, not only to the issue of unequal power, as Gilligan explicitly suggests, but to the more general issue of the distribution of benefits and burdens (the justification of inequalities not only of power, but of resources in general).[27] Care would speak to the issue of attachment to self, special relations, and strangers (persons as such) (see Held 1993). Whereas Frankena writes of a general disposition and directive to do good and prevent harm, one would speak of an attachment to, and a disposition to desire and act to further someone's good.[28] For both Frankena and Gilligan (in this thought experiment) justice, in contrast, would answer the question, whose good *should* we further? Both could argue that we experience issues about attachment and distribution first in our earliest interactions, but they arise across the field of social relations.

Second, justice and care as distinctive dispositions to feel, desire, and act in certain ways could be said to utilize distinctive vocabularies that express distinctive moral considerations. Both relate to harms and benefits, but justice speaks, for example, of what is *fair*, whereas care speaks of *concern*. Each virtue is associated with forms of expression that shape it in light of assumptions about the overall contours of human motivation and moral experience (Reeder 1994). For example, agents demand what is just in specific forms of expression, such as the language of rights. Even if we love only ourselves, or if there are social relations in which only this form of care can be assumed (e.g., some conceptions of commerce), we could still desire to be fair and to act fairly in relation to others.[29] Our sense of justice can be expressed in the language of rights, which we demand for ourselves and others. Feinberg argues, for example, that "respect for persons . . . may simply be respect for their rights" (Feinberg 1980a, 151). If "Nowheresville" lacks both rights and persons who are aware of them (1980b), then even if its inhabitants possess "benevolence, compassion, sympathy, and pity" (1980a, 143), it is morally deficient (1980a, 155). As Gilligan argues that rights without care are morally impoverished, so Feinberg insists on the indispensability of rights even where compassion and benevolence are present.

In a similar way, concern based on attachment can be expressed in a variety of ways according to the sort of situation in which it is experienced and reigning assumptions about moral experience. For example, in Thomson's abortion article such concern takes the form of a kindness or generosity, which even if required and not optional calls for only minimal cost to the giver. One ought not to fail to do for this fetus what one should do (Minimally Decent Samaritanism) for *anyone*. Giving at greater cost, however, extends Minimally Decent Samaritanism into Good or Splendid Samaritanism (Thomson 1997). To fail in MDS is to be "greedy" or "callous"; one is praised for doing more than MDS enjoins, but is not blamed for failing to be a Good or Splendid Samaritan.[30] Gilligan's care (in its fullest development), in contrast, comes to include the self, but nonetheless seems to demand more of the giver; the concept of care now has the connotation of a deep and possibly costly attachment to the good of the other. Moreover, the category of care is the *basis* of the special relation of woman and fetus; attachment is constitutive. Gilligan's concept of care thus represents a shift in general assumptions about motivation and experience.[31]

CARE AND THE DISTRIBUTIVE ISSUE

In the account I have given so far, as moral concepts, justice and care are distinguished in two ways: They speak to different problems, and they do so in different vocabularies that express different sorts of moral considerations. Let us look first at the thesis that only justice has the function of judging distributions. This seems not to stand up under inspection.

Care itself, especially in Gilligan's view, seems to have its own distributive guidelines. Justice can issue a verdict about which right hierarchically overrides which, for example, in abortion cases, but care says that no one should be hurt, and if hurt to someone is inevitable in "conflict" cases, it says do the most good or the least harm.[32] Has Gilligan in effect characterized care as utilitarianism—to do the greatest good (or least harm), counting all affected without bias? Has she covertly introduced a standard of fair distribution into care?

Gilligan could respond as follows: I do think care makes distributive judgments, but it is not utilitarian (see Tobias 1996). First, I do not believe that goods can always be commensurate, as some forms of utilitarianism presumably require; one may have to choose in some other way *what* sort of good to actualize (see Meilaender 1987, 96–98). Second, care does not necessarily demand that goods be distributed according to a utilitarian criterion (maximization, counting the effect on each without special weight or bias). Care begins in the love of particular persons. One does not necessarily allocate goods and evils according to a utilitarian sense of "impartiality"; one may have to choose in some other way *whom* to hurt.[33] In sum, care as a virtue is not equivalent in content to the "generalized benevolence" of utilitarianism.[34] If it uses the metarule, "do the most good/least harm," it does not necessarily add the rider, "counting all without bias," that is, impartially. Care may be partial, weighing the good of some more than others, yet still trying within these parameters to do the most good/least harm one can for all affected.

Thus Gilligan argues that the scope of care includes self as well as other, but she does not seem to say that care inherently requires an equal consideration of interests in a utilitarian sense. Care nonetheless has its own distributive patterns—one loves self, kin, and friend, persons in other special relations, and even any person in need. Care has its own reasons. It often seems to legitimate partiality while still trying as far as possible to maximize the good.

In sum, both fairness and care make distributional demands. It is not that we merely *have* various attachments and concerns that possess no *ordo* without the intervention of justice (as Frankena's beneficence needs the direction of justice). Both justice and care, in Gilligan's view, have their distinctive ways of answering distributive questions. This seems to me correct—we should not ascribe the distributive function only to justice. Care does not need justice for distributional direction, but it does need some such direction, and this is the grain of truth in the thesis that it needs justice; the point, however, is that it has its own distributive compass (see Card 1996).

But what is this compass? If we take our cares, our loyalties, our loves as having their own distributive patterns, even among themselves, these are apparently only prima facie. Love for family or friend, in a famous example, can conflict with love for country. Perhaps it is best to say that various constructions of care have different distributive compasses, just as conceptions of justice do.

THE VOCABULARY OF CARE

Let us look also at the suggestion that justice and care express different considerations. What is the difference in the substantive considerations that we appeal to under the headings of justice and care? Are their vocabularies as distinctive as I have suggested?

In judgments of fairness or justice, Gilligan would say, we typically appeal (beyond the formal criterion of consistency) to certain distinctive sorts of substantive criteria such as equality (e.g., of opportunity) and autonomy. In judgments of care, by contrast, we respond to need, and where we cannot meet all needs, we appeal to patterns of attachment. The fact that X is my friend is a reason that not only explains, but justifies (at least prima facie) my preference for X. In matters of justice, in sum, we appeal to rights; in matters of care, to attachment. In one strand of Gilligan's thought, justice and care are completely distinct, irreducible perspectives (Gilligan 1987).[35]

But this putative difference in vocabulary and criteria does not hold up, a critic could object. Need is often a criterion of justice, and judgments of justice can justify partiality (see Heller 1987; Outka 1974).[36] Judgments of care, it seems natural to say, should not be arbitrary or inconsistent.[37] Moreover, the critic might continue, to be fully caring is to respect the autonomy of the other. Gilligan argues that "justice" from a care perspective is respect for the difference of the other (1987, 24–25), but one could say that respect for autonomy and difference is integral to care itself.[38]

My sense is that these objections can be answered at least in part. Some sorts of considerations, we should acknowledge, are common to both judgments of justice and care, for example, consistency and need. But in some settings we seem to want to maintain important differences. Thus in a medical context, it is commonly said, even if empathy provides a reliable grasp of a patient's suffering, we are not necessarily entitled to act out of compassion and benevolence according to our view of the patient's good; we are required to respect the competent agent's wishes (Beauchamp and Childress, 1994).[39] And if empathy is unreliable (generally or in a particular case), the case for respect for autonomy is even stronger.[40] It might be that where there is mutual trust that persons will respect and treat each other fairly, we do not have to assert a right to autonomy or self-determination, a discourse of claiming or waiving our sovereignty. Thus we can amend Feinberg's thesis that rights are the constitutive feature of respect; but we can retain a sense of the distinctiveness of fairness and respect.[41]

Although some say that we don't "truly" love unless we respect, we often seem to acknowledge the genuineness of someone's love—they are not deficient in that regard—but feel that they have not treated us fairly in some way, for example, not respected our autonomy or difference. Others, we say, have a keen sense of justice, but fail to love. This is not to deny that both justice and care can have their own characteristic distortions—a rigid justice or a possessive love, for example. The point is that one can pass muster in one dimension but not in the other.

In sum, I would hold that the thesis that we have two entirely distinct sets of vocabulary and underlying considerations is false; the two virtues overlap somewhat. Nonetheless, there is a grain of truth in this thesis, as in the first.[42] The justice family in its various constructions often seems built on a notion of playing according to a set of rules. The notion of fair play seems central to many images of justice. To act fairly is to play by the rules, such as of a game, competition, or practice. To be treated fairly is to receive what one is due according to the rules (i.e., *suum cuique*, including merit or desert where appropriate), and the rules should be administrated consistently (i.e., like cases alike) (see Childress 1985, 228). A system of rules, moreover, can be construed as norms attached to certain roles and statuses; for example, parents have duties of justice to children, and persons as such have duties to other persons ("respect for persons").[43] As a virtue, then, justice would refer to a disposition to have certain emotions (to "hate" injustice and to "love" justice), to desire to be just, and to act to further justice.[44]

The care, benevolence, or love family in its various constructions refers to dispositions to feel, desire, and act on behalf of someone's good. Like facets of justice, forms of care or love are characteristically related to roles and statuses: care for someone as a friend, as a child, as a person. One has a disposition to be averse to someone's suffering and to like their flourishing, as well as a disposition to desire and act to further their good. A tradition or some reflective account—possibly critical and constructive as well as interpretive—will construe and relate a variety of concepts that pertain to this sort of disposition. For example, Vacek (1994) distinguishes various senses of "love" and relates these to concepts such as "benevolence." It seems that various traditions often make one or another concept (construed in a particular sense) the dominant focus of attention, for example, love in the Christian tradition, benevolence in some strands of Anglo-American philosophy, and care in Gilligan and others. "Care" can be thought of as an overarching virtue that organizes a family or cluster of related disposi-tions, such as compassion and benevolence (see Blum 1994, 264–65). My sense is that there is a recognizably similar family of concepts across at least some traditions; representatives of these traditions inherit and reshape normative constructions.

DISTINCTIVE WAYS OF SEEING ABORTION

The difference between justice and care does not lie, as Frankena suggests, in a division of labor such that the one pertains to distribution and the other solely to increasing good/lessening harm for those to whom one is attached. Both justice and care make distributive judgments. Although their vocabularies need not ever overlap, as Gilligan sometimes seems to claim, they do often seem to invoke different sorts of considerations expressed in distinctive ways.

Let us look at abortion to review where we have been. Gilligan roots the difference in the two perspectives in a contrast between issues of "equal-ity" and "attachment" (1987, 20). "Justice" images selves making claims and asserting rights against one another, whereas "care" focuses on how to maintain "relationship" (22–23). The abortion debate has been carried on, says Gilligan, from the perspective of and in the discourse of justice (23–24), with rights, respect, and moral status as the categories of the debate. But from the perspective of care, one looks at the issue differently: "The connec-tion between the fetus and the pregnant woman becomes the focus of attention and the question becomes whether it is responsible or irresponsible, caring or careless, to extend or end this connection. . . . To ask what actions constitute care or are more caring directs attention to the parameters of connection and the costs of detachment" (1987, 24).

What exactly is the difference Gilligan suggests? She suggests several contrasts that do not seem to work. First, it cannot be that *only* care responds to "need," for, as I noted above, need can be one sort of criterion of distributive justice. Second, it cannot be that *only* care grasps that the self is "by definition connected to others, responding to perceptions, interpreting events, and governed by the organizing tendencies of human interaction and human language" (Gilligan 1987, 24). To suggest that justice, even a "liberal" conception of justice that stresses individual rights, does not recognize the "sociality" of the self in these broad senses is mistaken.[45] Nor in the third place can the difference be that, whereas the agent making a judgment of justice assumes "one set of terms" in which to ask the question of fairness and to find "agreement," care respects difference and seeks only "understanding" (1987, 25, 31). Justice in many accounts seeks to recognize differences in situations and in points of view, and privileges those differences through notions of respect for autonomy; and after trying to understand, care in the end must also judge.

Gilligan suggests, however, a more basic contrast, as I noted: justice's concern for equality and autonomy in contrast to the attachments of care (1987, 31–32). Care is focused on attachment or the loss thereof, a severing of a certain sort of relation. It would seem a decision for abortion is a decision to sever or abandon ("attachment cannot be sustained"), but if one takes "responsibility" one keeps the "web of relationships intact" (1982, 59).

In contrast to attachment, justice is (among other things) having a right to decide what happens in and to your body. No one may injure you or use your bodily resources without your consent. Thus a Thomson's error, from a Gilligan's point of view, is not so much that a Thomson envisages justice in this way, but that he or she sees the woman-fetus special relation only as a matter of justice (a right to decide whether to be committed or not) and does not see this relation as attachment *ab initio*.[46] Attachment is not necessarily chosen; it can exist even when the pregnancy is unplanned. Thus for Gilligan, although a woman does have a right to decide what happens in and to her body, she also may have an unchosen attachment (see Cahill 1984; Farley 1981; Pope 1991). For Gilligan, one faces abortion from two perspectives: sovereignty over oneself (in relation to the rights of others) and attachment (not just to the fetus, but to self and others).[47] Being able to decide whether to commit one's body as life support is the *value* justice (so understood) is designed to preserve. Care, in contrast, as a moral category expresses the *value* of certain affective attachments (to self as well as other). In the end, justice and care stand for dispositions to preserve two sorts of values or goods.[48]

In sum, one contrast Gilligan wants to preserve—as do many of us—is between justice construed as a sort of autonomy and care conceived principally as affective attachment. Both require discretion in judgment, but as virtues both are integral to the moral life (care is not optional). The general view I take is this: "Justice" and "care" contrasts are in fact contrasts between an interpretation of values from different families. To tell what's going on, we have to "look and see."[49]

Justice and Care Related

I want to stay with the thesis that Gilligan's "justice" and "care" are constructions of two families of moral virtue. Various traditions and their associated theories explicate and relate these families in different ways. Traditions use the terms to construct a moral map and to deal with a number of issues (see appendix).

I want to reject in my account the idea that justice is relevant to situations where what counts is only that there are persons as such and that care is relevant only when personal histories are essential in one's judgment (see Gilligan 1982, 58–59).[50] Sometimes, although our judgments in a sense may still refer to particular persons, all that counts is that these persons are instances of a particular class—for example, they are noncombatants owed immunity from direct attack according to the just war tradition.[51] In other cases, I assume, our judgments make essential reference to particular persons (their histories and relationships)—for example, this person is not only my son or daughter, this person is Nick or Kate.[52] In my view justice, no less than care, applies in the second as well as the first sort of case.[53]

Consider a family situation in which one child of several has a chronic illness. Let us assume that within this set of special relations there is a parental duty of justice to provide resources to all of the children; it is a duty of equal attention, we might say, though it does not require identical treatment.[54] Let us also assume that in this family the parents care for their children; the parents have a deep attachment to and a disposition to further the good of these particular individuals.

What difficulties could arise here? First, the healthy siblings in this family could complain that although they are loved "as much" as the ill child—I interpret "as much" to mean in the same degree or with the same quality—they have in fact been *unfairly* shortchanged in the distribution of resources. Although they have not been deprived of what is absolutely basic, the devotion of resources of money, time, and effort to their ill sibling has meant that their parents have allocated to one child resources that would otherwise have been distributed across the children. The criterion of equal attention has not been met.

Second, the healthy children might believe instead that they have been treated fairly. Although the parents' attention to the ill child went beyond standard adjustments to special needs, the other children believe that in this case so long as basic needs are met, it is not unjust, for example, that what would have been college money for all went to provide medical care or simply a more tolerable existence for the ill child. Nonetheless, these children might complain that they are not *loved* as the ill child is. This is not a complaint about how they are cared for or taken care of, but it has to do with how they are *cared about*. It is not a complaint that the parents do not desire to act on their behalf, but it is a complaint about how they feel toward them, about the quality of their emotion or attachment. It is not a complaint that love, considered as some sort of quantifiable commodity, has not been equally distributed (although the complaint is sometimes expressed this way); it is a complaint that the love or care they receive does not have the depth or quality of the parents' devotion to the ill child. It is a complaint not so much about distribution, but about absence or lack. The parents themselves may well be conscious that they love one child in a different way, and they may worry about how that difference has an effect on the other siblings.

Is there any way to resolve these tensions? My sense is that there may be no metarule. Where care leads to an unequal distribution, one that exceeds any standard adjustment to special need, and on the assumption that parents should provide resources beyond bare essentials, the other children may well have a valid complaint that they were unjustly treated. And even if we suppose that the healthy children have not been treated unjustly, they could experience a deficiency in care. Although the parents have struggled mightily to do justice, the situation is such that they are more deeply attached to the ill child. Thus, in sum, whether care has led to an unjust distribution, or whether justice has been accompanied by a difference in care, success in one category does not seem to compensate for failure in another.[55]

I assume in any case that justice, which pertains in one dimension to persons as such, also has a role in relations to particular persons such as one's children. I have also argued elsewhere that care, which begins in relations between particular persons, can be "built on" in order to construct a universal and equal love for persons as such (Reeder 1998).[56] What is the relation between care and justice at the level of persons? The model I sketch here tries to capture the familiar form of thinking in some theological traditions (and in secular analogues) that posits an integration of love and justice at the heart of the moral life.[57] In imitation of the deity who is both loving and just, we should have a just love for all.[58] A foundational perspective (Shue 1996) could be construed as a compound of loving attachment and fairness.[59] The dimension of justice that pertains to persons as such combines with universal and equal love.

Thus Frankena grants that *agape* can include universality of scope, but insists that equality as a principle of distributive justice is a "qualification" of love of neighbor (1964, 220). He argues therefore for a "mixed" or "impure" agapism, a "synthesis" of love and justice (1973a, 58; 1973b, 33). I follow Outka (1972, 1992) in arguing that love in one of its senses takes the form of universal and equal "regard," and that it overlaps, but is not identical, with egalitarian justice (on Outka, see Childress 1985, 236–40).[60] Let me then suggest, as others have, combining agapistic love (care) as universal and equal regard and respect that is owed as a matter of justice.[61] How we approach persons as such will be a function of both *agape* and justice, within either a theological or nontheological framework.

The *agape*-justice combination could be the basis, moreover, for more specific principles of social justice that structure the life of communities (King 1986; Okin 1989).[62] Justice in the first instance is a broad sense of respect for persons; combined with an affective attachment to the good of all provides the basis for a second more determinate sense of justice as the structure of social practices.[63] This is not necessarily to suggest that more specific principles of social justice are deductively derived; general and specific judgments are dynamically related in an ongoing process of interpretation and "reflective equilibrium." The compound of care and justice, however, has a foundational function;[64] it establishes the normative framework of a way of life.[65]

CONCLUSION

In this paper I have begun to sketch justice and care as virtues. I have tried to escape the grip, as it were, of the "transcend and ground" vertical model in order to explore a horizontal model of nonidentical but overlapping virtues. My most general assumption is that both vertical and horizontal models construe and construct two broad families of moral concepts that appear in many traditions and are shaped in light of broader assumptions (see Childress 1985, 229). I have not presented care and justice as "voices" or "dimensions" of morality as such, but as virtues, or perhaps better as clusters of virtues. I have suggested that although "justice" and "care" in some constructions may carry connotations from patriarchal or liberal society, these virtues are not necessarily limited to these settings. I have noted some of the features that I would want to include under each virtue (or cluster), while pointing out that even on a horizontal model the content and relation of each virtue is often differently construed across traditions and authors. In trying to escape the vertical model, moreover, I have not tried to escape theological interpretations of justice and care (love). Indeed, it would seem natural on a theological account to see interhuman justice and care as images of divine qualities and relations. But one critical question will be the possible differences between theological and nontheological horizontal models.

Endnotes

1 I would like to thank the following who have offered criticism and counsel on these issues: Diana Fritz Cates, Andrew Flescher, Lauren Fine, Jennifer A. Herdt, Laura Jones, Matthew Kutny, Rosalind Ladd, Paul Lauritzen, Jung Lee, Karen Lebacqz, Chappell Marmon, Richard Miller, Philip Muntzel, Gene Outka, Ruth Smith, Donald Swearer, Linwood Urban, William Werpehowski, and Lee Yearley.

2 I have learned much from the voluminous debate surrounding Gilligan and feminist ethics. What I argue here draws in particular from Andolsen, Gudorf, and Pellauer (1987); Antony and Witt (1993); Benhabib and Cornell (1987); Blum (1994); Card (1991); Clement (1996); Cole and Coultrap-McQuinn (1992); Crysdale (1994); Farley (1981, 1993, 1996); Hekman (1995); Held (1995a); Kittay and Myers (1987); Lanagan (1991); Tanner (1996); and Tong (1997). See also, e.g., the *Hypatia* "Symposium On Care and Justice" (Deveaux 1995; Held 1995b; Narayan 1995; Tronto 1995). To go further with this project, as I have attempted to do in a longer version of this paper, one would need to consider many other sources recent and not so recent. My regrets for their omission.

3 By "independent" here I do not mean that views in this family do not make some assumptions about basic goods; the point is rather that the moral demand is not dependent on a full vision of human flourishing or ties of affection. Thus Gewirth's (1978) neo-Kantianism, for example, utilizes some assumptions about the good.

4 Gilligan could allow justice to include a general positive duty or right of aid, such as Gewirth (1978) posits, without altering her basic point: Care has been regarded as outside the sphere of morality as such or at least outside the sphere of moral requirement. See Kroeger-Mappes (1994) and Friedman (1995).

5 Cf. Beauchamp and Childress (1994) on beneficence and nonmalficence.

6 Hekman (1995) argues that Gilligan's work in effect proposes to supplant the "disembodied knower" of abstract principles with the "relational," culturally situated self. Gilligan herself later speaks of the self of liberal individualism—the "separate self"—as "intrinsically problematic," and claims that care is "primary and ... fundamental in human life." The "separate self and the selfless woman" are part of patriarchy (Gilligan 1995, 121–22). See also Keller (1986). See Smith (1988) on Gilligan, liberal individulaism, and the public-private dichotomy.

7 Gilligan would not want to endorse a reason-emotion dichotomy—care has a cognitive dimension—but it is difficult not to see this contrast at work in her early thought at least. See Michaels (1986) and M. O. Little (1995).

8 On care extended to anyone in need, see Kymlicka (1990, 271).

9 See Carse's (1991) useful analysis. See also Cannold et al. (1996).

10 Cf. Reeder (1998). I do not want, however, to say that care is a "natural" virtue and justice "artificial." Both care and justice are culturally constructed modes of relationship that have evolved in human experience; we attribute a second-order moral significance (valuation and commitment) to each. See O'Neill (1996b, 98–99), Baier (1987), Hursthouse (1991), Noddings (1984), and Schneewind (1998, 365–69) on Hume. I do endorse the general idea that capacities formed in early childhood are a precondition for justice and care. See Baier (1987, 42, 50) on Hume's view of the role of early experiences of self-control and cooperation. See Stocker (1987, 60–67) on virtues as both natural and moral.

11 Nagel says: "Sympathy is not, in general, just a feeling of discomfort produced by the recognition of distress in others, which in turn motivates one to relieve their distress. Rather, it is the pained awareness of their distress as something to be relieved" (Nagel 1971, 80).

12 See Nussbaum (1993, 332, n. 16), who says that an Aristotelian view of justice with its emphasis on "equity" and "particularity" will "support" and "be continuous" with care, and is a better account of justice than Gilligan's rather "Kantian" view that emphasizes "universal principles of broad generality." See MacIntyre (1988) on the contrast between "liberalism" and other views of justice. See also Taylor (1986) and Hursthouse (1991) for Aristotelian views of justice. Other voices, particularly from the theological traditions, would also join in criticizing a "liberal individualist" view of justice. See, e.g., Lebacqz (1987, 1996a, and 1997). See also Sharpe (1992), who connects "justice" to moral and political liberalism, and relates a care perspective to Aristotelian tradition.

13 Curzer suggests that a "voice" is "something more comprehensive and primordial than a virtue" (Curzer 1993, 180 n. 5), but I am reading Gilligan or perhaps constructing a Gilligan for whom justice and care are virtues.

14 See Foot, for example, on justice and on "charity" as attachment (1978, 44–45). I am assuming that a contemporary Aristotelian would think of justice as a disposition to feel as well as to desire and act; hence in this broad sense it is a virtue comparable to care. I am indebted to Diana Fritz Cates on this point.

15 Gilligan (1982) of course takes as her immediate target Kohlberg's theory of moral development. See also Peters (1973, 25–26), who says that the "Piaget-Kohlberg" theory "suffers ... defects of the Kantian approach. ... There is no probing of the motives that explain their [the subjects'] actions, no assessment of the intensity or level of compassion which suffuses their dealings with others. Yet this, surely, is developmentally most important; for what is the moral status of a man who can reason in an abstract way about rules, if he does not *care* about persons who are affected by his breach or observance of them." See also Bernstein and Gilligan (1990); Brown and Gilligan (1992); Gilligan, Rogers, and Brown, (1990); Gilligan and Wiggins (1998).

16 See J. Ladd (1998, 163–64) on Kant's distinction between justice and charity. Ladd argues that acts of beneficence that would be optional or supererogatory in themselves are mandatory in communal relations; thus we can speak of the care that is due, that someone is entitled to (164–65). O'Neill argues that the sense of "imperfect" obligation, which refers to the "indeterminacy of act descriptions," does not distinguish obligations of justice from obligations of charity; principles of justice are also underspecified and require discretion in particular cases (1989, 229–31; 1996, chap. 5 and passim). But she thinks that obligations of charity are not initially correlated with recipients and hence with rights, which can be claimed or waived. Thus duties of justice, although they need interpretation in particular cases, are correlated with recipients and rights from the outset and hence are "perfect," whereas charity is an "imperfect" obligation that requires "allocation" to certain givers and receivers. When the allocation is institutional, then the recipient has a right, e.g., to a particular service, but when an individual simply identifies a recipient—this starving person here and now—O'Neill does not speak of the recipient having a positive right. My view is that even this sense of the perfect/imperfect distinction breaks down. First, duties of justice obtain only under certain circumstances. For example, I have a duty not to harm others only under certain circumstances; in this sense duties of "justice" require an analogous sort of allocation. Second, my intuition is that under certain circumstances, above and beyond any institutional obligations—e.g., the lifeguard's—a stranger owes aid to a stranger to which the stranger in these circumstances has a right. Thus I would want to put both general negative rights and a general positive right to be rescued under the heading of justice, and contrast both with the negative and positive responsibilities of care or benevolence.

17 Gilligan later says that she "theorized both justice and care in relational terms" (1995, 125). See also Gilligan (1988 and 1993).

18 Two sources of the notion that care or love is gratuitous suggest themselves: the Protestant notion of salvation as an unmerited gift of grace, and the strand of Western liberalism that sharply distinguishes between duties of justice (even including a minimal positive duty) and optional ideals of charity.

19 I am concerned here to challenge the familiar notion that justice is required and "charity" optional. One can distinguish justice and care without suggesting that one is required and the other not; an "obligation" of justice is not the only form of moral requirement (O'Neill 1989, 1996). Moreover, I suspect, although I will not try to defend the view here, that there are certain absolutes, but that there are many other judgments of both justice and care that require discretion in regard to the who, what, when, why, and where of particular situations, and hence cannot be antecedently stated except as rules of thumb.

20 Gilligan (1982) sometimes evokes justice or rights to buttress the legitimacy of self-love, but she also makes the inclusion of the self part of the developmental process of care (Friedman 1993, 128, 142–43, 159).

21 Note that O'Neill's structure is similar to Thomson's: the duties of aid that are correlated with rights (claimable, waivable, and enforceable) are those created by contract, special relations, or "legal and political systems" (O'Neill 1996b, 147–48). Other required positive actions, such as rescue, are a function of imperfect obligation or virtue (cf. MDS). O'Neill also wants to distinguish those positive duties that are required from those that are supererogatory and thinks that justice extends to institutions and law (enforcement), whereas virtue is principally or "best" expressed in character (O'Neill 1996b, 201).

22 Wolgast wants a role for rights (and justice more generally), but favors a broader conception of morality. See, e.g., Wolgast (1987, 36–49, and chap. 6).

23 See Hekman (1995) on Gilligan and the "liberalism-communitarian" debate. See also Baier (1995a).

24 A full account would also address retributive and restorative justice. I am speaking here of distributive justice in a broad sense, which includes the justice of exchanges, or commutative justice.

25 Would Frankena say Gilligan tends to hold a "rule" view of justice and an "act" view of care? (see Frankena 1973a, 23–28, 34–43, 55–59; 1964, 207).

26 Frankena later identifies a sense of "caring" or "non-indifference," which simply signifies that one's reasons, if they are to be called moral, must have to do with what happens to sentient beings, including others (Frankena 1983, 68, 71, 74–75). See Fry (1989) on Frankena.

27 Gilligan (1982) associates justice or fairness with autonomy and equality (over against the power of the parent). One classical notion of justice ("like cases alike") does require formal equality, but even this notion of impartiality, as it is often called, allows for serious substantive inequalities; it does not entail a substantive sense of impartiality or equality, such as the "equal consideration of interests." (And there are various views of substantive equality, of course). More generally, substantive notions of desert and hierarchy also figure in classical conceptions of justice. On formal and substantive notions of justice, see Heller (1987).

28 See Kuhse on a variety of senses of "care." She discusses two senses in particular—concern and caring for—that parallel these central notions of attachment and a disposition to desire and act to further someone's good (Kuhse 1997, 145–47, 158). See Lebacqz (1996b, 88) for a similar distinction: being "moved" by the suffering of another and "being impelled to counteract the suffering." See also Noddings (1984) on "engrossment" and "displacement"; Reich (1995a) on the "family" of meanings of care and his distinction between "caring for or about" and "taking care of" (1995b, 331); Reich and Jecker (1995, 341–42) on the difference between care as "affective orientation and moral commitment" and beneficence as a principle of action; Friedman (1993, 174), who distinguishes "care about" and "care for"; and my (1998) distinction between "compassion" and "benevolence."

29 Under these circumstances, "benevolence," construed simply as a disposition to desire and act on behalf of the good of others, could perhaps be understood to be instrumentally motivated by self-interest (see Vacek 1994). See Held on contractualism in contrast to nurturing relations (1993, 184, 187–88, 195, 202, 211–14).

30 See Kymlicka on Good Samaritan principles (1990, chap. 2, n. 9). See also D. Little (1986, 1992).

31 Hekman wants to displace a "Cartesian, modernist subject" (autonomous, culturally disembodied) with a "discursive subject" that is "constituted by the play of linguistic forces, a subject whose moral agency is a function of that constitution" (Hekman 1995, 113). Even if one is in sympathy with this metaphysical direction, as I am, one difficulty is that the "relational self in this sense does not seem to entail any particular view of the good and the right; a metaphysical picture of the self in this broad sense is morally indeterminate. It does not even demand that one forsake the moral idea that there is a single test of duty, e.g., a Kantian appeal to universalizability, in favor of the view that there are a plurality of "voices" or considerations, Hekman's underlying normative thesis. The diversity of voices could signify that moral considerations in various cultures are fundamentally different, or it could signify that morality consists of a certain set of considerations interpreted in culturally distinctive ways.

32 Gilligan might even be read to say that although a decision of justice relieves one of guilt (although not of regret), care inevitably produces guilt in "conflict" cases. See Werpehowski on a conflict between a special fiduciary obligation and a broader duty to help/not harm (1986b, 12). Werpehowski rejects the idea that we can find a "neat balance or harmony" that would eliminate "moral costs" we "regret" (12, 16), but he makes clear that this is not to say that there are "genuine moral dilemmas" in which one would do wrong and incur guilt whatever one does (23 n. 36; 24 n. 50). On these issues see Santurri (1987).

33 See Kymlicka on limits (e.g., desert) in responding to "subjective hurt" (1990, 276–86). Kymlicka says that care rejects utilitarianism, but still focuses on "subjective hurt and happiness" (282).

34 The very idea of "counting as one," estimating the effect on all without bias, imposes a distributive criterion. Frankena argues, however, that Mill was wrong when he said that a principle of justice was "built into the principle of utility" (Frankena 1973a, 41–42). Utilitarianism or the "principle of utility" does require us to count "equal effects equally," but this is not yet a principle of justice (it leaves open, for example, whether to distribute a given amount of good to a smaller group according to a "greatest number" criterion). In my view, to count the effects without bias (one sense of impartiality) is already to impose a substantive principle of distribution, an interpretation of the equal consideration of interests, although other criteria are yet more determinate, as Frankena argues.

35 See Flanagan (1991, 214–17), for criticism of the idea of Gestalts.

36 Note, moreover, that notions of respect for persons as such can and must be responsive to particularity as they are put into operation; as Outka (1972, 1992) and others note, equal regard does not necessarily require identical treatment. Thus unlike Dillon, I do not think one has to shift from "Kantian respect" to "care respect" in order to justify "treating different persons differently" (Dillon 1992b, 116–19, 122, 125). On need as distinguished from equal access, see Childress (1985, 236–37).

37 On care as a principled approach with a concern for consistency, see Kuhse (1997, 121–22), who refers to Purdy (1998, 11). See also Vreeke (1991, 38–39).

38 See Cates (1997) on compassion's concern for difference. See also Piper, who uses "compassion" to refer to an appropriate linkage between empathy, sympathetic "fellow-feeling," and a " disposition to render aid or mercy" (1991, 743–44). (Compare my 1998 threefold distinction between empathy, compassion/sympathy, and benevolence.) Piper wants compassion to include a formal or metaethical sense of "strict impartiality," which rules out self-absorption or vicarious possession (735–36, 745–46, 751, 753–57).

39 Empathy in my sense (Reeder 1998) functions in relations of both justice and love. But compassion and benevolence (in my senses) I put in the love or care family. See Card (1996), and Lebacqz (1993, 1996b).

40 See Lebacqz (1996b) on the requirement to respect autonomy and the problem of the other's true good; see also Card (1996, 89–90), who insists that compassion and benevolence are not morally sufficient, but require some judgment of the legitimacy of the recipient's needs and aims; see Outka (1972, 1992) on the "blank check" problem; see also Cates (1997) on trying to understand while not abdicating to the other; on the need for other values beside caring in order to avoid exploitation, see Houston (1990); see O'Neill's distinction between "charity," which has to do with "agency-threatening needs," and "beneficence," which could extend to happiness (O'Neill 1989, 233); on morally problematic forms of care (undermining autonomy, chauvinistic, nurturing "suspect types of persons and projects"), see Flanagan (1991, 202, 226–27).

41 In "Analogues" (1992), I noted several features that have been used to identify justice as a type of moral consideration: (1) providing for a morally right distribution of certain goods; (2) having a distinctive vocabulary and content; (3) having a certain sort of justification (283–84). I also discussed the motivational assumption that mutual love is not sufficient (287) and that given these "subjective circumstances" justice is required. I argued that under certain utopian conditions justice could be superseded, but that "analogues" to justice would nonetheless be necessary. My view now is that even if a sufficiently robust form of mutual love could be assumed, one would still need justice as a distinctive type of moral consideration, although rights might be unnecessary. (See Hubin 1979 for an analysis and critique of Hume and Rawls.) When writing "Analogues," I was thinking of justice as a distinct form of practice with its own motivation that is necessary due to the relative absence or weakness of other-regarding affections. Thus it becomes possible to think of the "circumstances of justice," at least the "subjective" ones, being overcome and justice becoming otiose. One relates justice and love therefore in a "vertical" model. Love both transcends (justice as otiose under utopian conditions) and grounds (justice as the "approximation" of love in "history"). The change for me in this essay is to think of justice not as a remedy for defective affections, but as a type of moral consideration that is never otiose. On this account I suggest only that rights could be otiose. See Baier (1993 and 1995a); see Ramsey (1970) and Werpe-howski (1986a, b) on the idea of love "transforming" justice.

42 Friedman argues that justice should be part of "interpersonal mutuality," a "morally adequate caring" (Friedman 1993, 126–34). In particular, Friedman intro-duces the notion of desert—caregivers deserve to be taken care of in return—and emphasizes the idea of the "intrinsic worth of care-giving individuals" (159–60; 160, n. 53; 161). I see intrinsic worth (as respect) and desert as part of the family of justice conceptions, which can be integrated, in Friedman's terminology, with care.

43 I think Gilligan assumes the fairness as rule following sense of justice, and adds other still more determinate notions, such as *equality* in the sense of the equal consideration of interests, and *autonomy* as sovereign control expressed in contempo-rary concepts of rights. Her picture of justice contrasts with other conceptions, e.g., ones that emphasize hierarchy or communal good. Fletcher (1997) argues that fair play is an especially salient feature of a society where competition (in sports and life) is dominant; my sense is that fairness as rule-following goes much deeper; conceptions of justice begin to divide where different sorts of rules are seen as legitimate. Thus in Rawls's (1971) terminology (though not his exact usage), fairness as rule-following is a concept of justice that allows for different views or conceptions of justice (what the rules should be). See Sterba's (1995) use of the concept/concep-tion distinction.

44 Friedman notes that Gilligan needs a notion of justice that includes positive rights, but argues that a duty of justice toward strangers would not necessarily involve "emotion, feeling, passion, or compassion" (Friedman 1993, 135). I would agree that compassion is different, but I think that justice as a virtue has its own sort of emotion.

45 For the thesis that "liberal democracy" is compatible with an acknowledgment of our sociality, see Greenawalt (1988, 22). See also Reeder (1998).

46 Note that autonomy as moral or nonmoral choice by an individual is sometimes distinguished from justice regarded as a matter of the distribution of social benefits and burdens. See Smith (1984) and Beauchamp and Childress (1994, chap. 6). The latter suggest that justice pertains generally to situations in which benefits or burdens are "due," and "distributive justice" pertains in particular to "social coopera-tion." Taylor limits distributive justice to "some kind of collaborative arrangement" in a particular society, in contrast to a broader sense that would include inalienable rights (Taylor 1986, 35, 48–49). For various senses of justice, see Werpehowski

(1986a). As Werpehowski makes clear, justice can refer to actions, social practices, and virtue.

47 Both rape and nonnegligent contraceptive failure are instances for Thomson in which the woman does not freely commit herself to providing her body as a life-sustaining resource for the fetus. See Tong (1997, 146–48) on Gilligan's treatment of abortion. On Thomson's rights approach and an early contrast with Gilligan, see John (1984, 294 and passim).

48 Vreeke (1991, 36) argues that according to Gilligan, care's interest is in "whether the future relationship between the woman and the child can be of sufficient quality."

49 MacIntyre (1999, chap. 10) argues there is a virtue in relationships of giving and receiving, which is partly "justice" and partly "generosity." MacIntyre's Aristotelian-Thomistic account is a good example of how a tradition (or a representative thereof) interprets and relates the two families of virtues.

50 Unlike Kuhse, Singer, and Rickard (1998), I do not think we should engage in "re-characterizing the justice and care debate in terms of impartialist and partialist ethical perspectives," important as the latter contrast is. If impartiality is defined as the equal consideration of the interests of all persons as such, then it does stand in contrast to special relations. But if it is understood as the equal consideration of persons in a particular class, e.g., one's children, then it also applies within the context of special relations. Cf. Friedman (1993, 2–3). See Kymlicka (1990, 289–90; 290 n. 12) and Judish (1998) on the conflict between responsibilities to the stranger and the near and dear.

51 The ascription of noncombatant status could be taken either as a prima facie consideration or as a moral absolute.

52 Dillon (1992b, 110) argues that one is not required by "logical consistency" to love anyone "sufficiently similar" to one's beloved. But it also seems that I am also not required from justice to act in a similar way to anyone who is sufficiently like my son or daughter. On irreplaceable others, see Nussbaum (1990).

53 Some say (wrongly in my view) that *only* our status as persons as such is morally significant; we must not confuse this thesis, however, with the more specific judgment that in some contexts identities, relationships, or features such as sex or ethnicity should not be the basis of "discrimination" in the pejorative sense. Thus, in one context, the fact that a person has a particular ethnicity, for example, is not a valid ground for special privilege or burden; but in another context, having a certain ethnicity could be a morally significant feature of a certain sort of "special relation," e.g., national identity. See Friedman (1995, 73–74); and Kuhse, Singer, and Rickard (1998, 457–58).

54 Dillon argues that "care respect" is an "active sympathetic concern" for persons, not as persons, but as particular individuals (Dillon 1992a, 72–73; 77). Thus Dillon links Kantian respect with the abstract status of persons as such, and care respect with particularity (74–75). See also Dillon (1992b): care "is a kind of respect we owe to all persons, not just to our loved ones and friends" (107). Friedman (1995,

66–70) argues that fairness pertains to "personal relationships" as well as nonpersonal public ones, e.g., "an appropriate sharing . . . of benefits and burdens" (67), that it recognizes special forms of harm possible in intimate relations (see Outka 1980), and that it calls for just forms of marriage and family and just treatment of children by parents (Friedman 1995, 69). See also Okin (1989) and Card (1996). On justice taking into account particular identities, see also Kymlicka (1990, 272–74). See Stocker (1987, 67) on the distinction between relating to others personally, and impersonally "as place holders in moral principles."

55 I am indebted to Prof. Rosalind Ladd for many of these points; see R. Ladd (1996). See also Dancy (1992, 463–64); Held (1995b); Kuhse (1997, 174, 197); Narayan (1995).

56 On extending concern, see Held (1987) and Friedman (1993, 87–88). Friedman argues that the crucial difference in "voices" has to do with commitment to particular persons (a) in a way that is not generalizable (because persons are "unique") and (b) for their own sakes alone (Friedman 1995, 71). See Brown on "personal love" directed at a particular individual in contrast to "benevolence—a relationship that, in principle, could include any number of persons" (Brown 1987, 32–33, 97, 102). Card also stresses the personal/impersonal contrast, although she sees this as independent of a care/justice distinction (Card 1995, 81, 87). Note, however, that we do not necessarily deal directly with particular persons in all special relationships, e.g., co-nationals and co-religionists. Moreover, even where there are relations to particular persons, as MacIntyre notes, roles in one sense have to do with what "anyone" in the role should do (MacIntyre 1999, 148). See Benhabib (1992, chaps. 5 and 6); Cannold et al. (1996, 370–71); Galston (1993); Kuhse (1997, 140).

57 I do not intend to suggest, however, that there are only two virtues to which all others could be reduced. On more than two virtues, see Flanagan and Jackson (1993, 74–75), and Blum (1993a, 58). Friedman (1993, 143–44) notes that Gilligan does not hold that justice and care are the only virtues.

58 On Radcliffe's view of compassion, the concern to alleviate that follows upon recognition of suffering is partly based on respect for persons and partly on the recognition itself (Radcliffe 1994, 58).

59 Flanagan and Jackson are skeptical of the idea of integrating justice and care into one principle (although they want them to work in tandem), on the grounds that the moral life is variegated, and that we should abandon the idea of morality as a "unitary domain" (Flanagan and Jackson 1993, 83–84). See also Blum (1993a, 57). But to combine love and justice at the level of persons as such need not obscure the differences between these virtues. This combination is close I believe to what some contemporary writers mean by "right relationship," which is a caring justice or a just care; see for example Heyward (1995).

60 Curzer argues that the general virtue of care extends (in degrees) only to friends as particular persons, not to everyone (Curzer 1993, 54, 57–58). I do not argue the point here, but I want to say that the "general virtue" of care extends to everyone; there is a form of attachment that can extend to persons as such. Thus in my vocabulary (1998), "extensive" benevolence does not simply mean a disposition to desire and act for the good of others, but involves attachment (what I call compassion), and hence coalesces with what Curzer and others call care (Curzer 1993, 53–54). Therefore, in my view the general virtue of care, like the general virtue of respect, should be part of the role virtues of health professionals. I agree with Curzer, however, that it is not part of the role of health professionals that they become *friends* of their patients.

61 See Benhabib (1992, 199 n. 7) on Flanagan's and Jackson's (1993) three interpretations of Gilligan: incompatible alternatives, complementarity, and remedy-deficiency. See Richardson (1998) on Nussbaum's view of the relation between love and respect. On these matters, see Outka (1972 and 1992), and Vacek (1994). On senses of respect integral to care or *agape*, see Dillon (1992a), and Outka (1986).

62 See Lebacqz on structural injustice as a cause of suffering and compassion as a "bridge" between oppressor and oppressed that can lead to *social* justice (Labacqz 1993, 90, 92; see also Carse and Nelson (1996, 30). Lebacqz suggests that compassion is both a "projection" of what we would feel and a "direct knowledge of the suffering of another" (1993, 90–91): "Perhaps what allows me to receive the other is precisely my ability to remember and touch my own locus of pain" (90). But Lebacqz argues that we need not have had a "similar experience" to "receive the pain of the other unto ourselves" (1996b, 92–93). My view (1998) is that empathy (or "compassion," which includes empathy) should not be cast as either "projection" or direct "reception," but as interpretation that relies both on our experience (though not necessarily exactly similar to the sufferer's) and on input from the other. See also Benhabib (1992, 197–98); Cates (1997); Clark (1997); Ferreira (1994, 1997); Herdt (1997); MacIntyre (1999); and Pohl (1995).

63 Okin 1989 speaks of equal concern or benevolence in the "original position"; I would suggest equal concern and respect.

64 The dynamics of Reinhold Niebuhr's view of love and justice depend on taking ideal love as selfless concern for the good of others, and justice, even ideal justice, as legitimate concern for the self as well as others (1956 [1935]). Thus the virtues are principally correlated not as part of a set in ordinary life, but as utopia and history. Having posed these polar ideals and settings, Niebuhr then has to resort to the metaphor of "approximation" in order to relate them (Jackson 1992, 190). Although Niebuhr espoused a form of mutual love in which everyone apparently would selflessly seek the other's good and no one would be forgotten, it seems to me that the idea of selfless love reifies as an overarching ideal form of self-sacrifice that is putatively justified only in particular contexts (Outka 1992). It would even be possible to construe sacrificial love as a norm applying in many modes of temporal existence, as both prudential and witness pacifists do, for example, in the Christian tradition, without writing selfless love into the very idea of the love that will be realized beyond history. What will happen beyond history is that the good of all including the sacrificers will be secured in God. Hence, one can legitimately seek the good of all including the self, even while laying down one's life. On Niebuhr, see Jackson (1992) and Outka (1972). I have tried to combine here a "horizontal" model of justice and love as twin virtues with a "vertical" model that makes these virtues the basis of social justice. I think this is roughly speaking what King (1986), for example, held, and combined with both "prudential" and "witness" forms of pacifism. On King, see Williams (1990).

65 I would argue that *agape* (along with justice) is foundational in the sense that it establishes a framework within which special relations operate. This means at least that the negative and positive requirements of *agape* pertain to special relations; one is never to do less within special relations, as Outka (1972, 1992) argues, than *agape* toward strangers (persons as such) requires. But it could also be claimed that *agape* toward strangers takes precedence over special relations when they conflict. The first thesis seems much more intuitive to me than the second. See Reeder (1998, 61–63) and Wong (1989, 259) on the point that to argue that we first learn to love in special relations and then extend that love more broadly is not the same as the normative thesis that special relations take precedence over universal love. Wong notes, however, that the learning theme can be combined with other reasons for "priority." Note in any case that in my notion of a "transformative process" (1998) I did not wish to suggest that the love generated first in special relations is changed without remainder into universal love; my suggestion was that a new love is constructed that can be in tension with special relations. See Wong (1989). On these issues see Cates (1997); Judish (1998); and Outka (1992).

References

Andolsen, Barbara Hilkert, Christine E. Gudorf, and Mary D. Pellauer, eds. 1987. *Women's Consciousness, Women's Conscience.* San Francisco: Harper and Row.

Antony, Louise M., and Charlotte Witt, eds. 1993. *A Mind of One's Own: Feminist Essays on Reason and Objectivity.* Boulder, Colo.: Westview Press.

Baier, Annette C. 1986. Trust and Anti-Trust. *Ethics* 96/2: 231–60.

———. 1987. Hume: The Women's Moral Theorist? In *Women and Moral Theory*, ed. Eva Feder Kittay and Diana T. Meyers, 37–55. Totawa, N.J: Rowman and Littlefield.

———. 1993. Claims, Rights, Responsibilities. In *Prospects for a Common Morality,* ed. Gene Outka and John P. Reeder, Jr., 149–69. Princeton, N.J.: Princeton University Press.

———. 1995a. The Need for More than Justice. In *Justice and Care: Essential Readings in Feminist Ethics*, ed. Virginia Held, 47–58. Boulder, Colo.: Westview Press.

———. 1995b. A Note on Justice, Care, and Immigration Policy. *Hypatia* 10/2 (spring): 150–52.

Beauchamp, Tom L., and James F. Childress. 1994. *Principles of Biomedical Ethics,* 4th ed. New York: Oxford University Press.

Benhabib, Seyla. 1992. *Situating the Self: Gender, Community and Postmodernism in Contemporary Ethics.* New York: Routledge.

Benhabib, Seyla, and Drucilla Cornell, eds. 1987. *Feminism as Critique: On the Politics of Gender.* Minneapolis: University of Minnesota Press.

Bernstein, Elizabeth, and Carol Gilligan. 1990. Unfairness and Not Listening: Converging Themes in Emma Willard Girls' Development. In *Making Connections: The Relational Worlds of Adolescent Girls at Emma Willard School,* ed. Carol Gilligan, Nora P. Lyons, and Trudy J. Hammer, 147–61. Cambridge, Mass.: Harvard University Press.

Blum, Lawrence A. 1993. Gilligan and Kohlberg: Implications for Moral Theory. In *An Ethic of Care: Feminist and Interdisciplinary Perspectives,* ed. Mary Jeanne Larrabee, 49–68. New York: Routledge.

———. 1994. *Moral Perception and Particularity.* Cambridge, U.K.: Cambridge University Press.

Brown, Lyn Mikel, and Carol Gilligan. 1992. *Meeting at the Crossroads: Women's Psychology and Girls' Development.* Cambridge, Mass.: Harvard University Press.

Brown, Robert. 1987. *Analyzing Love.* Cambridge, U.K.: Cambridge University Press.

Cahill, Lisa S. 1984. Abortion, Autonomy, and Community. In *Abortion: Understanding Differences*, ed. Sidney Callahan and Daniel Callahan, 261–76. New York: Plenum Press.

Cannold, Leslie, Peter Singer, Helga Kuhse, and Lori Gruen. 1996. What Is the Justice-Care Debate *Really* About? In *Moral Concepts*, ed. Peter A. French, Theodore Uehling, Jr., and Howard K. Wettstein (Midwest Studies in Philosophy, vol. 20), 357–77. Notre Dame, Ind.: University of Notre Dame Press.

Card, Claudia, ed. 1991. *Feminist Ethics.* Lawrence: University of Kansas Press.

———. 1995. Gender and Moral Luck. In *Justice and Care: Essential Readings in Feminist Ethics*, ed. Virginia Held, 79–98. Boulder, Colo.: Westview Press.

———. 1996. *The Unnatural Lottery: Character and Moral Luck.* Philadelphia, Pa.: Temple University Press.

Carse, Alisa L. 1991. The "Voice of Care": Implications for Bioethical Education. *The Journal of Medicine and Philosophy* 16: 5–28.

Carse, Alisa L., and Hilde Lindemann Nelson. 1996. Rehabilitating Care. *Kennedy Institute of Ethics Journal* 6/1: 19–35.

Cates, Diana Fritz. 1997. *Choosing to Feel: Virtue, Friendship, and Compassion for Friends.* Notre Dame, Ind.: University of Notre Dame Press.

Childress, James F. 1985. Love and Justice in Christian Biomedical Ethics. In *Theology and Bioethics*, ed. E. E. Shelp, 225–43. Dordrecht, The Netherlands: D. Reidel Publishing Co.

Clark, Candace. 1997. *Misery and Company: Sympathy in Everyday Life.* Chicago: University of Chicago Press.

Clement, Grace. 1996. *Care, Autonomy, and Justice: Feminism and the Ethic of Care.* Boulder, Colo.: Westview Press.

Cole, Eve Browning, and Susan Coultrap-McQuin, eds. 1992. *Explorations in Feminist Ethics: Theory and Practice.* Bloomington: Indiana University Press.

Crysdale, Cynthia S. W. 1994. Gilligan and The Ethics of Care: An Update. *Religious Studies Review* 20/1 (January): 21–28.

Curzer, Howard J. 1993. Is Care a Virtue for Health Professionals? *Journal of Medicine and Philosophy* 18: 51–69.

Dancy, Jonathan. 1992. Caring About Justice. *Philosophy* 67: 447–66.

Deveaux, Monique. 1995. Shifting Paradigms: Theorizing Care and Justice in Political Theory. *Hypatia* 10/2 (spring): 115–19.

Dillon, Robin S. 1992a. Care and Respect. In *Explorations in Feminist Ethics: Theory and Practice,* ed. Eve Browing Cole and Susan Coultrap-McQuin, 69–81. Bloomington: Indiana University Press.

———. 1992b. Respect and Care: Toward Moral Integration. *Canadian Journal of Philosophy* 22/1 (March): 105–32.

Farley, Margaret. 1981. Review of Alan Donagan, *The Theory of Morality. Religious Studies Review* 7/3 (July): 233–37.

———. Feminism and Universal Morality. In *Prospects for a Common Morality,* ed. Gene Outka and John P. Reeder Jr., 170–90. Princeton, N.J.: Princeton University Press.

———. 1996. A Feminist Version of Respect for Persons. In *Feminist Ethics and the Catholic Moral Tradition,* ed. Charles E. Curran, Margaret A. Farley, and Richard A. McCormick, S.J., 164–83. New York: Paulist Press.

Feinberg, Joel. 1980a. The Nature and Value of Rights. In *Rights, Justice, and the Bounds of Liberty: Essays in Social Philosophy,* 143–55. Princeton, N.J.: Princeton University Press.

———. 1980b. A Postscript to the Nature and Value of Rights. In *Rights, Justice, and the Bounds of Liberty: Essays in Social Philosophy,* 156–58. Princeton, N.J.: Princeton University Press.

Ferreira, M. Jamie. 1994. Hume and Imagination: Sympathy and the "Other." *International Philosophical Quarterly* 34/1 (March): 39–57.

———. 1997. Equality, Impartiality, and Moral Blindness in Kierkegaard's *Works of Love. Journal of Religious Ethics* 25/1 (spring): 65–85.

Flanagan, Owen. 1991. *Varieties of Moral Personality: Ethics and Psychological Realism.* Cambridge, Mass.: Harvard University Press.

Flanagan, Owen, and Kathryn Jackson. 1993. Justice, Care, and Gender: the Kohlberg-Gilligan Debate Revisited. In *An Ethic of Care: Feminist and Interdisciplinary Perspectives*, ed. Mary Jeanne Larrabee, 69–84. New York: Routledge.

Fletcher, George P. 1997. The Case for Linguistic Self-Defense. In *The Morality of Nationalism,* ed. Robert McKim and Jeff McMahon, 324–39. New York: Oxford University Press.

Foot, Philippa. 1978. *Virtues and Vices and Other Essays in Moral Philosophy.* Berkeley: University of California Press.

Frankena, William K. 1964. Love and Principle in Christian Ethics. In *Faith and Philosophy,* ed. Alvin Plantinga, 203-25. Grand Rapids, Mich.: William B. Eerdmans.

———. 1973a. *Ethics,* 2d ed. Englewood Cliffs, N.J.: Prentice-Hall.

———. 1973b. The Ethics of Love Conceived as an Ethics of Virtue. *The Journal of Religious Ethics* 1 (fall): 5–33.

———. 1983. Moral-point-of-view Theories. In *Ethical Theory in the Twentieth Century*, ed. Norman E. Bowie, 39-79. Indianapolis, Ind.: Hackett Publishing Co.

Friedman, Marilyn. 1993. *What Are Friends For? Feminist Perspectives on Personal Relationships and Moral Theory.* Ithaca, N.Y.: Cornell University Press.

———. 1995. Beyond Caring: The De-Moralization of Gender. In *Justice and Care: Essential Readings in Feminist Ethics*, ed. Virginia Held, 61–77. Boulder, Colo.: Westview Press.

Fry, Sara T. 1989. The Role of Caring in a Theory of Nursing Ethics. *Hypatia* 4/2 (summer): 88–103.

Galston, William. 1993. Cosmopolitan Altruism. In *Altruism,* ed. Ellen Frankel Paul, Fred D. Miller, Jr., and Jeffrey Paul, 118–34. Cambridge, U.K.: Cambridge University Press.

Gewirth, Alan. 1978. *Reason and Morality.* Chicago: University of Chicago Press.

Gilligan, Carol. 1982. *In a Different Voice: Psychological Theory and Women's Development.* Cambridge, Mass.: Harvard University Press.

———. 1987. Moral Orientation and Moral Development. In *Women and Moral Theory*, ed. Eva Feder Kittay and Diana T. Meyers, 19–33. Totawa, N.J.: Rowman and Littlefield.

———. 1988. Remapping Development: Creating a New Framework for Psychological Theory and Research. In *Mapping the Moral Domain*, ed. Carol Gilligan et al., 3–19. Cambridge, Mass.: Harvard University Press.

———. 1993. Reply to Critics. In *An Ethic of Care: Feminist and Interdisciplinary Perspectives*, ed. Mary Jeanne Larrabee, 207–14. New York: Routledge.

———. 1995. Hearing the Difference: Theorizing Connection. *Hypatia* 10/2 (spring): 120–27.

Gilligan, Carol, Anne Rogers, and Lyn Mikel Brown. 1990. Epilogue: Soundings into Development. In *Making Connections: The Relational Worlds of Adolescent Girls at Emma Willard School*, ed. Carol Gilligan, Nora P. Lyons, and Trudy J. Hammer, 314–34. Cambridge, Mass.: Harvard University Press.

Gilligan, Carol, and Grant Wiggins. 1988. The Origins of Morality in Early Childhood Relationships. In *Mapping the Moral Domain*, ed. Carol Gilligan et. al., 111–38. Cambridge, Mass.: Harvard University Press.

Greenawalt, Kent. 1988. *Religious Convictions and Political Choice.* New York: Oxford University Press.

Hekman, Susan J. 1995. *Moral Voices, Moral Selves: Carol Gilligan and Feminist Moral Theory.* University Park: Pennsylvania State University Press.

Held, Virginia. 1984. *Rights and Goods: Justifying Social Action.* New York: The Free Press.

———. 1987. Feminism and Moral Theory. In *Women and Moral Theory,* ed. Eva Feder Kittay and Diana T. Meyers, 111–28. Totowa, N.J.: Rowman and Littlefield.

———. 1993. *Feminist Morality: Transforming Culture, Society, and Politics.* Chicago: University of Chicago Press.

———, ed. 1995a. *Justice and Care: Essential Readings in Feminist Ethics.* Boulder, Colo.: Westview Press.

———, 1995b. The Meshing of Care and Justice. *Hypatia* 10/2 (spring): 128–32.

Heller, Agnes. 1987. *Beyond Justice.* Oxford: Basil Blackwell Ltd.

Herdt, Jennifer A. 1997. *Religion and Faction in Hume's Moral Philosophy.* Cambridge, U.K.: Cambridge University Press.

Heyward, Carter. 1995. *Staying Power: Reflections on Gender, Justice, and Compassion.* Cleveland, Oh.: The Pilgrim Press.

Hoagland, Sarah Lucia. 1990. Some Concerns About Nel Noddings' *Caring. Hypatia* 5/1 (spring): 109–14.

Houston, Barbara. 1990. Caring and Exploitation. *Hypatia* 5/1 (spring): 115–19.

Hubin, Clayton D. 1979. The Scope of Justice. *Philosophy and Public Affairs* 9/1 (fall): 3–24.

Hursthouse, Rosalind. 1991. After Hume's Justice. *Proceedings of the Aristotelian Society* 91: 229–46.

Jackson, Timothy P. 1992. Christian Love and Political Violence. In *The Love Commandments: Essays in Christian Ethics and Moral Philosophy,* ed. Edmund N. Santurri and William Werpehowski, 182–220. Washington, D.C.: Georgetown University Press.

John, Helen J., S.N.D. 1984. Reflections on Autonomy and Abortion. In *Respect and Care in Medical Ethics,* ed. David H. Smith, 277–300. Lanham, Md.: University Press of America.

Judish, Julia E. 1998. Balancing Special Relations with the Ideal of Agape. *Journal of Religious Ethics* 26/1 (spring): 17–46.

Keller, Catherine. 1986. *From a Broken Web: Separation, Sexism and Self.* Boston: Beacon Press.

King, Martin Luther, Jr. 1986. *A Testament of Hope: The Essential Writings of Martin Luther King, Jr.,* ed. James Melvin Washington. San Francisco: Harper San Francisco.

Kittay, Eva Feder, and Diana T. Meyer, eds. 1987. *Women and Moral Theory.* Totawa, N.J.: Rowman and Littlefield.

Kroeger-Mappes, Joy. 1994. The Ethic of Care Vis-à-vis the Ethics of Rights: A Problem for Contemporary Moral Theory. *Hypatia* 9/3 (summer): 108–31.

Kuhse, Helga. 1997. *Caring: Nurses, Women, and Ethics*. U.K.: Blackwell Publishers.

Kuhse, Helga, Peter Singer, and Maurice Rickard. 1998. Reconciling Impartial Morality and a Feminist Ethic of Care. *The Journal of Value Inquiry* 32: 451–63.

Kymlicka, Will. 1990. *Contemporary Political Philosophy: An Introduction*. Oxford, U.K.: Clarendon Press.

Ladd, John 1978. Legalism and Medical Ethics. In *Contemporary Issues in Biomedical Ethics*, ed. John W. Davis, Barry Hoffmaster, and Sarah Shorten, 1–35. Clifton, N.J.: The Humana Press.

———. 1998. The Idea of Community, an Ethical Exploration, Part II: Community as a System of Social and Moral Interrelationships. *The Journal of Value Inquiry* 32: 153–74.

Ladd, Rosalind Ekman. 1996. Partiality and the Pediatrician. *The Journal of Clinical Ethics* 7, 1 (spring): 29–34.

Larrabee, Mary Jeanne, ed. 1993. *An Ethic of Care: Feminist and Interdisciplinary Perspectives*. New York: Routledge.

Lebacqz, Karen. 1987. *Justice in an Unjust World: Foundations for a Christian Approach to Justice*. Minneapolis, Minn.: Augsburg Publishing House.

———. 1993. Bridging the Gap: Pain and Compassion. In *The Future of Prophetic Christianity*, ed. Denise Larder Carmody and John Tully Carmody, 88–93. Maryknoll, N.Y.: Orbis Books.

———. 1996a. Justice. In *Dictionary of Feminist Theologies,* ed. Letty M. Russell and J. Shannon Clarkson, 158–59. Louisville, Ky.: Westminster/John Knox Press.

———. 1996b. The Weeping Womb: Why Beneficence Needs the Still Small Voice of Compassion. In *Secular Bioethics in Theological Perspective*, ed. Earl Shelp, 85–96. Dordrecht, The Netherlands: Kluwer Academic Publishers

———. 1997. Change, As in "How I've . . ." or They Don't Make Pants the Way They Used To. *Journal of Religious Ethics* 25/1 (spring): 25–32.

Little, David. 1986. Natural Rights and Human Rights: The International Imperative. In *Natural Rights and Natural Law: The Legacy of George Mason*, ed. Robert O. Davidow, 67–122. Fairfax, Va.: George Mason Press.

———. 1992. The Law of Supererogation. In *The Love Commandments: Essays in Christian Ethics and Moral Philosophy*, ed. Edmund N. Santurri and William Werpehowski, 157–81. Washington, D.C.: Georgetown University Press.

Little, Margaret Olivia. 1995. Seeing and Caring: The Role of Affect in Feminist Moral Epistemology. *Hypatia* 10/3 (summer): 117–37.

Lomasky, Loren E. 1995. Justice to Charity. *Social Philosophy and Public Policy* 12/2 (summer): 32–53.

MacIntyre, Alasdair. 1988. *Whose Justice? Which Rationality?* Notre Dame, Ind.: University of Notre Dame Press.

———. 1999. *Dependent Rational Animals: Why Human Beings Need the Virtues.* Chicago: Open Court.

Manning, Rita. 1992. Just Caring. In *Explorations in Feminist Ethics: Theory and Practice,* ed. Eve Browing Cole and Susan Coultrap-McQuin, 45–54. Bloomington: Indiana University Press.

Meilaender, Gilbert. 1986. Friendship. In *The Westminster Dictionary of Christian Ethics,* ed. James Childress and John Maquarrie, 240–41. Philadelphia, Pa.: Westminster Press.

———. 1987. *The Limits of Love: Some Theological Explorations.* University Park: Pennsylvania State University Press.

Michaels, Meredith. 1986. Morality Without Distinction. *Philosophical Forum* 17: 175–87.

Nagel, Thomas. 1971. *The Possibility of Altrusim.* Oxford: Clarendon Press.

———. 1972. War and Massacre. *Philosophy and Public Affairs* 1, 2 (winter): 123–44.

———. 1991. *Equality and Impartiality.* New York: Oxford University Press.

Narayan, Uma. 1995. Colonialism and Its Other: Considerations on Rights and Care Discourses. *Hypatia* 10/2 (spring): 133–40.

Niebuhr, Reinhold. 1956 [1935]. *An Interpretation of Christian Ethics.* New York: Meridian Press.

Noddings, Nel. 1984. *Caring: A Feminine Approach to Ethics and Moral Education.* Berkeley: University of California Press.

———. 1990. A Response. *Hypatia* 5/1: 120–26.

Nussbaum, Martha C. 1990. *Love's Knowledge: Essays on Philosophy and Literature.* New York: Oxford University Press.

———. 1993. Onora O'Neill: Justice, Gender, and International Boundaries. In *The Quality of Life,* ed. Martha Nussbaum and Amartya Sen, 324–35. Oxford: Clarendon Press.

Okin, Susan Moller. 1989. Reason and Feeling in Thinking About Justice. *Ethics* 99/2 (January): 229–49.

O'Neill, Onora. 1989. The Great Maxims of Justice and Charity. In *Constructions of Reason: Explorations of Kant's Practical Philosophy,* 219–33. Cambridge, U.K.: Cambridge University Press.

———. 1996a. Ending World Hunger. In *World Hunger and Morality*, ed. William Aiken and Hugh LaFollette, 85–112. Englewood Cliffs, N.J: Prentice-Hall.

———. 1996b. *Towards Justice and Virtue: A Constructive Account of Practical Reasoning.* Cambridge, U.K.: Cambridge University Press.

Outka, Gene. 1972. *Agape: An Ethical Analysis.* New Haven, Conn.: Yale University Press.

————. 1974. Social Justice and Equal Access to Health Care. *Journal of Religious Ethics* 2/1 (spring): 11–32.

————. 1980. On Harming Others. *Interpretation* 34/4 (October): 381–93.

————. Respect for Persons. In *Dictionary of Christian Ethics,* 2d ed., ed. James Childress and John Macquarrie, 541–45. Philadelphia, Pa.: Westminster Press.

————. 1992. Universal Love and Impartiality. In *The Love Commandments: Essays in Christian Ethics and Moral Philosophy,* ed. Edmund N. Santurri and William Werpehowski, 1–103. Washington, D.C.: Georgetown University Press.

Peters, R. C. 1973. *Reason and Compassion.* London: Routledge and Kegan Paul.

Piper, Adrian, M.S. 1991. Impartiality, Compassion, and Modal Imagination. *Ethics* 101 (July): 726–57.

Pohl, Christine D. 1995. Hospitality From the Edge: The Significance of Marginality in the Practice of Welcome. In *The Annual of the Society of Christian Ethics,* ed. Harlan Beckley, 121–36. Washington, D.C.: Georgetown University Press.

Pope, Stephen. 1991. Expressive Individualism and True Self Love. A Thomistic Perspective. *Journal of Religion* 71 (July): 384-99.

————. 1994. *The Evolution of Altruism and the Ordering of Love.* Washington, D.C.: Georgetown University Press.

Purdy, Laura. 1998. Feminist Healing Ethics. *Hypatia* 4/2 (summer): 9–14.

Radcliffe, Dana. 1994. Compassion and Commanded Love. *Faith and Philosophy* 11 (January): 50–71.

Ramsey, Paul. 1970. *Nine Modern Moralists.* New York: New American Library.

Rawls, John. 1971. *A Theory of Justice.* Cambridge, Mass.: Harvard University Press.

Reeder, John P., Jr. 1992. Analogues to Justice. In *The Love Commandments: Essays in Christian Ethics and Moral Philosophy,* ed. Edmund N. Santurri and William Werpehowski, 281-307. Washington, D.C.: Georgetown University Press.

————. 1994. Three Moral Traditions. *Journal of Religious Ethics* 22/1 (spring): 75–92.

————. 1998. Extensive Benevolence. *Journal of Religious Ethics* 26/1 (spring): 47–70.

Reich, Warren Thomas. 1995a. History of the Notion of Care. In *Encyclopedia of Bioethics,* vol. 1, ed. Warren T. Reich, 319–31. New York: Simon and Schuster MacMillan.

————. 1995b. Historical Dimensions of an Ethic of Care in Health Care. In *Encyclopedia of Bioethics*, vol. 1, ed. Warren T. Reich, 331–36. New York: Simon and Schuster MacMillan.

Reich, Warren Thomas and Nancy S. Jecker. 1995. Contemporary Ethics of Care. In *Encyclopedia of Bioethics*, vol. 1, ed. Warren T. Reich, 336–44. New York: Simon and Schuster MacMillan.

Richardson, Henry S. 1998. Nussbaum: Love and Respect. *Metaphilosophy* 29, 4 (October): 254–62.

Santurri, Edmund N. 1987. *Perplexity in the Moral Life*. Charlottesville: University of Virginia Press.

Schneewind, J.B. 1998. *The Invention of Autonomy: A History of Modern Moral Philosophy*. Cambridge, U.K.: Cambridge University Press.

Sharpe, Virgina A. 1992. Justice and Care: The Implications of the Kohlberg-Gilligan Debate for Medical Ethics. *Theoretical Medicine* 13: 295–318.

Shue, Henry. 1996. Solidarity Among Strangers and the Right to Food. In *World Hunger and Morality*, ed. William Aiken and Hugh LaFollette, 113–32. Upper Saddle River, N.J.: Prentice-Hall.

Singer, Peter, Leslie Cannold, and Helga Kuhse. 1995. William Godwin and the Defense of Impartialist Ethics. *Utilitas* 7/1 (May): 67–86.

Smith, David H., ed. 1984. *Respect and Care in Medical Ethics*. Lanham, Md.: University Press of America.

Smith, Ruth. 1988. Moral Transcendence and Moral Space in the Historical Experience of Women. *Journal of Feminist Studies in Religion* 4 (fall): 21–37.

Sterba, James. 1995. Justice. In *Encyclopedia of Bioethics*, ed. Warren T. Reich, vol. 3, 1308–15. New York: Simon and Schuster Macmillan.

Stocker, Michael. 1987. Duty and Friendship: Toward a Synthesis of Gilligan's Contrastive Moral Concepts. In *Women and Moral Theory*, ed. Eva Feder Kittay and Diana T. Meyers, 56–68. Totawa, N.J.: Rowman and Littlefield.

Tanner, Kathryn. 1996. The Care that Does Justice: Recent Writings in Feminist Ethics and Theology. *Journal of Religious Ethics* 24/1: 171–91.

Taylor, Charles. 1986. The Nature and Scope of Distributive Justice. In *Justice and Equality Here and Now*, ed. Frank S. Lucash, 34–67. Ithaca, N.Y.: Cornell University Press.

Thomson, Judith Jarvis. 1997. A Defense of Abortion. In *The Problem of Abortion*, 3rd ed., ed. Susan Dwyer and Joel Feinberg, 75–87. Belmont, Calif.: Wadsworth Publishing Co.

Tobias, Sarah. 1996. Toward a Feminist Ethic of War and Peace. In *The Ethics of War and Peace: Religious and Secular Perspectives*, ed. Terry Nordin, 228–41. Princeton, N.J.: Princeton University Press.

Tong, Rosemarie. 1997. *Feminist Approaches to Bioethics: Theoretical Reflections and Practical Applications*. Boulder, Colo.: Westview Press.

Tronto, Joan C. 1995. Care as a Basis for Radical Political Judgments. *Hypatia* 10/2 (spring): 141–49.

Vacek, Edward Collins, S.J. 1994. *Love: Human and Divine: The Heart of Christian Ethics*. Washington, D.C.: Georgetown University Press.

Vreeke, G.J. 1991. Gilligan on Justice and Care: Two Interpretations. *Journal of Moral Education* 20/1: 33–46.

Werpehowski, William. 1986a. Justice. In *The Dictionary of Christian Ethics*, 2d ed., ed. James Childress and John Macquarrie, 329–32. Philadelphia, Pa.: Westminster Press.

———. 1986b. The Professions in Context: Vocations to Justice and Love. In *Proceedings of the Theology Institute of Villanova University*, ed. Francis A. Eigo, O.S.A., 1–24. Villanova, Penn.: Villanova University Press.

Williams, Preston. 1990. An Analysis of the Conception of Love and Its Influence on Justice in the Thought of Martin Luther King, Jr. *Journal of Religious Ethics* 18/2 (fall): 15–32.

Wolgast, Elizabeth H. 1987. *The Grammar of Justice*. Ithaca, N.Y.: Cornell University Press.

Wong, David B. 1989 Universalism Versus Love With Distinctions: An Ancient Debate Revived. *Journal of Chinese Philosophy* 16: 251–72.

Yearley, Lee. 1990. *Mencius and Aquinas*. Albany: State University of New York Press.

APPENDIX
Some Senses of the Justice/Love Contrast
(Some in Gilligan and Some from Others)

"Justice," "Rights"	"Caring," "Love," "Benevolence"
(1) any distributive criterion (whose good?)	benevolence as such
(2) moral relations grounded in reason	moral relations grounded in emotion, e.g., compassion, sympathy
(3) moral relations expressed as shares, claims, what is owed or due; assertion; conflict	moral relations as expression of mutual trust; deference; cooperation
(4) social principle that expresses virtue	a fundamental *virtue*
(5) negative duty of noninterference	positive duty of aid
(6) *equal* regard	regard for *others*
(7) "impersonal," "impartial," "anyone," generalized other, stranger	inherently "personal," "partial," "someone," concrete other, special relations
(8) required	supererogatory
(9) *claim* of the other on the self	a *response* of the self to the other
(10) rights	responsibilities to those who are loved
(11) individual rights	collective good
(12) retributive justice	mercy, forgiveness, pardon
(13) abstract, general, hypothetical, repeatable	concrete, particular, real, unique
(14) absolutes	exceptions

(15) autonomy (separation)   interdependence (relation)

(16) law   narrative

(17) respect (status)   concern (attachment)

(18) agreement; regret   residual conflict; guilt

(19) argument, persuasion   communication, understanding

(20) hierarchy of considerations   no metarule

(21) restrain aggression   prevent aggression

(22) self-interested contracts   relations valued for themselves

(23) generalizations   imaginative connections between
                                               concrete situations

(24) social hierarchy   social inclusion

(25) reciprocity (*do ut des*)   giving and receiving

(26) conflict of self-interest and   indivisible good of self and other
     concern for others

(27) equality as identical treatment   equity as concern for difference

(28) duty (motive)   desire (motive)

(29) actions   character (virtue)

(30) rule-following   discernment

2

Care and Justice as Moral Values for Nurses in an Era of Managed Care

Barbara Hilkert Andolsen

Many nurses have eagerly embraced the ethics of care; they especially appreciate the way the ethics of care makes the activity of caring a practice central to human morality. For these nurses, the ethics of care seems to describe accurately the fundamental dynamic of their professional lives. In addition, for both its practitioners and the larger society, nursing has always been understood as an essentially feminine activity. The feminine ethics of care coheres nicely with nursing as a quintessentially feminine profession.

The ethics of care fits particularly well with a type of nursing called "primary care nursing." Under this system, the nurse's experiences at the patient's bedside make the ethics of care seem especially plausible as the basic ethical model for nursing. In the 1990s, however, fierce economic pressures forced a piecemeal restructuring of the health care industry. Hospital nurses report being hard pressed to care for a larger group of patients who have more serious medical problems. Recent economic trends have made it more difficult for nurses to live up to the moral ideal described by an ethic of care. In addition, some hospitals have attempted to substitute lower-cost, less-educated labor for part of their nursing workforce. Where hospitals are teaming nurses with unlicensed assistive personnel (UAPs), racial/ethnic and social class differences raise other ethical questions for nurses, nursing supervisors, and other hospital administrators.

In this essay, I investigate whether an ethic of care is still realistic for nursing professionals in an era of managed care. I argue that an ethic of care needs to be supplemented by attention to the value of justice in order to address all the questions arising from the reorganization of nursing labor as the health care system is restructured. In particular, the value of social justice allows us to ask urgent questions about the obligations of registered nurses (RNs) toward other members of the care giving team, especially toward UAPs.

A HISTORICAL PERSPECTIVE ON NURSING CARE

Although the ethical theory called the ethics of care is of recent intellectual origin, the challenges and constraints facing nurses who are dedicated to caring are not new. To understand the moral challenges that confront nurses both in their relationships with patients and patients' loved ones, as well as in their relationships with other hospital care givers, it is helpful to review some aspects of the history of hospital nursing in the United States.

Nurses have always been a crucial part of the labor force in modern hospitals. Hospital administrators have sought to obtain nursing labor on terms that meet potentially conflicting objectives: providing quality health care, achieving patient (customer) satisfaction, and controlling labor costs. Over the last century, staffing arrangements have gone through pendulum swings between labor patterns that involve high amounts of RN labor per patient and nursing team models where less-educated workers provided more routine bodily care for patients. The attempt by some hospitals currently to substitute UAPs for some RN labor is not an entirely new endeavor.

When the twentieth century began, a major segment of the labor force in U. S. hospitals was student nurses who were attending training programs at nursing schools affiliated with these hospitals. These students worked long hours and were expected to provide many services, including manual labor; for example, students mopped floors as part of their "training."

In 1923, the Goldmark Report recommended a series of reforms. It advocated that nurses be trained in college settings where they would be less vulnerable to exploitation as a captive labor force. Hospitals should be staffed by two groups that would divide the duties formerly done by student nurses. RNs who had completed their education at nursing schools, colleges, and universities would perform the professional duties associated with pa-tient care. A cadre of lower skilled workers, such as nursing assistants, orderlies, and housekeeping staff, would do more mundane tasks.

These recommendations fit nicely with a widespread economic theory, known as Taylorism, about the most cost-effective way to deploy labor. Taylorism advocated that any given work process should be broken down into its smallest units of activity; then each narrowly defined task should be assigned to those people with the minimum level of skill necessary to do the tasks properly. For example, when applied to nursing labor, a Taylorist approach indicated that RNs should prepare medications for distribution to patients because only they had the education necessary to verify that medications were administered in compliance with doctors' orders. Nursing assistants should help a patient use a bedpan. Housekeepers should mop the floors.

M. Catherine Lundy indicates that the American Hospital Association's drive in the 1930s to apply Taylorism to hospital labor stimulated the creation of the category of licensed practical nurse (LPN) as an intermediate category of nursing labor (Lundy 1996). Hospitals hired LPNs to handle a wide range of direct patient care tasks at lower cost. LPNs could take and record vital signs (temperature, blood pressure, pulse, and respiration), change dressings, or collect samples of urine or feces from patients, for example.

Because RN labor is the most expensive category of labor among nursing care deliverers, the economic interests of RNs are threatened by the substitution of lower-cost, less-skilled labor. Several sociologists have studied the ways in which nursing leaders and organizations of RNs have sought to protect RNs against the encroachment of less-skilled workers. In the 1930s, RNs did not have enough economic or political power to stop a trend toward the use of less-educated, lower-cost nursing personnel, so they responded by lobbying for state licensing regulations that reserved the most skilled tasks for RNs only (Lundy 1996, 163–64). For example, in some states only an RN may administer medicines or start an IV. Nona Glazer suggests that nursing leaders sought to prevent "the displacement of RNs by licensed practical nurses (LPNs) and nursing aides by restricting the training of these lower-grade personnel and by limiting their work to nontechnical health care tasks" (Glazer 1991, 352). Indeed, she reports that in 1948, the National Nursing Council rejected proposals for "a career ladder in which further education for nursing assistants could lead to the RN degree" (364). RNs used the argument, which is again being advanced, that the substitution of less-educated nursing labor for fully qualified RNs at the bedside threatened the health of patients (367). In many states, Boards of Nursing dominated by RNs gained control of the licensing process for LPNs, as well as for RNs.

By the 1950s, the American Nursing Association reported that LPNs had taken over so many routine patient care tasks that "bedside care was no longer the principal occupation of the professional nurse" (Lundy 1996,

164). In a team approach, nursing aides did the most basic, least technical physical care tasks. They helped patients to eat (if necessary), to bathe, and to use the bedpan or toilet. LPNs took a patient's vital signs, gave alcohol rubs, observed the patients' reactions to procedures and medications, and, in some states, distributed medications prepared by the RN. The RNs did the most technical patient care tasks and planned and supervised the more basic nursing services provided by aides and LPNs.

During the 1950s, some nursing leaders hoped that RNs would gain higher professional status and higher wages precisely because they were doing fewer routine physical care tasks. RNs spent a significant portion of their time performing important supervisory functions as the coordinators of nursing teams (Wagner 1980). This viewpoint reflected the social opinion that direct physical care was work of limited social worth; the mental work of delegation and supervision was more highly regarded.

By the late 1960s, however, the pendulum had swung back in the direction of greater RN presence at the bedside. Nursing leaders began to advocate a concept known as "primary care nursing." Many nurses desired more contact with patients than they experienced as leaders in a nursing team approach.[1] RNs were also concerned that, as licensed professionals, they might be held accountable for patient care errors made by subordinates. Hospital administrators were willing to consider the primary care nursing approach because they realized that organizing and monitoring the performance of subordinates in the nursing team was consuming excess RN labor. Hospitals were also concerned about accountability for errors in patient treatment. With the nursing team approach, it was sometimes difficult to determine who was responsible when something went wrong. For example, if a patient suffered when an adverse reaction to a drug went undetected, hospital administrators might not be able to determine whether the LPN or the RN was responsible. Had the LPN failed properly to observe and report signs of the drug reaction? Or had the supervising RN failed to respond appropriately to the LPN's information about the patient's condition? Faced with such problems, some nursing leaders and hospital administrators began to argue that a greater use of RN labor was actually more cost effective. They contended that RNs, who had a greater repertoire of skills, could respond more expeditiously to unpredictable patient needs. RNs could be deployed more flexibly (Brannon 1994).

So hospitals moved to a primary care nursing approach. Each nurse was assigned a small group of patients for whom she was primarily responsible during her shift. Because RNs were spending more time providing physical care for individual patients, nurses had the opportunity to get to know patients and their families in more depth, and to assume a greater share of the "emotional labor" of caring (Brannon 1994, 116). It is important, however, not to romanticize the nurse-patient relationship under primary care nursing. When hospitals switched to the primary care nursing approach, they reduced the size of their auxiliary staffs significantly. Thus, the remaining RNs had many more direct patient care tasks to perform. In some hospitals, RNs found themselves seriously pressed for time as they tried to meet the essential physical needs of their charges with little help from other hospital employees. Brannon indicates that "to ensure their completion of higher priority work, RNs omitted some of the tasks formerly performed by auxiliaries, shifted other tasks onto patients and their families, and structured work at the bedside to limit excessive patient demands" (168). Indeed, one nurse, who had experienced both the nursing team approach and the primary care nursing reform movement, told Brannon that "patients got more personal care, more TLC under team nursing. They got more back rubs, baths, the personal care tasks, including more opportunities to talk to someone" (168).

By the early 1980s, federal government officials were concerned about the escalating costs of health care services—costs paid by the federal government for older patients under Medicare. Therefore, the government adopted new policies for determining hospital reimbursement rates. These new prospective payment policies were designed to force hospitals to limit increases in the rates that they charged the government. In 1983, the federal government introduced the concept of DRGs, diagnosis-related groups. Under this approach, government bureaucrats determined an appropriate payment for the treatment of a specific medical problem (i.e., diagnosis), taking into account the average length of a hospital stay for its treatment. Thus the government announced *in advance* a standardized price that it would pay a hospital for treatment of a patient who received a particular "principal diagnosis."[2] In health industry jargon, the government reimbursed a hospital a fixed, predetermined fee based on the patient's DRG. Many HMOs and other third-party payers shifted to similar prospective reimbursement methods.

In order for a hospital to remain fiscally sound (or profitable) when many patients fell under prospective reimbursement methods, hospital administrators had to make a number of changes. Two strategies are of particular relevance to this discussion. First, administrators had to keep careful control over hospital costs, including labor costs. Second, they had to urge doctors to discharge patients from the hospital as quickly as possible. As a result of an emphasis on getting patients out of hospitals quickly, the patients who remained hospitalized were a sicker group compared to the hospital's patient census prior to the establishment of the DRG reimbursement system.

One nurse described succinctly the pressure created within a "primary care nursing" system by patient populations with a greater overall level of acute illness—the new patient mix fostered by the financial constraints of prospective payment systems. Discussing the situation at the start of the 1990s, she says:

> Five years ago, nurses would comment about a heavy patient case-load, trying to ensure that one particular nurse wasn't carrying more than one patient who required a particularly heavy amount of work. Today, all the patients are heavy. They have multiple problems or they would be in the community, being cared for in a home-care situation. These patients require intensive care, but they are placed on regular hospital care floors, and assigned in groups of seven, eight, nine or ten to a single nurse. (Storr 1996, 32–33)

Ironically, during roughly the same period, RNs demanded wages more nearly commensurate with their level of education and professional responsibilities. Himmelstein and others report than in the period from 1968 to 1993, the wages of RNs "nearly doubled"; in comparison, "the wages of most other [health care] occupations rose 25% to 50%" (Himmelstein, Lewontin, and Woolhandler 1996, 527). Increases in nursing pay substantially enlarged the significance of nursing salaries as a portion of hospital budgets in a period when the government, insurance companies, and employers who provided health insurance coverage were all trying to hold down rapidly rising health care costs.

One obvious way for administrators to cut nursing costs was to substitute cheaper, less-educated labor for RN labor. In some highly publicized instances, major hospitals realized substantial cost savings by cutting full-time positions for registered nurses while substantially increasing jobs for unlicensed aides. For example, at the UCLA Medical Center in 1996, "there [were] 650 full-time positions for nurses, down about 60 [over] five years"; simultaneously, positions for unlicensed workers known at this facility as "care partners" had expanded from "30 to 120" (Shuit 1996, A17). In 1994, the American Nursing Association surveyed its members to get a better idea of the employment picture for RNs in hospital settings. "Seventy percent of all respondents said their employers were cutting back on staffing by leaving vacant positions unfilled, 66 percent said their hospitals had already laid off nurses or were planning to do so, and 67 percent of registered nurses said the number of patients assigned to them had increased" (Fagin 1999, F7).

Thus, during the 1980s and 1990s, hospital administrators instituted a new version of the team nursing approach, with one important difference. The team is now more sharply polarized, with many RNs and a number of less-trained, lower paid unlicensed care providers, but relatively few intermediate-level LPNs. Despite some highly publicized cases in which hospitals laid off full-time RNs, it was actually nursing personnel with intermediate skills who suffered the greatest job losses during the period between 1981 and 1993. One reason why RN positions remained somewhat more stable was that an increasing percentage of patients in hospitals were acutely ill. When there are more seriously ill patients, more RNs are needed to provide the highly skilled nursing functions that only they are trained (and permitted by law) to perform. Still, "fewer nursing caregivers per patient [across the spectrum from nursing aide to registered nurse] are available today than a decade ago to provide care to a more acutely ill patient population" (Aiken 1996, 90).

RACIAL AND CLASS DIVISIONS IN THE HOSPITAL WORKFORCE

Racial and class divisions among women are pertinent to any analysis of ethical issues that arise in the nursing process. Among paid patient-care providers, European American women are over-represented at the higher, professional end, as RNs. African American women, Hispanic women, and Native American women are more likely to be found at the lower, nonprofessional levels, as LPNs, nursing aides, and UAPs. This long-embedded pattern does not appear likely to change in the immediate future. For example, a 1993 essay indicates that although minority group members made up 22 percent of the population in the United States, they provided less than 15 percent of the students enrolled in programs to train RNs (Sabatino 1993, 23).

In this section, I will concentrate largely on African American women, because fairly detailed information about their experiences in the health care field is more readily available. Based on limited information, it appears that the situation may be even more dire for Hispanic workers (Trevino et al. 1993). Native American workers are particularly unlikely to be found as RNs. They constitute less than 1 percent of the workers in that occupational category.

The health care industry has provided an important source of employment for African American women. First, the traditionally feminine professions such as nursing have been an important source of employment at the professional level for African American women. African American women are more likely now than women of European descent to be clustered in such feminine professions. European American women are moving more quickly into formerly male-dominated professional or managerial positions. Still, African American women who are health care workers are more likely to fill lower-level positions in the nursing labor structure. "African-American women are only 8% of the RNs but they are 15.5% of LPNs, 24% of the health aides and assistants" (Himmelstein, Lewontin, and Woolhandler 1996, 527).

There are important class differences among women in the health care system. A growing number of women are found at the higher levels as administrators and staff doctors. Nurses and social workers, who are predominantly female, find themselves in a middle level in the hospital class structure. Many female UAPs join others like housekeeping personnel at the bottom of the class structure.

Himmelstein and his colleagues see two simultaneous trends affecting the employment of African American women in hospitals. One is a trend away from hospital stays toward care in other, less costly settings such as nursing homes or patients' own homes. The other is a trend toward a higher percentage of administrators compared to other employees in hospitals. These two trends bode ill for African American women presently working in hospitals. As Himmelstein and his colleagues note: "1 of every 10 employed African-American women works as an aide, housekeeper, or food service worker in medical care, while few are health executives" (Himmelstein, Lewontin, and Woolhandler 1996, 528). I would add that many African American women are employed as aides in nursing homes and as home health care workers. However, lower level workers in these settings usually receive lower wages than their counterparts who work for hospitals. Home health aides and nursing home attendants are also less likely to be represented by unions.

THE NURSING PROFESSION AND THE ETHICS OF CARE

Patients in the hospital are dependent on others for care. Nursing personnel do much of the caring work in hospitals. Nursing care is multidimensional and many of these dimensions have important moral aspects. The moral significance of the care that is provided to sick people in hospitals, in other health care facilities, and in their own homes did not receive sufficient attention from ethicists until feminists created a moral theory called the ethics of care. Some commentators writing about nursing ethics found an ethic of care particularly well-suited for articulating the values of the nursing profession. One of the most important proponents of an ethic of care within nursing, Jean Watson, declared that "caring is the essence of nursing and the most central and unifying focus for nursing practice" (Watson 1988, 33). Sara Fry seconded that opinion when she declared that "caring ought to be the foundational value for any theory of nursing ethics" (Fry 1989, 89).

In this next section, I identify and discuss four distinct but interrelated moral dimensions of care within nursing practice. First, the best work on the ethics of care draws our attention to the physical work of caring that is too often ignored in ethical discourse. When focusing on care as work, I point briefly to nurses' important moral obligation to provide *competent nursing care*, that is, skillful technical nursing services. Second, there is a complex relationship between caring as a moral imperative for nurses and nurses' *positive, "caring" feelings* toward most, but not all, patients. Third, nurses who gain a more holistic knowledge of patients as they spend time providing hands-on care for those patients are well positioned to employ an ethic of care as *a specific style of moral reasoning*. Fourth, nurses as a professional group often assign a high priority to care as *a moral value*.

Competent Body Care

The ethics of care at its best draws the attention of ethicists to activities associated with physical care for vulnerable and interdependent human beings. The work involved in caring for the sick and the physically vulnerable has been virtually ignored by most thinkers in the field of ethics. Society has also accorded such work—not incidentally, a traditional form of women's work—limited social value.

Among theorists who discuss the ethics of care, Joan Tronto and I have (separately) insisted that ethicists need to examine closely the physical work involved in caring and how that labor is distributed. In an essay about caring for frail elderly people with chronic diseases, I stressed the moral significance of reliable and gentle physical aid in meeting the most mundane bodily needs of persons with disabilities. For example, it is a work with moral value to clean urine and feces from a frail body consistently, carefully, and gently. Helping frail elders to survive with as much dignity as possible requires a great deal of mundane work that should not be glossed over (Andolsen 1993, 134–37). Tronto also insists that the "direct meeting of needs for care," which "involves physical work," is a crucial component of the process of caring (Tronto 1993, 107). She is concerned that, in this society, people are too quick to believe that they have shown that they "care" for some vulnerable group when they write a check. Tronto is also concerned about the social exploitation that results when society refuses to consider specifically who does the physical work of care giving and at what cost to themselves. Importantly, Tronto has probed how the socially privileged often delegate the work of caring for sick bodies to working-class women—often women of color.

It is crucial that ethicists discussing the implications of an ethic of care for nursing not disregard the moral implications of the physical work of caring for the bodies of sick persons. Nursing personnel—from unlicensed aides to RNs—do something morally significant when they assess the physical and (other) human vulnerabilities of their patients as morally salient, and when they respond with practical care giving activity designed to meet the specific needs of those patients.

As RNs work to provide skillful nursing services to vulnerable patients, they are also responding to a legal and moral obligation to provide each patient with competent nursing care. Nurses employ critical technical skills as they care for the bodies of their patients. They also perform a series of nursing assessments as they care for these bodies. A skillful nurse is alert to signs revealing the patient's physiological and psychological state and the more general state of a patient's well-being. The moral connection between professional competence and the ethical responsibility to care is too rarely articulated in the nursing ethics literature.

Here, I am making a point about nurses' moral responsibility to provide competent nursing care, similar to a point made by medical ethicist Edmund D. Pellegrino about doctors. He asserts that professionals such as doctors (and, by extension, nurses) have a duty to provide competent care that flows directly from their claim as professionals to have mastered a unique body of professional knowledge. Pellegrino says, "to begin with, the act of medical profession is inauthentic and a lie unless it fulfills the expectation of technical competence. If the special knowledge upon which the act of profession is based is wanting, then the whole relationship begins with a lie" (Pellegrino 1989, 80).

The special professional knowledge of nurses includes a variety of skills, such as the ability to administer an injection or the ability correctly to insert a urinary catheter. In hospitals, patients give themselves over to nurses with the expectation that RNs have the professional knowledge and skill to provide competent nursing services.[3] If nurses do not have the intellectual knowledge or technical skill to provide adequate nursing services for their patients, they fail to uphold the professional moral imperative to provide competent care.

One of the greatest ethical concerns that RNs express about the restructuring of nursing labor in hospitals in the 1990s is that nurses are charged with caring for too many seriously ill patients at the same time. Hence, time, and so their ability to meet the professional ethical imperative to provide competent nursing care is compromised. Financial pressures undermining the ability of nursing personnel to provide competent care are an international phenomenon. One British patient told researchers investigating nursing care in the United Kingdom's National Health Service Hospitals a horrifying story. A few days after having undergone two major operations, the patient was supposed to be helped to take a bath in a nearby bathroom. The patient reports: "I was lowered into the bath on a chair, *then I was forgotten*. I was too weak to pull the cord [for assistance]" (Anderson 1998, A22, emphasis added). Leaving such a seriously ill patient alone in the bath is incompetent nursing practice. Moreover, it is simultaneously a violation of a professional ethical obligation to provide competent care and a violation of a broader ethic of care.

A serious moral question facing RNs as a professional group is what types of collaboration with UAPs are consistent with RN duties to provide competent nursing care. Which patterns of UAP labor make a nurse complicit in a violation of the moral duty to provide competent nursing care for patients? Nurses frequently express concern that unlicensed personnel do not have the training to do a sophisticated assessment of the patient's state while assisting the patient with basic activities such as eating or bathing. Concern that the quality of patient care is being undermined by administrative decisions about staffing raises questions of institutional ethics, not just professional ethical questions about the responsibility of nurses to exercise careful judgment when assigning tasks to UAPs.

Caring Work and Caring Feelings

Nurses often find their caring labor to be satisfying work because they have warm, compassionate feelings for their patients. A positive emotional bond between patient and nurse fuels the nurse's caring labor. However, the relationship between emotion and care is a complex one for nurses, who as hospital employees do not necessarily feel positively toward all the patients for whom they are assigned to provide care labor.

An ethic of care recognizes a positive role for emotion in the moral life. Care givers are often emotionally moved by the needs of the recipient of care. None of the advocates of an ethic of care endorses a moral system rooted in shallow sentimentality. However, Nel Noddings in particular draws our attention to caring actions that are rooted in an *emotional* recognition of the moral worth of the recipient. Moreover, she contends that caring activities should be undertaken with "an attitude that warms and comforts" the recipient (Noddings 1984, 19). According to Noddings, actions that are done in a "perfunctory" or "grudging" way fail in an important sense to convey caring (12, 20).

The moral ideal of caring integrates positive emotions with a commitment to care that results in caring actions. The *ideal* of a caring nurse is one of a professional who conveys a generous, compassionate, and warm concern for the patients who are entrusted to her or his care. The ethic of care gives us language to offer moral praise for nurses' emotional pull toward patients that manifests itself in spontaneous concern and comfort offered to those patients. However, I suggest that nursing as caring *work* also challenges us to assess realistically the ambiguity of caring as a positive affective state. The moral responsibility of nurses toward "difficult" patients shows that there is a complex relationship between morally admirable "caring" and positive affective states. It is too simple to suggest that nurses have somehow failed to fulfill their moral duty if they do not have a warm, generous emotional response to some patients.

For example, a group of nurses found it hard to provide skillful nursing services for a young male patient because of his sexually provocative behavior toward the nursing staff. The young man asked blunt, intrusive questions about the nurses' sex lives while they were in his room performing essential nursing procedures. When a nurse came to provide routine morning care, she would invariably find that the patient had deliberately shifted his bedding to expose his erect penis. In a fairly short period, almost the entire nursing staff tried to avoid going into the young man's room. Fortunately, a highly skilled "float" nurse volunteered to take charge of the provocative patient's bedside care.[4] She set firm limits on behavior that she would tolerate. This nurse was able to help the patient act more appropriately and to assist him in confronting the sexual anxieties connected with his illness in a much more positive way (Stockard 1991). The nurse who volunteered to care for the exhibitionist patient was a "caring" professional who came to share a rapport with her difficult patient. However, it is understandable that other staff members felt angry and resentful about the sexually harassing behavior of this difficult patient. I suggest that the moral lapse displayed by the other nurses was *not* a failure to summon up warm and generous feelings about the patient while he was engaging in harassing behavior. Instead, their moral failing was allowing their understandable, negative feelings to interfere with their duty to provide competent nursing services for the patient.

An honest analysis of caring as a professional duty for nurses reveals that an attitude of moral concern for the well-being of the patient is *not* dependent on a feeling of warm personal regard for the patient (see Mahony 1998). A morally virtuous nurse can provide high quality care, that is, skillful nursing services, for a patient even when the nurse does not "care for" the patient's personality traits or when the nurse disapproves of the patient's moral character. Nurses can (and ought to) struggle to maintain a stance of fundamental respect for the patient even when the patient's behavior is emotionally repulsive. The moral ideal of care for nurses encompasses a praiseworthy warm emotional concern for patients. However, that ideal is tempered by a realistic appreciation of most nurses' mixed feelings toward difficult patients.

An Ethic of Care as a Method of Moral Reasoning

When dealing with an ethic of care in a nursing setting, it is important to notice the intersection of physical care for the body, recognition and sharing of emotions, and ethical reflection. It is, in part, the bedside work of nursing personnel that provides the opportunity for nurses to come to understand their patients' moral situations, their feelings, and their values in a personal way. One nurse commenting on the crucial role that nurses play as patient advocates says that, "the difference nurses can make is really because we are closer more often to people, *because of the physical care we give*" (Zalumas 1995, 116, emphasis added). Especially under the primary care nursing model, nurses are at the patient's bedside checking vital signs, administering medications, monitoring intravenous fluids, and so on. While doing all those things, nurses have many opportunities to be attentive to the needs, feelings, and values of their patients. Philosopher Peta Bowden emphasizes the legitimate source of moral knowledge that nurses achieve through the "relative continuity and intimacy of their relationships with patients" (Bowden 1997, 135). That intimacy is, in part, established through the nurses' physical ministrations to the bodies of their patients.

The form of knowledge about patients that is available only to those who spend consistent time caring for the bodies of those patients is often ignored or dismissed in medical ethics. Throughout the health care system, those with more education and a higher professional status tend to minimize the value of the ethical insights gained by subordinates whose jobs entail more mundane physical care giving. In turn, subordinates argue that precisely because they spend more time doing direct patient care, they gain important knowledge about patients' physical states, emotions, and moral views. However, subordinates complain that their knowledge of patients is not sought by superiors who have less patient contact. Nursing aides and home health care aides complain about nurses who, in turn, complain about doctors (Glazer 1988, 130).

Some commentators on nursing ethics appreciate the ethics of care especially because it provides a language to discuss the value of the more individualized, personal knowledge that nurses gain at patients' bedsides. Nurses, particularly proponents of primary care nursing, have gravitated toward the ethics of care because it is holistic, individualized, and relational. An ethic of care requires that the care giver pay close attention to the unique needs, interests, and values of the care recipient. Ethicist Helga Kuhse explains aptly how a nurse practicing a caring approach apprehends the patient as a unique person. She says such nurses "are more likely to be receptive to the needs of patients, where the patients are recognized as *particular others*, that is, as individuals with special needs, beliefs, desires and wants, rather than a malfunctioning organism" (Kuhse 1997, 150). Advocates of this style of moral decision making recommend that care givers attempt a comprehensive review of the concrete circumstances of the care recipient, taking into account all relevant dimensions of the context in which care giving takes place.

An ethic of care is a relational ethic. Within a relational framework, the moral values that ought to be accorded primacy in a given situation are determined in the interaction between care giver and care recipient. The notion that moral principles are recognized as binding within a particular set of relationships fits well with the emphasis during the 1970s and 1980s in nursing ethics on the duties of the primary care nurse as patient advocate. The nurse, it was said, is the health care worker who has the best opportunity to gain insight into the particular configuration of moral values that matter most to a specific patient. Therefore, the nurse can and should demand that the patient's specific moral views be respected when health care providers make moral decisions about health care services for a particular patient. One version of the patient advocate model stresses the uniqueness of an individual patient's moral perspective. This stance challenges theories of moral decision making that claim to establish, through independent rationality, a hierarchy of objective moral values and then to make a rational decision about which moral principle ought to govern a patient's treatment.

Another strength of the ethic of care as a relational ethic is its explicit acknowledgment that human beings as moral subjects are always involved in extended patterns of relationship. The interlinking sets of relationships in which persons are embedded have a bearing on moral obligation. The foregrounding of relationships in discussions about the ethics of care provides a theoretical basis for nurses to assert their own important moral insights developed through their time-intensive relationships with hospital patients. The ethics of care also allows nurses to voice their concerns about the impact of medical decisions not only on the patient, but also on the patient's loved ones.

Time is necessary to build up the detailed knowledge about patients and their loved ones that is required to implement an ethic of care style of moral reasoning. I note, for example, that stories in the nursing literature that illustrate an ethic of care style of decision making often involve the relationship between a nurse and a patient who is hospitalized for an unusually long time (Parker 1990) or between a nurse and a patient who have come to know each other throughout a series of repeated hospitalizations (Cooper 1991).

There is a tendency, I suggest, to romanticize the nurse as the caring moral decision maker at the bedside. Technology, the midlevel position of nurses in the hospital hierarchy, and economic restructuring of the health care system make the situation of the RN as the caring moral agent at the bedside a more complex one.

Technological equipment, which may offer important benefits in patient care, sometimes creates barriers to morally fruitful human contact between a nurse and a patient. Nurses who began their careers at a time when fewer technological devices were used in patient care report important differences in human contact between nurses and patients. Reflecting on her experience in the 1950s, one nurse says that "the nurse really had almost direct patient contact then. You did not have the machine between the nurse and the patient so much" (Zalumas 1995, 57). Another nurse working in an intensive care unit admitted to Zalumas, "You can walk to the foot of the bed and know everything you need to know. You don't have to touch the patient. Sometimes I find people not even bothering to talk to the patient because he is intubated and he doesn't really respond, so guess what—neither does the nurse" (81).

The middle status position of nurses in the hospital bureaucracy makes their execution of an ethic of care more difficult and complex. As Condon comments, "because of the impersonal goals of bureaucratic systems, care givers in institutions are frequently thwarted in their efforts to provide personalized holistic care; their low status in the hierarchy intensifies this problem" (Condon 1992, 15). Although Condon describes nurses as having a low status, the reality is that nurses are in the middle status position in the hospital hierarchy—ranking below administrators and doctors, but ranking above LPNs, aides, and housekeeping personnel. Bowden notices but does not develop fully the moral potential of nurses' position in the hospital bureaucracy. She realizes that nurses working in a properly struc- tured health care system could facilitate "collaborative caring"; the position of nurses contains "the ethical potential to communicate between different members of the 'team' and to encourage co-operation and accommodation among those involved for the sake of the patient's well-being" (Bowden 1997, 126). In order to fulfill this function, nurses would have to receive professional respect from doctors and hospital administrators. Nurses would also have to show an appreciation for the moral wisdom offered by workers who rank below them in the hospital hierarchy.

Hospital nurses continue to have encounters with patients that are charac- terized by relatively more physical intimacy and often more continuity than the relationships between staff physicians and patients. However, with severe financial pressures to limit hospital stays to the minimum necessary to deliver highly technical health care services, nurses' opportunities to come to know each patient as a unique individual are under serious pressure. Many patients, even patients with serious illnesses, are hospitalized for much shorter lengths of time these days. If physical care is rendered under circumstances of sharp time constraints, then it is less clear that physical care, a sharing of emotion, and the development of special ethical insights can be smoothly integrated into the nursing labor process. As nurses provide essential physical care for many seriously ill patients, they must concentrate on delivering care as quickly as possible in order to "move on" to the next patient. Patients may be less likely to share emotions during a brief, perhaps noticeably rushed, encounter. Under the stress of providing essential physical care for a larger number of seriously ill patients, it becomes more difficult for a nurse to remain genuinely attentive to the physical, emotional, and ethical needs of each patient.

The Moral Value of Care

The ethics of care is a style of moral reasoning that emphasizes unique moral decisions arrived at through careful examination of the particular values of the parties involved and their unique circumstances. However, an ethic of care also suggests that care as a moral value should be central in human activity, or at least in a variety of human activities involving fairly intimate personal contact, such as parenting, teaching, or nursing. Thus, Noddings creates an ethic that has a crucial dispositional component. She asserts that "an ethic of caring locates morality primarily in the *pre-act consciousness* of the one-caring" (Noddings 1984, 28, emphasis added). In other words, it is the *prior recognition* of another as worthy of care and a firm commitment to act so as to promote the good of the one-cared-for that are particularly important in an ethic of care.

Noddings's understanding of the ethic of care is rooted in the realization that human beings "want to be moral in order to remain in the caring relation and to enhance the ideal of . . . [themselves] as one-caring" (Noddings 1984, 5). Noddings argues that one of the most important experiences in human life is the experience of being cared for in a loving way. Our youthful experiences of being cared for are a tangible good; we long to preserve ourselves as persons involved in caring relationships. As we mature, we realize that we must—and that we want to—become persons who care for others as an indispensable part of remaining involved in caring relations. Noddings's depiction of the moral agent naturally attracted to the ideal of the self as a caring person fits closely with the professional and social ideal of the nurse as a caring individual.

The dispositional dimension of the ethic of care resonates strongly with the ethical experiences of nurses, although the nursing ethics literature does not always specifically identify this dispositional or attitudinal aspect as a separate dimension of an ethic of care approach. Codes of ethics for nurses have always stressed an attitude of concern for the patient—a commitment to advance the welfare of the patient. Helga Kuhse indicates helpfully that "caring . . . is not primarily concerned with tasks and processes, but is a mode of being, a virtue, or a stance or attitude towards the object of one's attention" (Kuhse 1999, 147).

The virtue of caring involves a firm disposition to advance the unique interests of the recipient of care. As a value, care is similar to but distinct from the value of beneficence. In a medical setting, both care and beneficence focus on advancing the "good" of the patient. However, beneficence can be a detached, paternalistic value. A beneficent health care provider may strive to make a rational, objective decision about what is best for the patient. Moreover, a beneficent provider might well strive for consistency when identifying and promoting the good for a group of similarly situated patients. For example, a nurse in a neonatal unit might come to the conclusion that it is in the best interest of all neonates with similar severe neurological injuries to allow them to die.

In contrast, an ethic of care stresses that the caring response is determined in a concrete way for each unique patient within that patient's particular network of relationships and given that patient's unique needs and desires. A caring nurse strives to do the caring thing for this specific neonate and his or her specific loved ones. What it means to do the caring thing for this particular neonate is a customized response. The nurse's caring response to one newborn has limited relevance when deciding the caring response to the next neonate.

THE ETHICS OF CARE AND OF JUSTICE

An ethic of care approach in nursing seeks customized moral solutions to ethical difficulties that arise while caring for patients. A nurse following an ethic of care places limited value on the consistent application of moral principles—let alone rigid adherence to bureaucratic proscriptions—when deciding how to respond to a patient's predicament. Both Carol Gilligan (1982) and Noddings contrast a caring style of moral reasoning with a deductive, principle-based approach. Those who follow the work of Gilligan frequently use her terminology, which differentiates between an ethic of care and an ethic of justice.

A principle-based style of moral reasoning emphasizes a careful procedure for moral decision making. This mode of moral reasoning stresses the consistent application of abstract moral principles ranked in a hierarchical order according to a carefully justified lexical ordering scheme. As Gilligan pictures this principle-based style of reasoning, the emphasis is on a specific type of procedural justice. Procedural justice, as described by Gilligan, requires a sophisticated ability to adjudicate rationally among conflicting (individual) rights. This so-called ethic of justice approach privileges the quality of impartiality as a characteristic of sound moral decision makers. The decision maker ought to determine the relative moral weight of conflicting rights *without being compromised* by undue self-interest or swayed by morally irrelevant personal characteristics of the parties involved. Thus detachment, coupled with high-order abstract reasoning skills, is especially prized in the approach that Gilligan calls an ethic of justice. This approach might more appropriately be called principlism.

It is important to avoid the temptation to view an ethic of care and an ethic of justice (or principlism) in a rigid dualistic fashion, that is, as mutually exclusive options. Numerous empirical studies show that many people spontaneously use both approaches when asked to respond to a hypothetical ethical dilemma. Moreover, both styles of moral reasoning are used by both women and men, although men are sometimes more reluctant to voice "caring" reasoning spontaneously (Johnston 1988). Of particular relevance to this essay, Mary Carolyn Cooper found that a small group of nurses, when asked to reflect upon difficult cases from their own experiences, "relied on traditional moral principles, such as respect for persons, patient autonomy, beneficence, or fidelity, and at the same time relied on the moral response of care" (Cooper 1991, 24).

It is unfortunate that Gilligan set the terms for a discussion of the ethics of care in a way that misnamed and marginalized the value of justice. Gilligan restricted justice to a mode of moral reasoning that privileges impartiality and consistency and concentrates on adjudicating between conflicting individual rights. Justice is a more complex norm. One important component of justice is distributive justice. Under conditions of relative scarcity, justice challenges us to discern how some good ought fairly to be apportioned among those who need it. Kuhse reminds us that distributive justice is an inescapable norm for most nurses who work in hospital settings. She points out that "clinical nurses care not only for *one* patient, but for many patients. This raises the question of balancing the various patient interests involved. How should nurses allocate their time and energy between [or among] patients?" (Kuhse 1997, 159–60). Much of the literature on nursing and the ethics of care does not acknowledge that professional nursing services are inevitably in finite supply and that decisions about how to distribute that good among patients have to be made.

The ethics of care, as it has been developed so far, does not provide detailed guidance about whom to care for when several people urgently require the care of a single care giver at the same time. This reflects in part Gilligan and Noddings's stress on caring as a particular response to the needs of the one-cared-for within a unique caring relationship. According to this view, it is impossible to create rules in abstraction from a particular moment of caring that adequately specify in advance how scarce care ought to be apportioned. In a situation where there are conflicting demands for care—not all of which can be met—an ethic of care seems to point in the direction of a form of moral intuitionism. The care giver discerns in a unique way—in response to the specifics of the situation—which recipient among several vulnerable ones needs the care giver's help most.

I would point out that centuries of discussion of the norm of distributive justice could provide more guidance about how to decide who ought to receive nursing care as a scarce good. For example, many ethicists who apply distributive justice as a norm for the health care system have challenged the fairness of distributing basic services on the basis of the patient's ability to pay. Yet hospital nurses, along with many other health care providers in the United States, are deeply involved in a health care system that often apportions basic, non-emergency medical care based on ability to pay. The category of distributive justice also stimulates us to consider what basic forms of medical care ought to be accessible to all members of our society. It is harder to imagine how a universal package of "basic" health care services (including nursing services) would be determined using an ethic of care approach, with its emphasis on the uniqueness of each recipient of care.

It has been rare for proponents of the ethics of care to discuss the relationship between care and distributive justice as moral values. It has also been rare for those advocating an ethic of care to explore the relationship between an ethic of care and social justice. An ethic of social justice seeks to articulate the conditions necessary for just relations within a social institution or throughout the whole society. A crucial feature of most feminist analyses of social justice is a moral critique of interlinking social systems marred by gender, race, and class oppression. Discourse on social justice prods us to articulate questions about who controls the institutional power necessary to shape the context in which patient care is provided. A comprehensive view of justice involves not merely who gets what resources, but also who participates in what ways in the process of deciding about the allocation of social resources (Young 1990). Although any detailed discussion of power is beyond the scope of this paper, it is important for those concerned about nursing ethics to give explicit attention to social mechanisms that give nurses greater institutional power to shape morally responsible patterns of patient care.

Unions and professional organizations for nurses are key elements in this discussion. As one nurse says, "Union activity is the only means I have found to improve hospital situations. It's the only way I've seen any success in fighting these staffing changes" (Storr 1996, 35). Such concerns about the power of nurses to participate in the determination of how nursing care is distributed could arise from within an ethic of care. However, within the ethic of care there is, I contend, a strong temptation to focus most of the discussion at the more immediate, more personal level of contact between care giver and care recipient.

Some discussions in the nursing ethics literature do acknowledge the moral complexity of caring as a norm for nurses, as long as nurses provide care within health care systems and larger societies that are marked by unjust gender exploitation. The problem of exploitation of women in the nursing profession is a long-standing one. Cooper mentions a tantalizing bit of this history in a brief comment in an essay that appeared in the *Journal of Professional Nursing*. There, Cooper refers to "the history of working-class nurses committed to the experience of caring within a context in which neither the commitment to relational caring nor the nurse's virtues of selflessness and obedience were intrinsically valued by the dominant ideology of the time" (Cooper 1989, 10).

Social justice language challenges us more explicitly to focus ethical attention on the exploitation of nurses as care givers who are increasingly pressed to provide humane care under economic conditions that make relational caring a work of supererogation. Condon has an urgent point when she insists that "an ethics of caring that ... [seeks to avoid] features of oppression and exploitation will also depend upon the emergence of caring as a political philosophy capable of transforming institutions and the politics within which nursing is practiced" (Condon 1992, 18). However, "caring as a political philosophy" has yet to be well spelled out. The work that explores the political implications of care most thoroughly so far is that of Joan Tronto (1993). Tronto insists that we need a politics that takes as fundamental the reality that one of the most basic activities of members of society is caring work on behalf of human beings and the earth itself. Politics ought to order our communal activities in a manner that facilitates necessary caring work and that prevents the exploitation of care givers. However, Tronto indicates that care and justice are *both* values central to our common life. She states that "the problem of determining *which needs* should be met shows that the care ethic is not individualistic. . . . Obviously a theory of justice is necessary to discern [on a society wide basis] among more and less urgent needs" (Tronto 1993, 138).

MORAL RESPONSIBILITY TOWARD UNLICENSED ASSISTIVE PERSONNEL

No work on the ethic of care for hospital-based nursing has yet examined sufficiently the intersecting responsibilities of nurses toward patients and toward other members of the health care team, particularly toward those whose jobs rank lower in the occupational hierarchy of the hospital. In one sense, this is an unsurprising, although regrettable, gap in the literature on nursing and the ethics of care. The vulnerability of the acutely ill patient understandably draws our attention to the nurse-patient relationship.

Focusing on the vulnerable patient as the recipient of care follows an analytic trend in the literature on the ethics of care. The examples of caring relations found in some of the most influential work on the topic focus on interpersonal relationships in which the one who is receiving care is in a position of significant vulnerability. In the literature, the recipient of care is usually highly dependent upon the care taking labor and the caring intentionality of the care giver. Carol Gilligan did research with pregnant women who were making abortion decisions about the survival of their completely dependent fetuses. Noddings focuses on the mother-child relationship and the teacher-student relationship. The nursing ethics literature focuses primarily on the nurse-patient relationship and to a lesser extent upon the relationship between the nurse and the loved ones of a patient with a serious, perhaps life-threatening illness. Because the vulnerability of these dependent recipients of care rivets our moral attention, moral claims of other parties may recede too far into the background.

Another reason that moral obligations toward UAPs receive scant attention from ethicists is that, in the United States, we find it difficult to discuss moral problems associated with race and class. UAPs hold jobs that require limited education and that provide low pay and low social status. These are working-class jobs. In medical ethics, as in ethics more generally, moral issues associated with working class occupations are often ignored. UAPs are more likely to be persons of color who have few other job options. As noted above, African American women are 8 percent of RNs, but 24 percent of health care aides (Himmelstein, Lewontin, and Woolhandler 1996, 527).

The relative racial composition of the nursing workforce and the UAP workforce raises social justice questions.

The American Nurses Association (ANA) has recognized one social justice question raised by the stratified racial patterns within the category of nursing personnel. Why are members of socially disadvantaged racial and ethnic groups finding it harder to obtain jobs as RNs? The ANA is on record as committed to the training and employment of a more ethnically and racially diverse group of nursing professionals. In a 1994 position statement, the association stated: "The principle of justice applies to nurses as providers . . . of care. ANA is committed to addressing the need for racial and ethnic diversity among nurses" (American Nurses Association 1994).

Perhaps the only bioethicist to have paid attention to nurses' moral obligations to UAPs is Amy Haddad. She tells RNs: "Simple human respect reminds us that each person has incalculable worth and deserves our care and attention. Making a real effort to understand the nursing assistant's role and to gain an adequate knowledge of her training can help you put her talents to good use" (Haddad 1998, 22, 24). In other words, RNs as supervisors of UAPs have a moral obligation to assign them satisfying tasks. At the same time, the RN must refrain from asking UAPs to perform nursing tasks for which the UAPs are not sufficiently trained because doing so exploits the UAPs, puts the RN's license at risk, and potentially imperils the welfare of the patient.

To the extent that nurses follow a strategy of fighting for legal restrictions upon the activities of UAPs, nurses may contribute to the exploitation of workers farther down the hospital labor chain. Sociologist Nona Glazer has analyzed how nursing leaders and nursing associations and unions—motivated by a desire to protect jobs for RNs—have blocked channels of upward mobility for unlicensed subordinates (Glazer 1991). When nursing jobs have seemed threatened, some nursing associations have opposed training programs aimed at helping aides and LPNs to become RNs. Glazer reports that in 1970, the National Nursing Council sponsored a report that "rejected a career ladder in which further education for nursing assistants could lead to the RN degree" (364).

The American Nurses Association is presently reassessing the relationship between UAPs and RNs. Although they have not adopted a particular position on this issue, they have enunciated some principles to govern the relationship, including:

IT IS THE NURSING PROFESSION that defines and supervises the education, training and utilization for any unlicensed assistant roles involved in providing direct patient care; . . .

IT IS THE RN who supervises and determines the appropriate utilization of any unlicensed assistant involved in providing direct patient care; and

IT IS THE PURPOSE OF unlicensed assistive personnel to enable the professional nurse to provide nursing care for the patient. (American Nurses Association 1992)

Thus, the focus in the 1992 document remains upon maintaining RN control over the activities of UAPs, not on respecting the moral claims of UAPs to satisfying work, just salaries, and respectful treatment in the hospital workplace.

A conflict over jobs is a difficult moral situation because both RNs and UAPs need work as a source of income and as a means to personal fulfillment. It is morally wrong for nurses to place unwarranted barriers in the way of upward mobility for unlicensed assistants, primarily as a means to protect jobs for RNs as the health care system is restructured. Nurses can avoid complicity with the exploitation of UAPs as care givers only if they are actively involved as a profession in promoting greater opportunity, greater respect, and more just wages and working conditions for care givers who rank below them in the hospital hierarchy.[5]

Nurses and others involved in the health care system could adopt a much more supportive stance toward LPNs and UAPs, helping them to gain more satisfying, better paying jobs. An example of the type of action that is possible is the Ladders in Nursing Careers Program (LINC) sponsored by the Robert Wood Johnson Foundation. The program offers personnel already working in hospitals in lower level jobs financial help to get further education in nursing. Donors pay the costs of tuition, books, and so on. The hospitals where the recipients work agree to pay the participants a full-time salary while the participants work part-time and take nursing courses full-time. "All participants are either minority or low-income individuals" (Taylor 1993, 66). This is one example of how UAPs could be treated more justly.

CONCLUSION

The ethics of care is a moral approach that has great affinities with nursing practice. However, economic pressures that are driving a massive restructuring of the health care system are making an ethic of care more problematic as the central moral paradigm for nurses who work in hospitals today. As nurses struggle to care for a larger group of acutely ill patients, many of whom remain in the hospital for shorter periods, it is difficult to live up to the ideal of an ethic of care as a holistic, relational ethic.

Nursing care, like other health care services, is in finite supply. An ethic of care provides limited guidance about how nursing services ought to be distributed among a large group of patients, all of whom would benefit from good nursing care. Questions of distributive justice cannot be subsumed under the rubric of an ethic of care.

Importantly, because nursing care takes place within relationships and institutions marred by injustice along multiple axes of gender, race, and class, an ethic of care does not provide all the moral wisdom that nurses need. An ethic of care must be enriched with the value of social justice. Social justice warns against the exploitation of nurses who struggle to provide humane care under severe constraints within today's restructured hospital settings. It also warns nurses against the temptation to protect their own professional status and jobs at the unfair expense of socially vulnerable UAPs.

Endnotes

1 Because (during this period) registered nurses received relatively low wages in comparison to their professional qualifications and duties, and because hospital nurses had few opportunities for advancement, promoting high job satisfaction among their nurses was one of the few means hospitals had to retain experienced nurses. Therefore, hospital administrators needed to be concerned if the registered nurses in their work force were growing dissatisfied with the team nursing approach (Krall and Prus 1995, 74).

2 The DRG system does allow for consideration of major complicating factors in a specific patient's case. Examples of factors that increase the reimbursement rate to a hospital are the presence of serious additional medical problems or the advanced age of the patient.

3 One of the serious difficulties with hospitals' use of a variety of types of UAPs is that it is difficult for the patient and the patient's loved ones to know what level of care they may reasonably expect from a UAP.

4 A float nurse moves among units of the hospital to provide additional nursing services on the units that are experiencing unusual, increased demand.

5 Haddad touches on the issue of fairness when she asserts that one reason that UAPs should not be assigned more technical nursing tasks for which they are not trained is because UAPs do not receive the higher levels of pay commensurate with the use of those more advanced skills.

References

Aiken, Linda, Julie Sochalski, and Gerard Anderson. 1996. Downsizing the Hospital Nursing Workforce. *Health Affairs* 15 (winter): 88-92.

American Nurses Association. 1992. Registered Nurse Utilization of Unlicensed Assistive Personnel. http://www.nursingworld.org/readroom/position (February 26, 1999).

————. 1994. Ethics and Human Rights. http://www.nursingworld.org/read room/position (February 26, 1999).

Anderson, Digby. 1998. Work Without Virtue, or the Decline of Professionalism. *Wall Street Journal*, Oct. 29, A22.

Andolsen, Barbara. 1993. Justice, Gender, and the Frail Elderly: Reexaming the Ethic of Care. *Journal of Religious Ethics* 9 (spring/fall): 127–45.

Bowden, Peta. 1997. *Caring: Gender-Sensitive Ethics*. New York: Routledge.

Boyer, Jeannine Ross, and James Lindemann Nelson. 1990. A Comment on Fry's "The Role of Caring in a Theory of Nursing Ethics." *Hypatia* 5 (fall): 153–58.

Brannon, Robert L. 1994. Professionalization and Work Intensification: Nursing in the Cost Containment Era. *Work and Occupations* 21 (May): 157–78.

Condon, Esther. 1992. Nursing and the Caring Metaphor: Gender and Political Influences on an Ethics of Care. *Nursing Outlook* 40 (January/February): 14–19.

Cooper, Mary Carolyn. 1989. Gilligan's Different Voice: a Perspective for Nursing. *Journal of Professional Nursing* 5 (January/February): 10–16.

————. 1991. Principal-Oriented Ethics and the Ethic of Care: A Creative Tension. *ANS: Advances in Nursing Science* 14 (December): 22–31.

Fagin, Claire M. 1999. Nurses, Patients and Managed Care. *New York Times,* March 16, F7.

Fry, Sara T. 1989. The Role of Caring in a Theory of Nursing Ethics. *Hypatia* 4 (summer): 88–103.

Gilligan, Carol. 1982. *In a Different Voice: Psychological Theory and Women's Development*. Cambridge, Mass.: Harvard University Press.

Glazer, Nona Y. 1988. Overlooked, Overworked: Women's Unpaid and Paid Work in the Health Services' "Cost Crisis." *International Journal of Health Services* 18 (November 1): 113–19.

————. 1991. "Between a Rock and a Hard Place:" Women's Professional Organizations in Nursing and Class, Racial and Ethnic Inequalities. *Gender and Society* 5 (September): 351–72.

Haddad, Amy. 1998. Ethics in Action: Nursing Assistants, *RN* 61 (November): 21–22, 24.

Himmelstein, David, James Lewontin, and Steffie Woolhandler. 1996. Medical Care Employment in the United States, 1968 to 1993: The Importance of

Health Sector Jobs for African Americans and Women. *American Journal of Public Health* 86 (April): 525–28.

Johnston, D. Kay. 1988. Adolescents' Solutions to Dilemmas in Fables: Two Moral Orientations—Two Problem Solving Strategies. In *Mapping the Moral Domain: a Contribution of Women's Thinking to Psychological Theory and Education*, ed. Carol Gilligan et al., 49–71. Cambridge, Mass.: Center for the Study of Gender, Education, and Human Development.

Kuhse, Helga. 1997. *Caring: Nurses, Women and Ethics*. Oxford, U.K.: Blackwell Publishers.

Krall, Lisi, and Mark Prus. 1995. Institutional Changes in Hospital Nursing. *Journal of Economic Issues* 29 (March): 67–82.

Lundy, M. Catherine. 1996. Nursing Beyond Fordism. *Employee Responsibilities and Rights Journal* 9 (June): 163–71.

Mahony, Chris. 1998. Patients Behaving Badly. *Nursing Times* 94/39: 26–29.

Noddings, Nel. 1984. *Caring: A Feminine Approach to Ethics and Moral Education*. Berkeley: University of California Press.

Parker, Randy Spreen. 1990. Nurses' Stories: The Search for a Relational Ethic of Care. *ANS: Advances in Nursing Science* 13 (September): 31–40.

Pellegrino, Edmund D. 1989. The Primacy of the Act of Profession. In *Ethical Issues in the Professions,* ed. Peter Y. Windt et al., 76–84. Englewood Cliffs, N.J.: Prentice-Hall.

Sabatino, Frank. 1993. Culture Shock: Are U. S. Hospitals Ready? *Hospitals* 67 (May 20): 23–25, 28.

Shuit, Douglas P. 1996. Hospital Nurses Feel Pain of Health System's Restructuring. *Los Angeles Times,* July 1, A1, A17.

Stockard, Stephanie. 1991. Caring for the Sexually Aggressive Patient: You Don't Have to Blush and Bear It. *Nursing* 21 (November): 72–73.

Storr, Janie. 1996. A Nurse's View. In *Abandonment of the Patient: The Impact of Profit-Driven Health Care on the Public*. ed. Ellen Baer, Claire Fagin, and Suzanne Gordon, 31–36. New York: Springer Publishing Co.

Taylor, Kathryn S. 1993. LINC Program Helps Valued Employees Pursue Nursing Careers. *Hospitals and Health Networks* (September 20): 66.

Trevino, Fernando M., Ciro Sumaya, Magdalena Miranda, Laudelina Martinez, and Jose Manuel Saldana. 1993. Increasing the Representation of Hispanics in the Health Professions. *Public Health Reports* 108 (September/October): 551–58.

Tronto, Joan C. 1993. *Moral Boundaries: a Political Argument for an Ethic of Care*. New York: Routledge.

Wagner, David. 1980. The Proletarianization of Nursing in the United States, 1932–1946. *International Journal of Health Services* 10/2: 271–90.

Watson, Jean. 1988. *Nursing: Human Science and Human Care, A Theory of Nursing*. New York: National League for Nursing.

————. 1990. Caring Knowledge and Informed Moral Passion. *ANS Advances in Nursing Science* 13 (September): 15–24.

Young, Iris Marion. 1990. *Justice and the Politics of Difference*. Princeton, N.J.: Princeton University Press.

Zalumas, Jacqueline. 1995. *Caring in Crisis: An Oral History of Critical Care Nursing*. Philadelphia: University of Pennsylvania Press.

3

The Need for Integrating Care Ethics into Hospital Care: A Case Study

Christine E. Gudorf

This case focuses on the interaction of doctors and hospital staff with my son, Victor, and his extended family during his five months in the intensive care unit (ICU) and ventilator units. Victor was admitted with Guillain-Barre Syndrome (G-B), which stopped all voluntary and involuntary movement, including lungs and heart, leaving only a quarter eye blink. The case shows that systemic applications of biomedical principlism are deficient in providing elements of good medical care (see DuBose, Hamel, and O'Connell 1994).

The case also supports using Carol Gilligan's research findings to propose an ethic of care that functions as a corrective to, rather than an alternative for, an ethic of principles (Gilligan 1982). Although some sections of *In A Different Voice* seem to suggest that feminine care and masculine principles are bases for alternative methods of decision making (155–62), Gilligan ultimately understands them as requiring integration.[1] Gilligan situates her work within the theory of Nancy Chodorow, who attributes differences between the sexes, including different sex-based approaches to moral decision making, "not to anatomy, but rather to the 'the fact that women, universally, are largely responsible for early child care'" (Chodorow 1974, in Gilligan 1982, 7).

Understanding an ethic of care as a feminine alternative to a traditional masculine ethic of principles is problematic because any adequate ethic, including one based on care, must respond to principles such as justice. In the same way, an ethic of principles must produce not only justice, but also care, if it is to respect human sociality and respond adequately to religious imperatives such as neighbor-love. Admittedly, the need for integrating the approaches in Gilligan's work would be clearer if she had distinguished traditional approaches to moral decision making in women from critically reconstructed feminist forms of women's morality in which the socio-critical element has forced some integration of modern Western masculine approaches (principlist) with more traditional Western feminine approaches (care).

What are often presented as examples of a principlist ethic are usually models that stress compliance with principles, but also respond to the individual patient. In Victor's case, for example, the medical staff, whose professional stance is rooted in a principlist ethic that underlies their professional training, nevertheless understand the practical product of their stance to be care for the patient. After the presumption that a principle-directed institutional system actually produces adequate patient care was challenged by the patient and his family, the staff became increasingly uncertain and uncomfortable.

The patient and his family primarily addressed treatment decisions in terms of care—for example, by being open to the use and display of emotion within decision-making processes—but we also struggled to integrate the principle of justice into our conceptions of care. This process of integration was and is a difficult one, in part because our society has for so long understood reason and emotion as inimical, teaching us to suppress one or the other, depending upon our role and social location. In this case, some family members, especially I, had dual, and from some perspectives, conflicting, roles and locations. I was the mother of the patient, called to give personal care and provide advocacy, but I was also an ethicist with twenty years of experience in teaching, writing, and consulting in bioethics. In addition, at the time my son fell ill, I had just enrolled in a graduate sociology seminar in qualitative research methods. For practical reasons, my observation point for the course assignments immediately became my son's ICU cubicle. While my mother-self was often reduced to silent sobbing in the hall or seething anger at careless staff members, my ethicist/sociologist-self was more distanced and evaluative, counting, comparing, and analyzing.[2] Throughout the ordeal, my ethicist/sociologist persona informed my actions as a mother, although I make no claims for adequate or consistent integration. At another level, the ethicist/sociologist persona provided me with a more distant stance that offered some relief from emotional turmoil. Other family members who came to care for Victor, especially two of my sisters (one a nurse practitioner and another a hospital CEO), as well as a sister-in-law who is a veteran X-ray technician, also experienced this double perspective.

I do not present my or my family's approach as having adequately or equally integrated personal care and commitment to principle, but only as more adequate than either a "pure" ethic of care or a "pure" principlist ethic.

MORAL THEORY, PRINCIPLISM, AND CARE

In insisting on the need to integrate care and the use of principles, I reject the feminist assumption that an ethic of care, as lifted from Gilligan's work, is in itself morally adequate. I also reject more traditionalist assumptions that an ethic of care adds little or nothing that is necessary or appropriate to principle-based moral theory. Lawrence Kohlberg and Jurgen Habermas, for example, have denied that Carol Gilligan's research on the ethics of care is even about moral theory. They maintain that her research is about evaluations of virtue and character in personal relationships—about the good life—but not about moral theory (Habermas 1990; Kohlberg 1984, 340–41; see also Benhabib 1992, 182–90). Kohlberg and Habermas propose that moral theory concerns justice and the shape it should take in society. They see Kohlberg's work as being about justice because it revolves around the use of abstract universal principles. Principlist bioethics, from their perspective, is also about justice because it involves the application of universal moral principles to broad social issues, such as equal access to health care and professional training, the allocation of scarce medical resources, and policies on abortion, life support, and euthanasia. Gilligan, they insist, discusses individual preferences within personal relationships, which are ancillary to real moral theory, which is universal.

In a parallel vein, Edith Wyschogrod's *Saints and Postmodernism* poses saints and moral theory as different tools for teaching morality. Wyschogrod prefers saints as exemplars to the teaching of moral theory. She maintains that moral theory helps people understand what is moral without motivating them to be moral, whereas the lives of the saints contain both an implicit, and often an explicit, imperative to imitate saints' moral activities, which motivates hearers (Wyschogrod 1990, 49–60).

An essential difference between saints and moral theory is the role of alterity in each. Moral theory, Wyschogrod insists, refers to an other who is generalized; the generalized other may even be based on one's self (as in the golden rule, for example). As we read in accounts of saints' lives, the others with whom the saints interact are often not fully enfleshed characters, but only caricatures; yet the point of each story is that the saint responds to others fully in their uniqueness and individual need, even at the cost of suffering to the saint (Wyschogrod 1990, 3–5, 35–60, 85). Wyschogrod, then, sides with Gilligan's ethic of care over against Kohlberg's (and Habermas's) focus on moral theory and justice. In both an ethic of care and the lives of the saints, it is the need to address suffering with compassion, with attention to the other's specific needs, that motivates action, and not abstract understandings of just communities. Saints are not devoid of reason, nor are those who rely on moral theory devoid of compassion. But for saints, reason is a tool of compassion, not the primary cause of action, whereas for moral theory, compassion is a motivator, but not the primary guide for action.

One of the results of feminism's dictum that the "personal is political" has been the realization that justice is an imperative in personal as well as social interaction. Moreover, care is an imperative that is no more limited to interpersonal relationships than justice is to social ones. In addition, justice is not exhausted by its rationalized description in principles, nor care by an emotional complex of feelings. Both care and justice, in their fullest sense, involve rationality and emotion and can be concretely enacted. I disagree with Wyschogrod that saints are always superior to theory; I see important functions for both saints and moral theory and so, as with care and principles in Gilligan, argue for retaining and mixing both approaches. From the perspective of Christian ethics, issues of character, virtue, and human relationships are essential aspects of morality. We are all called to be saints. Morality is about being truly human. The truly human is not defined solely by moral principles like justice, or even patient autonomy, but by all the different ways we care for the other, ourselves, and our world.

One problem in the implementation of principle-based bioethics, as we shall see, is that patients are objectified in terms of categories. Patients become "the hip replacement in 302" and the "Guillain-Barre in 401." The very space of the hospital is organized into categories. There is one space for emergency patients, another for critical care patients, and others for surgical, maternity, and neo-natal patients. Although such organization is efficient—and efficiency is an important value, given the finiteness of health care resources—efficiency is not our only, or even our primary, value. Efficiency could demand putting all our resources into prevention and letting the sick die untended. Efficiency is only a second order value, useful in making primary values such as justice or compassion more effective. The principle of respect tends to be reduced in institutional settings to signed consent forms.[3] It is unable to compensate for the effects on care of justice understood as treating like cases alike, which inevitably leads to patients being treated as members of larger categories all due the same care. Problems usually arise at the boundaries of categories around patients who "belong" in more than one category or not quite in any category.

THE CASE

This is a case study of Victor, a 27-year-old male hospitalized December 26, 1995, with Guillain-Barre Syndrome. G-B is caused by a relatively common virus to which only people with stressed immune systems are vulnerable. The chronically ill and elderly, those recovering from flu and other diseases, pregnant women, people with transplants and HIV-positive people are typical G-B patients. In G-B, the body perceives the sheathing on the nerves as invading. The body reacts by destroying the sheathing. Symptoms begin with tingling and numbness in the hands and feet, which progress up the arms and legs toward the trunk, ending voluntary movement and distorting sensation. In most cases, symptoms stop at the trunk, and after weeks or months the paralysis begins to recede in precisely the reverse order from its onset. A few cases are more severe, paralyzing the muscles in the face, head, and entire trunk, including involuntary muscles such as lungs and, in rare cases, heart. Recovery takes many months; even in ordinary cases patients can require two to five years to regain complete movement and coordination (Heller 1986). Some severely affected patients die, especially the elderly and chronically ill whose compromised immune systems make them vulnerable to G-B in the first place. About 10 percent of G-B patients emerge with some permanent neurological disability in the extremities, especially feet and hands.

Victor was probably vulnerable to G-B due to his immune-suppressed status following a successful kidney transplant two months earlier. That same immune suppression made his G-B extremely severe. He remained totally paralyzed except for the slight eye blink, fully dependent upon a ventilator to move his lungs and, at random intervals, a pacemaker to initiate heartbeats, for five months. During five additional months of less acute hospital care he began to breathe independently and to slowly regain movement. After those ten months he left the hospital for a year and a half of outpatient therapy, which restored him to normalcy, apart from some permanent foot drop and hand palsy.

CONCERNS ABOUT JUSTICE

Victor and our family's interaction with the staff was not moved solely by emotional concern for Victor's needs and well-being, but was concerned as well with broader social justice. At Victor's birth, doctors said that he would need dialysis or a transplant or both to survive childhood. Although that crisis took twenty years longer to arrive than predicted, the family debated for years whether or not to pursue dialysis or a transplant, given the common and often chronic complications that accompany both treatments— treatments that also absorb such a disproportionate share of the nation's, not to mention the world's, limited health resources. We followed the statistics on how many children could be immunized, how many could be cured of tuberculosis, how many more lives could be saved by redirecting the personnel, training, and dollars involved in dialysis, transplantation, and permanent immunosuppression (drugs for Victor run $25,000 per year). We concluded that health care policy should change: Transplants should be experimental, not standard treatment, until the ratio of health benefit to cost is considerably better.

At the same time, however, we were convinced neither that social policy is changed through individual refusals of transplants, nor that it was appropriate for us as parents to deny a transplant for our son. There was simply no way for us to justify to Victor a decision to refuse options that could keep him alive and relatively independent in the naïve hope that the social costs thus saved would be reallocated to save larger numbers of threatened lives. What kind of parental love could do this? Perhaps it was moral cowardice on our part, an unwillingness to allow Victor ever to ask whether we would have chosen differently for his brother who was not adopted. For whatever reasons, we have been political and financial supporters of health care reform aimed at expanding access, providing preventative care, and greater equalization of health care nationally and internationally. But we ultimately decided—not without some discomfort—that this did not morally oblige us to refuse for Victor all benefits not universally available, especially when such a decision was a death sentence, and especially when it was not our lives, but our child's life, at stake. We were relieved that the decision for or against dialysis and transplantation was delayed until Victor was an adult and able to choose for himself.

One could argue that demanding that all the needs of a high-needs patient are met is unjust in that it inevitably detracts from the care due other patients. Although the fact of Victor's being on immunosuppressants for his kidney transplant did complicate the treatment for G-B paralysis, every part of the care we demanded for him was *ordinary* care framed not in terms of results, but of actions. Family demands for improved care included demands that hospital staff: (1) give Victor the medications ordered for him, rather than those of neighboring patients; (2) check the *Physician's Desk Reference* for adverse drug interactions before ordering new drugs; (3) use normal sterile technique (applying alcohol swabs before injecting anything into the lines connected to Victor's body); (4) follow normal nursing assessment procedures so that problems (e.g., an accidentally clamped catheter line) are detected early in each shift; and (5) implement effective safety measures (e.g., make sure that the ventilator disconnection alarm in the ICU works). Although the volume of care required in Victor's case was great, and his paralysis and immunosuppressed status made the consequences of staff failure to provide care severe, no part of his care was extraordinary in the sense of the burden of care being disproportionate to the health benefit expected. His care was aimed at recovery; his high-needs condition was neither permanent nor terminal.

The emphasis in medical care, certainly in physician training, has been on extraordinary care—on high tech treatments and instruments—and on transforming, through frequent use, successive types of technologically extraordinary treatment (experiments) into ordinary treatment. In terms of U.S. medical care today, none of the treatments provided Victor were technologically extraordinary, nor were they extraordinary in the sense of requiring care disproportionate to the expected health benefit. The transplant had been extraordinary, although many transplant surgeons see kidney transplants as ordinary, and only multiple organ transplants as extraordinary today. The immune-suppressant drugs to maintain the transplant might well be extraordinary in terms of the burden of their cost to many families, but Victor was already receiving these; their cost was not borne by this hospital or these doctors. Although the ventilator and the pacemaker had been extraordinary in the past and still would be extraordinary in some parts of the world, there was an entire floor of ventilator patients at Victor's hospital, and pacemakers are the norm in many U.S. senior citizen centers. Most Americans would consider it immoral for insurance companies and hospitals to allow, for example, pneumonia or heart attack patients to die on the grounds that a ventilator or a pacemaker is extraordinary and therefore need not be supplied.

The structural situation in which hospital staff felt unable to deliver the care demanded was one impacted by managed care. Managed care was initiated by insurers, both public and private. It reinforces problematic tendencies in principle-based bioethics by utilizing diagnosis-based categories of patients, and setting the limits of reimbursement for type and length of care based on the average case with that diagnosis. In managed care, insurance companies use their large pool of patients to intimidate hospitals and doctors into accepting lower and lower levels of reimbursement for reduced stays and restricted treatments based on the average patient with a particular diagnosis. Patients who require less than the average amount of care for their condition recover and are discharged without exceeding the limits of insurance coverage. Those who require more than the average amount of care reach the limits of coverage. Unless they have private resources to cover the costs of extended care that the insurer denies, they are discharged earlier than their condition warrants, pay the difference themselves, or the hospital loses money on their continued care. Hospitals can no longer raise the general charge per service to cover their losses on un- or under-insured patients because insurers set the amount paid for each service, as well as the duration of coverage.

There is, then, severe financial pressure on hospitals to treat and discharge all patients within the diagnosis-based limits of insurers, and to cover the costs of those they cannot discharge for fear of liability by cost economies such as staff reductions. For-profit hospitals have the additional motive to produce profit, which, because managed care has already taken any fat out of budgets, is most often achieved through cutting staff. Since the advent of managed care the proportion of for-profit, rather than nonprofit, hospitals and nursing homes has increased at a tremendous rate. Because managed care relegated many categories of former hospital patients to out-patient services, the needs of patients at each level of hospital care have increased. The nurses at this hospital made bitter jokes about the fact that, compared to fifteen years ago, the patients that are outpatient used to be in medical-surgical units, those in the medical-surgical units used to be in the ICU, and the ones in the ICU used to be in the cemetery.[4] Over the previous three years the nurse/patient ratio in the ventilator unit had gone from one nurse and one aide for four patients (1+1/4) to one nurse and one aide for eight patients(1+1/8), and on some (night) shifts one nurse and two aides for sixteen patients (1+2/16). As aides were forbidden to order, mix, or administer medications or touch the IV or feeding lines, and most patients needed medications every four to six hours (which for ventilator patients go into feeding or, more rarely, IV lines),[5] nursing care took a beating.

The situation was at least as serious with respiratory technicians. The likelihood of ventilator patients getting pneumonia goes up 10 percent for every week spent on a ventilator. Victor's suppressed immune system was expected to succumb to frequent pneumonia. As both treatment for and prevention of pneumonia, respiratory technicians were to give Victor a special inhalant and pound his sides, chest, and back for half an hour every six hours. Sometimes harried, overworked technicians chose to give Victor his third or fourth treatment during severe pneumonia and skip the one preventive treatment in another ventilator patient without pneumonia; other technicians skipped Victor to give the other patient his/her only ordered treatment.

A number of people both on the hospital staff and outside it have suggested that we should have been content with less than the level of care ordered or needed if giving all the care ordered took care from others. Although I agree that it was not just to make nurses and technicians choose between patients, responsibility for forcing such choices does not rest with high-needs patients or their families, but with the administration that decides staffing levels. We fully understood that the problems in care were a result not of lack of concern by individual staff, but of understaffing and overwork of staff. For this reason the family took over large parts of Victor's care from the first week in the ICU. For ten months we spent 18–24 hours per day, seven days a week, with Victor. We did all the bathing, bed changing, range of motion exercises, eye drops, nose and mouth suctioning, filling of the enteral feeding machine, readjusting of room temperature, calling of the cross-town lab for cyclosporine levels twice a week, and a variety of other tasks. We complained of staffing levels to administrators, but we also complained to staff of their most egregious mistakes, such as giving Victor another patient's medications.

By comparison, it is not the responsibility of children in orphanages to lower their demands for food below their need level in order to relieve the staff of the awful necessity of choosing whom to starve; rather, it is the responsibility of the administrators of the orphanage to find more food or transfer orphans to institutions that have more food. The only exception would be if a society as a whole were so short of resources that no orphanage or institution could find sufficient food. When that is the case, then a careful weighing of costs and benefits is necessary; services should be cut to those who have the lowest chances of surviving or are most able to survive and recover without them—and not those who have the highest needs at the moment.

Furthermore, if the hospital has set staffing levels so low that it cannot manage high-needs patients, then it has a responsibility to acknowledge this and should either refuse to admit, or should transfer, those patients who present such needs. Instead, this hospital at the point of diagnosis in the emergency room claimed to be the equal of the downtown university hospital, and immediately began to set up a medical team for Victor involving neurologists, nephrologists, pulmonologists, surgeons, cardiologists, and infectious disease specialists, thereby assuring the family that it understood the specialized care necessary. These doctors must have—or at least should have—known that because this hospital did not do transplants, its lab could not test cyclosporine levels, its doctors did not know any of the common drug interactions with post-transplant drugs, and outside of surgery its nurses did not always utilize full sterile techniques. It was irresponsible to admit this patient, who was still days away from requiring any form of emergency care and could easily have been sent to the university hospital. In this age of medical specialization, failure to make appropriate referrals should be a clear violation of the principle of beneficence within a principlist approach to bioethics, although I have never heard that case made.

All medical practitioners learn new skills and techniques by practicing on patients—which are what teaching hospitals are all about. Such practice, however, should always be under the direct supervision of experienced staff. The desire of this hospital's medical staff to be involved in this interesting and challenging case should not have overridden their responsibility to exhibit beneficence toward the patient. To determine what is due a patient only in terms of present institutional policies, ignoring possibilities for more just and adequate policies, is wrong; it serves to place institutions above the demands of justice and to have all the demands of justice fall on individuals already under constraints.

PRINCIPLISM AND CARE IN STAFF COMMUNICATION

By the second day of hospitalization the family communicated with the patient by an elaborate system. By blinking his eyes to the recitation of the alphabet, Victor indicated one letter at a time, slowly forming words and sentences. For the first few months this communication entailed a great deal of running by family members, because Victor lay on a bed that rotated every two minutes from one side to the other at an angle almost perpendicular to the floor. To keep the patient on the bed, foot-high cushioned panels were anchored to the bed around the outline of the patient's body. This prevented seeing the patient's face from any one position for longer than about seven or eight letters of the alphabet. In order to watch for Victor's blink, the family member had to run around the end of the bed from one side to the other and jump up on a stool on either side of the bed. The development of this method of communication by family and the unwillingness of staff, except for a handful of nurses, to use the laborious process even after Victor was moved to a flat air mattress helped place family members in the middle of communication between patient and staff.

A charting exercise that I performed in the ICU uncovered a pattern in the staff's verbal communication with the patient.[6] A staff member who needed to touch his body or bed first identified himself/herself and then briefly explained what he or she was doing. Nurses who came into the room to put medications either into the first line into the stomach (PEG) or the second line into his intestine (PEJ) always said, "Victor, I am putting some medicine into the PEG/PEJ." If they thought he might be asleep (for many months his eyes did not completely open when awake or close when asleep), they said, "This is _____, Victor, and I am putting medicines in the PEG/PEJ." Respiratory technicians who came to check the numbered readouts on the ventilator or to take water from the cups that drained the condensation in the tubes were generally silent; but if they came in to attach a cylinder of mist to the tracheal appliance (four or five inches from Victor's chin), they always identified themselves and what they were doing, even when it was clear from his eye movements that Victor was alert. Aides who came in to put supplies in the closets never spoke to the patient, and most nurses who brought supplies in did not, either. Maintenance people were almost always silent, and when they did speak, they spoke to family members and not to the patient.

Total Staff Entries Into the Patient's Room over a 40-Hour Period: 74

24 (32%)   Entered and left silently
19 (25%)   Greeted patient ("Good morning, Victor")
9 (12%)   Uttered rhetorical questions, expecting no response ("How are you today?")
21 (28%)   Asked yes/no question(s); waited for yes/no blink ("Did you sleep well?"). Ten of 21 (13%) asked more than one question using yes/no blink response
3 (4%)   Spelled answers to questions with patient to allow patient more than yes/no response ("Where's the pain worst?")[7]

The majority of doctors abided by the unwritten rule that touching the patient's body or bed required speech, but they seldom entered the patient's room. Most of Victor's more than forty doctors (ten different specialties, with three to six doctors per specialty) did their real work at the nurses' desk with the chart, where they checked the lab results, the nurses' notes on heart rate and blood pressure, feeding levels, stool output, and so on.

Some did not speak to the patient or his family for weeks at a time, especially after the first month. The doctors who did interact with Victor did so more or less as their specialty required. The GI doctors and the surgeons who put in the tracheotomy, feeding lines, and pacemaker showed up only to obtain consents. Neurologists, on the other hand, needed to examine the patient in ways that required patient feedback: "Can you move/feel when I touch you here, Victor? One blink for yes, and two for no." They thus tended to talk with the patient more. Pulmonary doctors had the next highest level of physician interaction because they periodically had to test for any regeneration of lung capacity: "Can you inhale at all, Victor?"

The physicians' concepts of patient care appeared not to have a personal component, but to be concerned instead with scientific competency. When some other more personal concept of care seemed necessary, doctors were quick to point out that the hospital system relegated such care to others. Doctors cared by ordering the best treatments possible, not by interacting with the patient. Not one of over forty physicians over a five-month hospital stay either inquired about the patient's frame of mind or anticipated any patient questions, concerns, or fears over changes in symptoms or treatments. Only two of the neurologists and one of the nephrologists (in the context of persuading me to speak at his church) ever initiated discussion about patient or family concerns. One of those two neurologists was concerned that the family's involvement was raising unfounded hopes of recovery in the patient and his family. When asked, however, he could cite neither studies nor experience of similar situations on which to base his prediction.

On the other hand, the responsibilities of nurses, as well as their training and the personal orientation of many of them, encouraged them to understand patient care in more personal terms. At each shift change, the new nurse assessed the patient—took vital signs, checked all incisions and lines into the patient's body, observed color and general condition. Assessment began with the courtesy formula, "Hello, Victor, my name is _____, and I am your new nurse. How are you feeling today?" The use of such a formula is, I suggest, a requirement of an ethic of care in nursing. Until the nurse learned of the single blink (yes), double blink (no) formula, she would continue with a "Your color looks good," or "You look a little down." Only two or three nurses out of thirty were silent following their introduction at assessment.

All three entries in the chart above involving spelling were made by the same nurse. In five months in ICU/ventilator units, nurses were the only staff to spell with the patient, and only four of them did so. Most of the first and second shift nurses did communicate by asking Yes/No questions and waiting for blinks. One of the four who spelled was a float who worked as Victor's nurse only a few nights; two of the remaining three were in the ICU, and one was the veteran nurse in the ventilator unit.

On the ventilator floor, the nurse technicians were generally cheery and talkative as they gave baths and brought linens, but for some reason were usually silent when they took blood pressures and temperatures every four hours (unless the patient might be asleep, in which case they began with the courtesy formula). Various technicians spoke to the patient as required by the nature of their work—they all either touched his body (respiratory, physical, and occupational) or else required his active participation (recreation and speech). Respiratory technicians, however, were often silent when they entered the room only to check the readouts on the ventilator.

Doctors were the only personnel who broke the rule: some stood at Victor's bedside, even touched his body, and did not address him. Most doctors bypassed and excluded Victor altogether when they needed information about his condition or consent for further diagnostic or treatment procedures, even surgery. Doctors on rounds regularly demanded of the nurses, and, in their absence, of family: "Did he sleep well last night? When was his last bowel movement? How is he tolerating the new pain meds?" These questions were routinely asked across Victor's conscious body, with no apparent concern for his self-perception. Doctors would wait impatiently while family communicated with Victor, even when the question required only a yes/no answer, as though doctors could not interpret single or double eye blinks.

No group of personnel spoke to the patient as often as the nurses for a variety of reasons. The nurses were assumed by the doctors to know the current status of the patient in terms of pain, energy, sleep, color, and vital signs. When I interviewed Nurse Carol, she noted that when she began nursing she stuck by the doctors on rounds in order to answer their questions. But now (25 years later), when the patient is alert and she has no pressing concerns for the doctor, she disappears during rounds so that the doctors have to interact with the patient if they want answers. Another reason why nurses communicate so much more is that nurses are charged with the overall care of the patient, whereas each of the other hospital staff has responsibility for only a narrow area of patient care. Although a respiratory technician can claim to have no responsibility outside the lungs and the trachea, there is no aspect of the patient that is *not* within the nurse's care. This includes, at least in the minds of many nurses, monitoring patient mental health.

In my interview of him on the speaking valve in month five, Victor identified four nurses whom he felt had cared about him as an individual. To him this meant that they were not only competent in their ordinary nursing tasks, but that they adapted their own and floor practices to meet his particular needs. He did not assume that their care for him as an individual patient involved a personal friendship with him; he pointed out that he could express gratitude for their care, but he was not in a position to form peer relationships such as friendships with staff.

One of his special nurses, Carol, was an otherwise crusty woman in her late fifties who went beyond even the call of any ethic of care. One night, having cared for Victor through a particularly painful and scary shift, Carol came to him before she went home, unfastened the chain from her neck, and said, "Here, I'm leaving you my guardian angel to watch over you until I get back tomorrow." She fastened it to an IV pole over Victor's head. Victor interpreted Carol's action as a vow that she would remain committed to looking out for his interests. Another incident involved a Muslim respiratory technician who came into the ICU in the middle of a long, dark, terrifying night after family left at 1 a.m., checked the ventilator, came up to the bed, and said, "Victor, I am Ali. I hold your hand. Rest, you are safe. Allah will take care of you whatever happens." He stayed for half an hour. For Victor, this too was a helpful religious intervention.

Not every religious overture was understood as compatible with care, however. Victor painstakingly spelled out an account involving a pair of young, pretty nurses who, noticing the crucifix left by his visiting former pastor and the many religious cards on the wall, asked if he was a Christian. Seeing his blink, they advised him that if he would just accept Jesus fully, he would recover, and they promised that they would pray for him at the big Nurses for Jesus conference the following week. For Victor, this was not helpful.

Three of Victor's special nurses adopted him as their patient—from that point on, whenever they worked, he was assigned to them. There was no disputing their choice; in both the ICU and the ventilator unit, Victor's case was by far the most demanding. Even the most efficient and lucky of his special nurses had to work in tandem with family members to provide all the necessary care. Out of this ongoing commitment, the special nurses, and from time to time a few of the other nurses, took up Victor's cause with the doctors. None of the nurses ever felt able to challenge a doctor's medical judgement, even when the grounds for their disagreement were medical. But many of the nurses did get sufficiently bold with the doctors, who of course had no knowledge of the nurse/patient/family relationships, to pressure a doctor who was ignoring weight loss or adding a new drug that the nurse knew was incompatible with cyclosporine (the immunosuppressant). The nurses would call the doctors: "I know you have consulted with the nutrition department, but the family is still convinced that Victor is continuing to lose weight—what should we do about it?" or "The family insists this drug is incompatible with cyclosporine—should I ask the nephrologist to consult with them about it?" Sometimes this was enough—the doctor would order a bed scale, or consult with another specialist about a more compatible medication. At other times, the nurses had to make such interventions again and again.

The greater orientation of nurses to an ethic of care, and the lesser sway of the principlist stance among them, at least in this case, was due not only to the different responsibilities of nurses, but also to their training. The medical literature on G-B, for example, focuses on disease progression and pharmacological treatments of the disease itself. The nursing literature covers these matters, but in addition addresses pharmacological and non-pharmacological treatment of patient anxiety, depression, and pain management (Anderson 1992; Barrall-Inman 1995; Mascarelle and Hudson 1991; Pfister and Bullas 1990; Ruiz-Rodriquez 1994; Thilagarani 1994).

Whatever the cause, nurses were not as inclined as doctors to let the system be responsible for care, but frequently attempted to intervene personally to improve care. Some nurses, for example, waged a constant battle with the doctors over the retention of pain medications, often wheedling the neurologists (the most patient sensitive) to support them against the other medical specialists. The underlying issue was nutrition. Due to the racing heart and hypertension caused by the G-B virus, Victor's metabolism demolished huge quantities of calories every day despite his immobility. His multiple doses of over 40 different medicines every day had to be pulverized, mixed in water and poured into the feeding tubes. Two days out of three the medications would clog the line for 2–12 hours, stopping enteral feeding, even after the surgical addition of a second feeding line to the intestine. Nurses and family requested a bed scale, which revealed that after eight weeks, Victor, admitted at 154 pounds, weighed only 87 pounds. The doctors were shocked that the formulas they had worked out for maintaining nutrition had been so far off base. They had assumed that their orders accurately anticipated both the care given and the results achieved, that the chart—their map—was identical to the concrete territory of Victor's body. Their response to news of his weight was to stop all "unnecessary" medications to increase food absorption. The first to go were pain medications.

G-B is intensely painful. The virus causes the nerves to send pain signals to the brain—sensations of icy fire, of cramp, of knifelike pain throughout the body. G-B patients usually receive four types of medication for pain: a narcotic, an anticonvulsant to calm the nerves, an antidepressant, and a mood elevator. The nurses agreed that some medications had to be moved from the feeding tubes to free them for food, but argued that pain medications, instead of being discontinued, should be given via shots. Even though it is generally better in long term care to give medications through the gut than in IV or IM (intramuscular) form, this, they argued, was not a case to be bound by general principles. Pain medications were the ones most available in IV or IM form, and should be given in that form, not eliminated altogether. The family weighed in on the nurses' side. Victor himself painstakingly spelled out that eliminating pain medications would not help his weight situation, because when his pain increased, so did his blood pressure and heart rate, which necessitated extra medications and increased his metabolism further. The nurses concurred—heart rate and blood pressure always rose the last hour or two before pain medications, and dropped significantly with pain medications.

The neurologists agreed, but were outvoted by the other doctors. They were only able to retain Tegritol, the anticonvulsant, which they argued had a medical as well as an analgesic function. The doctors stuck to the medical principle: medications to the gut in long-term cases. The first night without pain medications, nurses became so alarmed by Victor's blood pressure and heart rate that they were unwilling to take responsibility, and repeatedly called the doctor on call, demanding his presence. Twenty-four hours later, Victor was receiving all his pain medications either IV or IM. Liability and convenience considerations were more persuasive than personal care considerations.

CONSENT: PROCEDURES AND MEANING

When doctors wanted consent to a new surgery or treatment, they called me out of the room and explained why it was necessary. They uniformly expressed irritation when I insisted they make the argument to Victor because he would have to approve any decision. They repeatedly replied that he could not make decisions because he was on pain medications. What they meant was that these medications disqualified him as the person who signed the consent form. I was accused of being unwilling to accept responsibility—one doctor called me a pain in the butt when I restated my refusal to sign a permission for them to do any surgery to which Victor did not agree. Victor was 27 years old, intelligent, conscious, and had been making serious medical decisions for himself for nine years.

Part of our refusal was based on our realization that the golden rule was not sufficient here. Choosing for him what my husband and I would want others to choose for us was not fair to Victor. We felt that if we were he, we would not be willing to hurt any more, to undergo more treatments, to keep on hoping. But Victor was committed to living, and he was willing to endure high levels of pain, discomfort, and risk in order to secure a future for himself. He was not likely to deny doctors any treatment or surgery that they felt might save his life.

Our insistence on forcing the staff to interact directly with Victor was also a way of keeping him involved in life and in his care, and of helping him see himself as an agent, a decider, not a lump of flesh to be manipulated at will. More than one doctor protested that he could not speak to Victor. "What could I say?" or even "I can't tell him this!" they said, revealing more than they knew about their feelings of inadequacy.

One of the incidents that clarified for us how doctors understood the relationship between communication and consent occurred late in the fifth month, when Victor's lungs began weakly and periodically to "turn on" for an hour or so. The pulmonologist had lowered slightly the level of ventilator breathing two days in a row to support these involuntary breaths. Hope was rising that maybe Victor had turned the corner. Then on the third morning, we inadvertently heard from a respiratory technician that the pulmonologist had reversed the previous day's order. When I saw the pulmonologist in the hall later that day, I stopped him, noted that Victor was depressed about the change, and asked if he could please explain to Victor the reason for the change of order. The normally quiet pulmonologist defensively shouted, "We don't need to get consent for adjustments to the ventilator! We can do that at any time!" I tried to explain that I was not complaining, that the general consent to treat certainly included changing ventilator settings; I was only asking that he give Victor an explanation. He replied that he did not want to set a precedent (!), that patient care and decision making were the doctor's, and they did not have to explain every step they made to the patient.

Victor's nurse on the next shift let me read the chart. The doctor had suspected that Victor's lung was filling up again, and did not want to strain it further. The nurse suggested that this pulmonologist—the favorite of nurses and technicians because he rarely left the hospital when on call—had shouted out of discouragement at Victor's slow progress, and discomfort with the lack of rigid division between hospital staff and family, which made it more odious to be unable to report progress. Whatever upset him, the sentiments expressed revealed an attitude of professional ownership of information about the patient's body that excluded even the patient.

POWER AND COMPETENCE

The competence of hospital staff is an issue for a principlist ethic, as well as an ethic of care. The principle of justice, for example, requires accepting responsibility commensurate with the power one exercises. A number of incidents over the course of five months demonstrated where lines of power and command were drawn within the hospital, as well as the problems that bureaucracy creates for care.

Doctors' orders took precedence over every form of authority in the hospital except bureaucratic procedure. For example, when Victor was placed on the ventilator, the doctor ordered him immediately placed on tube feedings (he had been NPO [nothing by mouth] for 24 hours). The nurses replied that the hospital pharmacy would not send the cans of food for 36 hours because it was then 45 minutes past the 2 p.m. deadline before which pharmacy supplies for the next day must be ordered. So Victor fasted another day and a half. In a similar vein, when the first cyclosporine levels came back from the outside lab at an improbably high, even lethal, level, the doctor ordered that a new level be taken immediately. The nurse explained that it was after 5 p.m. on Friday; she was only allowed to send blood to the outside lab on Monday, Wednesday, and Friday. The doctor changed the order to the following Monday.

In Victor's case, the doctors had overall control over the activities of hospital staff, but they generally refused to take responsibility for anything other than their own activities. For example, Victor's aunt Connie, an ICU neo-natal/transplant nurse-practitioner at Loma Linda Research Center in Los Angeles, pointed out to the head of the medical team (a specialist in infectious diseases) many failures in sterile technique, all of which were potentially fatal to immunosuppressed patients (Green and Claiborne 1989). The doctor insisted that this was a nursing issue; there was nothing he could do. Similarly, I told the nephrologist that one reason for wildly inconsistent cyclosporine levels was that the nurses were not drawing the blood for the test eleven and a half hours after the morning dose of cyclosporine (through trough technique), but were instead drawing it at varied times. The nephrologist put me off, saying that he knew there were some problems in that these nurses were not trained as transplant nurses, but he had no authority over them.

Two weeks later this same doctor asked the nurse who happened to be drawing blood for the cyclosporine level how long since the last dose of cyclosporine. She replied that she had no idea, but that she was careful to follow proper trough technique and give each dose exactly 30 minutes after drawing the blood. Instead of drawing blood eleven and a half hours after the last dose of cyclosporine (ordered for every 12 hours), and then 30 minutes later giving the next dose, the nurses were drawing the blood whenever it was convenient, and giving the next dose 30 minutes later. Lab results reflected how much cyclosporine was in the bloodstream 16 hours after a dose one day, 6 hours another day. Now the nephrologist interfered in nursing by calling an immediate meeting of nursing managers at which he insisted that in-service training on correct trough technique be done on every shift, beginning immediately. This intervention gave the lie to earlier disclaimers of power within the institution. These incidents also illustrate how easy it is to push responsibility on complex, impersonal systems and fail to use one's power in those systems to insure care.

MISTAKES IN CARE AND THE PROFESSIONAL-FAMILY DIVISION

Physicians were the most resentful toward family involvement in Victor's treatment, though a few nurses and technicians were also, and even some staff who were most helpful and generally supportive of our involvement and interventions had moments when they, too, felt resentment. A number of incidents led family to think that a major cause of their resentment was our recognition of occasional staff failures of competence. All these personnel, but especially the doctors, expected to be seen as competent healers. From the very beginning, however, the complications of Victor's case, under-staffing, and the lack of expertise with transplant patients made the staff vulnerable to incompetence.

In the third day on the ventilator in the ICU, one of the leads to the heart monitor snagged on a hook at the foot of the roto-rest bed and stretched, restricting the tubing to the ventilator. As the bed continued to rotate, the ventilator tubing popped off the tracheostomy, and I could neither stretch it far enough to reconnect, nor figure out how to reverse the bed's rotation. The ventilator alarm went off. I assumed it would bring the nurses running, so I proceeded to breathe into Victor's trachea opening and then shout for help as I ran to the other side of the bed to breathe again into the trachea appliance. No one came. After four or five minutes I dashed out to the nurses' station shouting for help. Two nurses finally came running from another cubicle, but neither knew how to stop the bed rotation. While they tried I continued to breathe air into the trachea, running from side to side. The pulmonologist arrived about ten minutes after the alarm sounded, dove under the bed, unplugged it to disengage the rotation, and then reattached the tubing to the trachea.

Had I not been present, Victor would have died. His blood oxygen got dangerously low despite my mouth-to-trachea resuscitation. The pulmonologist lectured the nurses and the respiratory technicians on Victor's extreme vulnerability—unlike other ventilator patients, he had no respiration without the ventilator. He also demanded that the nursing coordinator begin in-service training that afternoon for all ICU nurses on how to operate the rotating bed. It was that evening that we contacted family members about flying in to help us keep a vigil.

Less than a week later there was an incident with the infectious diseases specialist who headed the team. He prescribed a hypertension medicine that Victor knew interfered with the immunosuppressant because he had had to discontinue it after the transplant. My husband asked the doctor to check the *Physicians Desk Reference* or ask the nephrologist, which he did, apologizing profusely and prescribing a different hypertension drug. With the help of one of Victor's nurses who checked each new drug ordered for counter-indications in the *PDR*, we were able to change four later drug orders by other doctors as well.

The next incident was almost five weeks into the ICU, when the hospital administration decided that as Medicare had reduced its payment level, Victor must be ready for step down care in the ventilator unit. The doctors were initially reluctant, but a week later they gave in to management's daily argument that the emergencies were past, and it was now just a waiting game to see whether he could be kept alive until the nerve sheathing reformed. The nurses were horrified at the proposed move, knowing that the level of care in the ventilator unit would be even lower than the ICU for nursing and respiratory technicians. Nurses and family protested, but were overruled. On his first day in the ventilator unit, his heart monitor alarm went off as his heart went from 200 beats per minute to 20, then zero, and then, after a 20-second pause, restarted. Ten minutes later it happened again, with a 40-second pause. There were neither doctors nor pacemakers in the unit. The nurses screamed for help, but a third stoppage commenced before a doctor from the ER arrived and ordered Victor back to the ICU and hooked to a stationary pacemaker until one could be surgically implanted.

The most persistent problem—persistently embarrassing for the staff and persistently terrifying for us—was blood pressure (BP) monitoring. Victor's BP could not be taken on his left arm because, for dialysis, a vein and an artery there had been joined to form a fistula. A BP cuff on that arm could blow the fistula and cause him quickly to bleed to death. This was not a problem in the ICU, where he wore a cuff on his right arm that automatically took his blood pressure at regular intervals, but in the ventilator unit, family had to stop nurses and aides every day from putting the cuff on the left arm, regardless of the fact that the danger was noted both on the chart and on the door. We made a four-foot-square poster that said "NO Left Arm BP" and hung it over his bed. It made no difference. Each staff person we stopped replied, "Oh, that's right," but tried again the next day. Victor kept track of the BP monitoring schedule, and refused to let family go to the restroom or to the vending machine if it was anywhere near BP time. Finally, one of his special nurses, Carol, and I took a fat black magic marker and wrote on his left arm "NO BP," and redarkened it every day or two. These dangerous attempts then subsided to once or twice a week, usually on the night shift.

What turned out to be the most serious incident happened late in the fifth month. I arrived at 6:30 p.m. to hear my distraught sister-in-law explain that Victor had developed terrible abdominal pain midmorning, which had gotten worse and worse. The doctor had been in twice, Victor had had three additional shots for pain, and they thought he was developing a bad kidney or bladder infection. The urine test would not be back for a few hours. I walked to his side, saw that his color, BP, and heart rate were sky high. He spelled out "Bad pain—fix." When I checked the color of the urine in the bag (infections make the urine cloudy), I saw that the line to the bag had a clamp on it. Unbelieving, I ran out in the hall where three doctors and the nurse were conferring, and asked, "Is there some reason why Victor's catheter is clamped off?" No one answered, so I ran back in with all of them following, and released the clamp. Within 30 seconds the bag overflowed. In a minute Victor's color went from scarlet to normal, and his blood pressure and heart rate began dropping. Within two minutes the floor was awash with urine, his pain was gone, and his BP and heart rate were down.

Joanne, his nurse on the 7–3 shift, had clamped the line to take a specimen and forgotten to unclamp it. Neither she nor the doctor who was called for Victor's pain thought to look at the catheter. The problem should have been caught at shift change when the 3–11 nurse did her assessment, which involves checking all the lines from the patient, but distracted by his acute pain, she put off assessment.

Within a week, almost certainly as a result of the urine reflux into the kidney forced by the clamp, an incurable kidney infection usually caused by reflux showed up on tests. It continues to slowly kill the transplant kidney.

Discovering inadequacies in Victor's care had unforeseen costs. Nurses who had made mistakes tended not to take Victor as a patient again, even when they had been competent regulars for him and had gotten along extremely well with him and us before. Joanne, the nurse who clamped the catheter, had been a regular, but transferred to a surgical floor without returning to the ventilator unit. Al, the head nurse during that incident, apologized later that night for what he freely volunteered was an egregious failure of care on the part of two nurses, himself, the head nurse on the first shift, and the doctor on call. But he never again took Victor as one of his patients.

Doctors in these incidents responded with a combination of physical avoidance and unwillingness to inform Victor or us of test results. (This hospital never informed us about this infection, though a later review of their labs in the chart revealed that they knew from the beginning, for over a month before he transferred to the rehab hospital.) The avoidance seemed to have multiple sources. One was concern over legal liability, although we never considered suit and we offered to release them from liability. Doctors also became both frustrated and embarrassed at their inability to report progress or to predict short- or long-term outcomes. G-B is not a comfortable disease for contemporary medicine because there is no cure. There is not even much of a treatment. Medicine merely tries to substitute for functions lost to the disease, and waits out the virus.[8] After a month, it was obvious that doctors saw Victor's failure to improve as a reflection on their skill as healers.

Incidents where the doctors or the personnel implementing their orders seemed incompetent only added to doctors' embarrassment and frustration. Serious mistakes caused embarrassment and discomfort for individual nurses who responded with avoidance, but the nurses as a whole tended to respond with a special commitment to provide the care needed. A transcript of Victor's first session on the speaking valve in the fifth month gives some sense of this:

Respiratory Tech Mike: [Inserting the Passy-Muir speaking valve.] Well, Vic, what do you have to say for yourself?

Victor: [Coughs for a minute or so, then squawks] I'm worried, always worried.

Nurse Patty: What are you worried about? Why?

Victor: About everything. Am I getting all my medicine? Am I getting it right? Will I get an infection and die? Will I lose my new kidney and have to go back on dialysis? I have to watch everything, and I still can't be sure.

Mom: Sure of what?

Vic: That they are doing everything right. They are so busy. I'm scared.

Nurse Nancy: What do you have to watch?

Vic: That you are all doing things right. Even the little things. When I first came to this vent unit Mom wrote on my left arm in big black letters "NO BP" because the nurse's aides kept trying to take it there. The fistula would blow, and I would bleed to death. Mom said they'd all learn quickly, but that was ten weeks ago, and last week my Aunt Connie put the sign back on my arm after she came out of the bathroom and saw the aide ignoring the sign over the bed, strapping a cuff on my left arm while I slept. That was only the first problem, not the worst.

Nurse Patty: But aren't things better now?

Vic: This week one nurse was ordered to use suction to remove the gas from my stomach and instead he hooked the suction drain to the line to my intestines, and sucked out all my food and medicines to the trash before my mom noticed. He argued with her that he had done it right; they got the nurse manager and found he had it wrong. By the time it was fixed, it was too long to know how many meds had been lost. I sat here all day waiting for my [transplant] kidney to begin rejecting. Yesterday the new night nurse put all my meds in the drain line, not the line to the intestine. She ignored my head shaking and Dad's questions. I can't live like this! And the drain line! Two nights ago a new nurse turned up the suction on the drain line, and a few hours later my mom sees fresh blood clots in the line. So she told Carol, who set it back lower. This morning when Mom came in she saw lots of dried clots in the drain line; somebody had set the pressure back up higher while I was asleep. I have enough feeding problems; I don't need an ulcer, too! [Sobbing loudly.]

Nurse Patty: Calm down, Victor. [Tearfully] Is there anything else you need to say?

Vic: My Aunt Connie [smiles through his tears], the dragon, as Mike says, is a neo-natal transplant nurse-practitioner. She said last week that with any patient all intravenous ports should be sterilized with alcohol before needles are put into them, and with immune-suppressed patients, even the ports of the Foleys [catheter bags] should be sterilized before emptying because it is a direct line to my kidney. Nobody here sterilizes the Foley ports, and only a few even sterilize the central IV port, which runs right to my heart! Nobody bothers to rinse the cyclosporin from the mixing glass with more cranberry juice so that I get it all, unless my family stands over them. I know you were not trained as transplant nurses, and maybe these things don't matter for ordinary patients, but they do for me. I am helpless. At your mercy. I am only 27 and want to have a life. Please be more careful. If you are careful, I can survive. [Bursts into tears. The rest of the room— nurses, aides and respiratory technicians—is completely teary.]

Respiratory Tech Mike: Anything for us techs, Vic?

Victor: [Smiling through tears] Well, you know how much I hate it when you pound on my ribs. But every one of the last seven pneumonias happened after I missed the pounding or the tech forgot to put the pneu bed back on lung rotation after the treatment, and the bed stayed off all night. [The pneu bed is inflated, and bumps inflate that roll the patient to the right side, flat on back, and the left side for 20 minutes every hour.] Last week my Aunt Connie said that of the four times a day that the pounding was ordered, I had zero times two days, one time on two days, and two times a day the rest. That's partly my fault; I've asked to put it off when I'm very tired. But I need it.

Respiratory Tech Arturo: When we're busy and you ask to postpone your therapy, we usually can't get back to you, especially at night.

Victor: Just please remember how vulnerable I am to infection. I'm not 75 like most of the people up here. I want to get out, go home, go to work, fall in love and have kids [tears]. I lay in that bed day and night worrying that one of you, rushing to get all your meds and labs and treatments done, will kill me by accident and never know it.

Nurse Inez: [In tears] Victor, we will have a staff meeting. Your aunt and your mom had a meeting last week with Tania [the nurse manager] about some of these concerns. None of us knew that you worried so much about them. That's why you got so upset last night, isn't it? Carol gave you Elavil to put you to sleep, and you kept demanding the other 10:00 meds—even Carol you don't trust enough to go to sleep and let her take care of them, do you? Even with your mom here!

Victor: I trust Carol almost as much as Mom. Last night Carol told me she was the only RN on both units. That meant that if somebody went bad, she would have to be with them, and an aide would take over my meds—and I don't trust any of them to get 'em right. If you do talk—could you ask all the nurses to tell me which meds they are giving me when, so I know what I've had and not had? Some don't like to tell us—but we have figured out the regular ones. I feel safer knowing.

Nurse Patty: That's easy enough. How about we mark the sites of the stomach drain and the intestinal line? We could mark the PEG "drain" and the PEJ "food/meds." [Others nod.]

Victor: Good. Thanks. [The speaking valve is removed.]

Health care workers need to feel competent at their jobs. The fact that already threatened lives depend upon their competence makes competence more important for them than it is for most workers. For doctors whose highly specialized training instills standards of near-perfection upon which their institutional authority is based, incompetence undermines their authority as well as their self-respect. For nurses like Joanne, who are not only trained to standards of precision but also to personal care for patients, feelings that they let Victor down were intolerable, even after he sent a message that he understood the incident was an accident and hoped she would return. When the staff came to hear Victor speak for the first time, as reported above, none of the issues he brought up were new. But every staff member present was affected by his pleas, and for his last two weeks in the ventilator unit, staff—including many who had not been present—made extra efforts to get things right and regularly asked him if particular aspects of care were improved. Significantly, none of the doctors, even three of his doctors who were in the unit during the session, joined in.

CONCLUDING ANALYSIS

Although there were great variations within each of the specific health care professions involved in Victor's care, it would be difficult not to discern a pattern—in fact, a spectrum—among them. Groups of staff differed in terms of the degree of communication with the patient, willingness to adapt unit/hospital policy and procedures to meet Victor's particular needs, and degree of concern for the whole patient (including mental health). On these points the various groups of hospital staff arranged themselves on a spectrum that could be characterized as extending between the poles of biomedical principlism and the ethics of care.

No group of staff fully embodied either of these poles to the exclusion of the other. For example, one of the pulmonologists, the one who exploded at being asked to explain the change in ventilator settings, once remained in the unit for 30 hours straight, for half of which he was not even the doctor on call, when Victor and another patient were in crisis. On the other hand, one nurse insisted that floor policy said that medications could be given within a three to four hour window, so there was no need to adjust the nurses' break schedule to give Victor's cyclosporine within the hour. But in general, the doctors and hospital administrators represented one end of the spectrum. Both groups exhibited a strong tendency to rely on deductive models of patient care. The doctors relied on biomedical ethical principles in ways that allowed them, for example, to treat Victor the same as a comatose patient because he was similarly incompetent to sign consent forms. For doctors, medicine is a scientific body of knowledge with a set of principles to be followed, such as the one that says that medications go to the gut in long-term patients.

For hospital administrators, the guiding principles were financial. Medicare's payment schedule became the set of principles that they thought should govern care. For example, because Victor was one day short of the required 60-day interval between his transplant hospitalization in Ohio and his G-B hospitalization in Florida, he was admitted in what was the eleventh day of a Medicare 60-day cycle of fully covered care. Neither we nor the hospital knew this until the second month. Upon obtaining this information from Medicare, a hospital administrator came to the ICU and told the doctors that the move to step down care must begin ten days sooner. Neither doctors nor hospital administrators thought that personal care was appropriate for them to give; it was the province of nurses, who have such lesser institutional power that they can easily be overruled, as they were when they protested the inadequacy of stepped down care. For doctors and administrators, the information flow ran from bottom to top, where they decided what was important and what not, and then issued orders that ran downward.

Respiratory technicians were in the middle of the spectrum. They tended to give personal care, one example of which was that on the ventilator unit, care providers chose their own patients, and three technicians consistently chose Victor. One brought Victor videos and more than once stayed after his 7–7 shift to watch one, allowing me to get a couple hours of extra sleep. Because technicians manipulated the patient's body, they were accustomed to adjusting treatments depending upon different levels of voluntary movement, of musculature, and of types of tubing running in and out of the patient's body. They all used the eye-blink system extensively for questioning, although none of them spelled to allow Victor to "speak." Yet none of the respiratory technicians would ever directly question the order of the pulmonologist, even when they as a group agreed that an order was mistaken or even dangerous. More than once they bit their lips at a doctor's order, then made arrangements among themselves to ensure that for the next shift or two, one of them was always near that patient in case of emergency.

Respiratory technicians seemed the biggest victims of the hospital's understaffing. Not only were the shifts understaffed, but technicians were also under constant pressure to work overtime, at least two back-to-back 12-hour shifts a week, and sometimes three. None of them ever worked less than 60 hours a week; they constantly shared stories of angry wives and children who complained that their overtime ruined family plans, that they were never home. More than once administrators chased down a technician in Victor's room to request a double shift. "Hell, no!," responded Arturo once. "I haven't seen my kids in a week!" (Arturo worked 7 a.m.–7 p.m., lived an hour away, and had three children under five.) The administrator insisted that there was no one else, that everyone else was either out of town or had just pulled a double, and that neither his patients nor his colleagues would appreciate being shorthanded. In the end Arturo agreed, cursing the hospital's refusal to hire more technicians because overtime was cheaper than paying benefits to new workers. Still, he concluded that "you have to be loyal to the system you're a part of."

That remark was instructive, and conveys the feelings of many technicians who sometimes felt pulled in two directions. On the one side were

professional loyalties, which included not only loyalty to professional principles, but also to fellow respiratory therapists, the pulmonologists they worked
with, and the specialized health care system of which the hospital was a
part. On the other side were personal desires to help patients, which reflected
both the initial desire that took them into health care, and the personal
responsibilities and commitments they had made to particular patients in the
course of treating them. In an interview at the end of Victor's hospitalization,
Natalie, the youngest of the respiratory technicians, was asked to explain
why she had referred to Victor both as her favorite patient and as the worst
patient in the unit. She explained that he had never been the sickest because
he had always had a chance to survive, as some of the sickest elderly did
not. But though he was the most cooperative and appreciative, his care
was full of problems because of the understaffing, so that frequently the
procedures worked out for other patients didn't work for him and had to
be changed. "And that makes us all tense," she said.

The nurses represent the group most influenced by an ethic of care.
Nurses who were predisposed to or developed a personal commitment with
Victor rendered a qualitatively different kind of care that was more adequate
not merely for supporting his emotional well-being, but for providing safe,
medically effective care.

One of the best indications that an ethic of care needs to be coordinated
with a more systemic, principle-based model of treatment is the catheter
incident. Had the head nurse and incoming nurse on the afternoon shift
followed normal assessment procedures, instead of being totally absorbed
in sympathy for Victor's pain, the clamp would have been discovered much
earlier, and the kidney possibly saved. Effective care requires not only
generalized procedures like assessment, which reflect professional principles,
but also the personal attention to the individual patient that the nurses
showed in their willingness to work with Victor and his family to reverse
dangerous drug orders. These reversals prevented numerous additional
drug complications.

Kohlberg and Habermas would object to locating these medical specialties on a spectrum between principlism and care poles. They would view
comparing doctors and nurses as similar to comparing apples and oranges
(Kohlberg 1984, 229–30, 360; Young 1990, 106–7). Doctors and nurses have
different care functions within a rationalized system of health care; the role
of doctors is to be scientific experts, and the role of nurses is to bring those
scientific decisions to the body of the patient, and thus to be more personally
involved. The adequacy of each type of care is thus evaluated on different

scales. There are different moral values attached to the professional socialization of doctors and nurses. Patients get their just due when all of the different staff fulfill their particular assigned duties within the organizational framework. Moral theory, whether carried out in terms of Habermas's communicative ethics (Habermas 1984; 1990, 178–80), Rawl's theory of justice (Rawls 1972), or even Benhabib's discourse ethics,[9] would reflect on how the social framework for justice should be theoretically constructed in order to secure justice for, among others, patients and staff. Each of them, like Kohlberg himself, assumes that the goal is to arrive at a theory of the just society that will then be implemented—and stops there, as if the real work is done when the theory has been agreed upon and transformed into procedural rules by social discourse. The perspective of those who desperately need justice suggests that the task is unfinished.

An ethic of care approach understands that the needs of the particular patient before one at any given time are the touchstone, the guide, for adapting any theory or any system's rules and procedures. The ethic of care is not an alternative to a system that implements a theory of justice. The rationalized division of labor, the organization of space, and the established procedures of the system may remain, but they become provisional, and must always be assessed in terms of their adequacy for each particular patient. The nurses in this case study were caught between these two approaches. By the end of Victor's stay, some represented a more or less principled ethic of care, some nurse managers stuck with the systemic procedural approach and the principles of bioethics that accompany it, and most vacillated between them, depending on what was at stake at the moment.

Victor's nursing staff was 80 percent female, his doctors 100 percent male, and his respiratory technicians 94 percent male. Sex did not seem directly to determine orientation to care or principlism; some male nurses were among the most care-oriented, and the female respiratory technician was the least care-oriented. But it is possible that sex-linked stereotypes of the different health care professions influenced who was attracted into which profession.

The contemporary hospital system has melded medical specialization to hierarchy in ways that have replicated patriarchy, but are slowly becoming more diverse.[10] Specialization is one hallmark of modernity that is further developed and exalted in postmodernity. Although it has greatly enhanced knowledge in medicine, it has, along with the bureaucracy necessary to manage a field of specialized niches, also enhanced the potential for mistakes due to miscommunication, complex orders requiring acute coordination, and overconfidence. The hierarchy in hospitals is structured with specialists at the top, and those with the most holistic but general knowledge, nurses, at the bottom. This internal class system is most strongly resented by the nurses, who are unable to act in many situations without a direct order from a physician. For example, when an IV infiltrated and Victor's arm blew up like a balloon, the acutely frustrated nurse could not stop the swelling by removing the needle for ten hours, until one of the eight doctors she called returned her calls and authorized its removal.

The nurses who best represented an ethic of care in this case were not merely pursuing a personal relationship with the patient, or acting out beliefs about the good life. They were struggling to deliver the justice owed this patient by this hospital in this society's health care system, which was not organized to provide that justice. They delivered justice significantly better than other elements of the system because they allowed their concern for this particular patient to open them to his alternative perspective on the systemic provision of care.

Endnotes

1 Gilligan proposed that the concept of rights and the assumption underlying justice (that self and others are equal) calls into question the opposition of passion and duty and the ideal of selflessness: "Among college students in the seventies, the concept of rights entered into their thinking to challenge a morality of self-sacrifice and self-abnegation. Questioning the stoicism of self-denial and replacing the illusion of innocence with an awareness of moral choice, they struggled to grasp the essential notion of rights, that the interests of the self can be considered legitimate. In this sense, the concept of rights changes women's conceptions of self, allowing them to see themselves as stronger and to consider their own needs. When assertion no longer seems dangerous, the concept of relationships changes from a bond of continuing dependence to a dynamic of interdependence. Then the notion of care expands from the paralyzing injunction not to hurt others to an injunction to act responsibly toward self and others and thus to sustain connection. A consciousness of the dynamics of human relationships then becomes central to moral understanding, joining the heart and the eye in an ethic that ties the activity of thought to the activity of care" (Gilligan 1982, 149). Gilligan is arguing that although a pre-feminist female moral perspective may have focused on care to the exclusion of more rational approaches, a female moral perspective informed by the feminist movement for women's rights integrates justice and care.

2 Research done for this seminar included 40 hours of charting daytime staff interactions with the patient; 26 hours of taped, transcribed verbal interactions among staff, patient, and family; four hours of taped transcribed interviews with

three staff care givers and the patient; and over 800 hours of participant observation notes. My tape recorder was unobtrusive because it was part of a boom box on which we often played the Baroque music Victor found soothing. The staff knew I was a teacher, and so assumed my typing on the laptop or taking notes was for my teaching.

3 Patient autonomy is perhaps the central problematic concept in bioethics, as it reflects an understanding of personhood that is nonrelational. Iris Marion Young writes: "Critical theoretical accounts of instrumental reason, postmodernist critiques of humanism and of the Cartesian subject, and feminist critiques of the disembodied coldness of modern reason all converge on a similar project of puncturing the authority of modern scientific reason. Modern science and philosophy construct a specific account of the subject as knower, as a self-present origin standing outside of and opposed to objects of knowledge—autonomous, neutral, abstract and purified of particularity. They construct this modern subjectivity by fleeing from material reality, from the body's sensuous continuity with flowing, living things, to create a purified abstract idea of formal reason, disembodied and transcendent. With all its animation removed and placed in that abstract, transcendent subject, nature is frozen into discrete, inert, solid objects, each identifiable as one and the same thing, which can be counted, measured, possessed, accumulated and traded" (Young 1990, 125). Patient autonomy is supposed to protect the interests of patients within the health care system, but the ease with which it is reduced to signed consent forms illustrates Young's point, and supports my argument that care giver relationships with patients provide more protection than such a concept in moral theory.

4 Interview with Nurse Carol.

5 In addition, in the ventilator units where oral feeding is impossible, most medications must be separately crushed, mixed with water, and injected into the enteral feeding tubes; some short-term patients receive intravenous feeding.

6 During five eight-hour day shifts, for a total of 40 hours, I charted 74 staff entries into the patient's ICU room as seen in the chart following this note. Staff included doctors, nurses, aides, respiratory therapists, occupational and speech therapists, maintenance staff, and bioengineers.

7 Victor may have had much more communication than most severe G-B patients. Sue Baier's *Bed Number Ten*, written with Zimmeth Shomaker (1986), details the experience of a Texas woman who spent ten and a half months paralyzed with G-B on a ventilator with no communication with either staff or her family, who were limited to a 15-minute visit every other day.

8 There is evidence that intravenous immunoglobulins or plasmaphoresis (removal of a few pints of blood plasma) may, for unknown reasons, slightly speed the beginning of recovery in roughly half of cases. Even with first the IV/IG treatments and then plasmaphoresis, Victor remained at the low point months past the norm.

9 Benhabib's discourse ethics not only improves on the rationalism of Rawls by requiring real discourse with others, it also improves on Habermas by expanding morality beyond justice. Although she understands the encounter with others as

being prior to theory, however, she does not elaborate the limits to theory and remains focused on its construction (Benhabib 1992, 148–202).

10 I have no idea why none of Victor's doctors were female. In Ohio, a number of his doctors have been female; in Miami, we encountered no females in the ten different specialist practices that treated him.

References

Anderson, S.B. 1992. Guillain-Barre: Giving the Patient Control. *Journal of Neuroscience Nursing* 24/5: 158–62.

Baier, Sue, and Mary Zimmeth Shomaker. 1986. *Bed Number Ten*. New York: Holt, Rinehart, and Winston.

Barrall-Inman, R.A. 1995. Question and Answer: Guillain-Barre Syndrome. *Journal of the American Academy of Nurse Practitioners* 7/4 (April): 155–59.

Benhabib, Seyla. 1992. *Situating the Self: Gender, Community and Postmodernism*. New York: Routledge.

Chodorow, Nancy. 1974. *The Reproduction of Mothering*. Berkeley: University of California Press.

DuBose, Edwin, Ron Hamel, and Laurence J. O'Connell, eds. 1994. *A Matter of Principles? Ferment in Bioethics*. Valley Forge, Penn.: Trinity Press International.

Gilligan, Carol. 1982. *In a Different Voice: Psychological Theory and Women's Development*. Cambridge, Mass.: Harvard University Press.

Green, A., and E. Claiborne. 1989. A Nursing Challenge: Cytomegalovirus in the Transplant Recipient. *Focus on Critical Care* 16/5: 249–54.

Habermas, Jurgen. 1984. *The Theory of Communicative Action. Volume I: Reason and the Rationalization of Society*. Boston: Beacon Press.

———. 1990. *Moral Consciousness and Communicative Action*, trans. Christian Lenhardt and Sherry Weber Nicholsen. Boston: MIT Press.

Heller, Joseph. 1986. *No Laughing Matter*. New York: Putnam.

Kohlberg, Lawrence. 1984. *Essays on Moral Development*, vol. 2. San Francisco: Harper and Row.

Mascarelle, J.J., and D.C. Hudson. 1991. Dissimmune Neurological Disorders. *AACN: Clinical Issues in Critical Care Nursing* 2/4: 675–84.

Pfister, S.M., and J.B. Bullas. 1990. Acute Guillain-Barre Syndrome. *Critical Care Nursing* 10/10: 68–73.

Rawls, John. 1972. *A Theory of Justice*. Cambridge, Mass.: Harvard University Press.

Ruiz-Rodriguez, M.C. 1994. Care of the Patient with Guillain-Barre Syndrome. *Enfermeria Clinica* 4/5: 238–41.

Thilagarani, N. 1990. Nursing Care of Guillain-Barre Syndrome. *Nursing Journal of India* 85/7: 147–48.

Wyschogrod, Edith. 1990. *Saints and Postmodernism*. Chicago: University of Chicago Press.

Young, Iris Marion. 1990. *Justice and the Politics of Difference*. Princeton, N.J: Princeton University Press.

PART II

CARE AND EMOTION

4

The Emotions of Care in Health Care

Edward Collins Vacek, S.J.

The world of medicine is charged with grandeur and gore, with relief and regret, with triumph and tragedy. The world of medicine is propelled by noble aspirations and narcissistic ambitions, by curious minds and power-seeking preoccupations, by bored salary-seekers and compassionate do-gooders. The world of medicine, in short, is filled with emotion.

Emotions pervade the lives of professional care takers, and emotions impact the kind of medical care they give (Gordon 1996, 273). But when cost-accountants do their bottom-line reckoning, they pay little attention to the affections that activate, inspire, and sustain medical care giving. They also ignore the emotions that degrade medical care. The malaise that has come over many health professionals derives in part from trends in medical ethics and economics that treat emotions as expendable road-kill along the highway to a rational, cost-effective medical "delivery system" (McCormick 1998). As Richard Gunderman notes, the virtues appropriate to good medicine are "most difficult to retain sight of when practicing the virtues of a good consumer" (Gunderman 1998, 12). As a consequence, the emotions of care tend to be overlooked in the contemporary reorganization of medical practice.

The role of affection in the practice of medicine is usually neglected by philosophers and theologians, and so I devote the largest section of this essay to a discussion of the nature of emotions and their role in health care. I will argue that affectivity is essential for the moral practice of medicine. I will also address some popular worries that emotions impede medical care.

MEANINGS OF "CARE"

What is care? Its meaning is anything but clear. When we say that a sleeping baby doesn't have a care in the world, we are speaking of an enviable absence of problems. When we say that a man is depressed and doesn't care about anything, we are speaking of a worrisome lack of emotion. And when we say that adults do not care for anyone (except perhaps themselves), we are making a severe moral judgment.

The meaning of "care" in "health care" is similarly complex. In part, it refers to a commendable attitude or virtue. When we say that a doctor really cares about his or her patients, we are praising her. But when an accrediting agency files a report saying that the care given in a barrio clinic is substandard, the agency likely is referring not to anyone's attitude, but to such things as sterilization procedures, drug availability, or equipment failures. Of course, such failures may reflect a lack of an attitude of care, but that need not be so. Indeed, the investigator might say that the clinic's staff cares very much for its poor patients, but might still insist that the staff just does not have the resources or the training to provide adequate care. "Care," in this sense, refers to standard benefits. I begin my analysis with this meaning of care. I will progressively add to it in order to display the complexity of this rich notion.

Care as Benefit

Adequate care means adequate benefits, benefits that meet human wants or needs. (In this essay, I prescind from veterinary medicine.) When people approach a health professional, they are usually seeking some sort of cure or palliation; or they want some improvement that only such professionals can provide, such as a shorter nose or straighter teeth. Medical care, of course, includes more than bodily care. When a hospice nurse holds the hand of a dying patient, the comfort offered is a genuine human good. Thus, to offer "care" to someone means, at least in part, to provide them with some human benefit.

Care-as-benefit is relative to what would be good for a particular patient. Life-prolonging CPR for a patient in the last stages of terminal cancer ordinarily is not good care. However, care-as-benefit is also relative to what typically happens in good medicine in a particular area of the world. The surgeon who is successful 90 percent of the time when others are only 50 percent successful gives excellent care. Still, this standard of excellence may not benefit a particular patient. We would be at least hesitant to say that a patient received excellent care if she died while being operated on by the best brain surgeon in the field. Conversely, most of us would rather have an incompetent surgeon cut the "wrong" part of our brain, if, contrary to standard medicine, this slip somehow cured our Parkinsonism. But, then, we would probably be ambivalent about whether we had received "good care." We might say that bad "care" (in terms of current standards) produced good "care" (that is, the benefit we needed).

Care as Benevolence

Not all benefits are benevolently given. A nurse may hasten to give pain-relievers to the ever-complaining patient, not because he wants to help her, but just to shut her up. The nurse might even, in a testy moment, wish her dead. But he acts for his own comfort. Conversely, not all benevolent desires lead to beneficent acts. A night orderly might very much want to help an elderly patient stop choking, yet he might not have a clue how to bring that about. Indeed, his clumsy, but well-intentioned efforts might cause serious harm.

A fully human form of care includes not only doing good, but wanting to do that good. Human beings have lots of reasons for doing good. Some of those reasons are morally good, some morally evil. For example, professionals may help out of a Kantian sense of duty, or they may help because they want to take away business from a struggling competitor and thus destroy his practice. Of course, if we are sick, we want the cure that is care-as-benefit, quite apart from the professional's motive, but usually we also want to be helped by people who truly want to help us. We want them to be benevolent toward us. Their personal concern is important to us not only because they are then more likely to benefit us, but also because each of us wants to be the focus of another's goodwill. Their benevolence typically is an affirmation of our own worth and dignity.

Even when professionals are primarily motivated by medically extraneous desires such as money, power, or prestige, they may still, in an odd sort of way, be benevolent. That is, they might genuinely want our good even when their more basic reason for doing good is to enhance their reputation or to demonstrate the effectiveness of their new drug. Benevolence simply means that we want the patient's good. It does not exclude other good (and bad) motives. Indeed, we usually act with mixed motives. Jesus was pictured as raising Lazarus partly out of friendship, but chiefly "so that you may believe" (Jn 11:15, 33, 35).

The scope of care-as-benevolence can be limited. A medical supply salesman can genuinely care about his customers without being interested in whether their marriages are doing well or the summer heat is oppressive. He cares that they get the right supplies. A medical professional might broadly care about her patients, but most immediately she cares about and for their health. Because many aspects of patients' lives can affect their health, she will be somewhat concerned about other matters, but ordinarily how people fare in the stock market and where they get their haircuts are not part of health care. Professionals are concerned about the whole person, but usually their specific acts of benevolent care refer only to a limited area for a limited period of time. Jesus cured a demoniac and then sent him on his way (Mk 5:18–19).

Care as Responsibility

When we entrust an heirloom to the "care" of a curator, it becomes his or her responsibility to see that it is kept in good condition or perhaps even put in an improved condition. Similarly, when a physician assumes care of patients, they become the physician's responsibility. We rightfully expect the physician to be concerned about them, to make sure that procedures are being carried out on their behalf, and to monitor whether treatments are in fact effective. The etymology of "care" is "anxiety" or "worry." For a physician to care means that he or she is worried about patients' health prospects. Their fate is a matter of special concern for the physician; the worse they get, the more worried and involved the physician must be.

The response of care may take several forms. At its most impersonal, we feel a need for remedy as "something should be done" (Noddings 1984, 81). Less impersonally, we feel it as "someone should do something." Most personally, the experience is one of "I should do something." The "someone should do" turns into "I should do" when we accept the role of care taker, at least until it becomes clear that nothing further can or should be done. For example, upon hearing a child in pain, we ordinarily expect that his parents will experience a demand to do something. They are his care takers. On the other hand, if the child is hopelessly ill, all may experience a "something should be done," but they may sense that only God can answer this appeal.

When we experience care-as-responsibility, we are inclined to pay attention to anything that may be relevant to the fulfillment of that responsibility. We act "carefully." Care givers have a special obligation to listen to their patients and to be responsive to their personal concerns. Careful medical professionals are rightly expected to note small details that most people miss as these details may indicate illnesses or other problems. Being responsible, professionals then respond in light of these details. Otherwise, they can rightfully be accused of negligence. They have a duty to be "careful."

Beyond paying close attention, however, care-as-responsibility also implies a commitment. Health professionals commit themselves to help patients overcome or deal with their burdens. These professionals enter a "special relationship" with the people who are "in their care." Each patient is no longer just one of six billion people on this planet. He or she is "my patient."

Care as Affection

Affections have both outward and inward aspects. When we care for someone, we show "concern, consideration, affection, devotion" toward the one cared for (Waerness 1996, 234). Our focus is on the other. At the same time, we let the other "make a difference" to us. When a boss says to subordinates, "I don't care what you think," he indicates that the subordinates' views make no difference. When the boss says to them, "Tell me what you think," he may only be asking for information or ideas that could be useful, but which he will ignore if not useful. When, however, the boss says, "I care what you think," he indicates that, even if he cannot act on their advice, they and their views are valuable to him.

The personal engagement involved in care-as-affection ranges from nearly none to almost complete engrossment. For example, we might say, "Yes, of course, I care about the thousand people who died yesterday in a flood in China, but I'm not going to let that prevent me from going out to the party tonight." On the other extreme, most of us have had someone to whom we could say, "I care for you so much that my life would not easily go on without you." If we are deeply religious, we want to care above all for God. That is, we focus on God, while at the same time we want God and our relationship to God to make a night-and-day difference in how we live.

In between minimal notice and supreme devotion, care usually includes "liking" someone. We enjoy being with them. The responsibility we have for a patient need not be a heavy burden; rather, it can be a self-fulfilling pleasure. This pleasure often results in preferences among patients. Thus, a psychiatrist might say that of all the patients on the ward, the one she cares for most, that is, the one she most delights in seeing, is an old man who was badly damaged in World War II. She may be able to provide little care for him in the form of beneficial treatments, but she will miss him when he dies because she has great affection for him.

Care for the Sake of

The notion of care is further filled out when we ask for whose sake we are caring. In almost every human encounter, the answer will be multiple and mixed. Reflection reveals at least three different emphases. We act altruistically, self-interestedly, and communally.[1]

An altruistic care affirms someone for his or her own sake. In health care we may meet patients whom we would never want as friends, but toward whom we feel compassion. Such patients may even be a "bother," or their cases may be so routine as to offer us little intellectual or emotional enrichment. Still, we care for them with an altruistic care when we affectively affirm them as persons and want their betterment for their own sakes and not for our own benefit (even if we may also benefit).

A contrary impulse to put distance between ourselves and disagreeable patients is understandable. The impulse to forget others when fatigue, boredom, or frustration take hold is also normal. But each of us, to greater and lesser degrees, is capable of a countervailing movement of self-transcendence. In altruistic care, this ability overrides alienating impulses and makes the very sickness, vulnerability, and even disagreeableness of patients an invitation and challenge to care for them. We want to aid them even though we seem to "get nothing out of it."[2] We come to their aid even when this requires "costly care" from us.

At other times, we care for others in view of some benefit or pleasure we derive (Blum 1980b, 24–27). We have "favorite patients" who are charming or otherwise endearing. We like being with them because we are enriched by them. Or we meet patients whose illness stretches our medical knowledge and thus are interesting to work with. We genuinely care for such patients and want their good, but we are focally motivated by what such eros-care does for us. Few people would stay long in health care work without the satisfactions of this eros-care.

We also care as part of our membership in various groups. For example, we care as a responsible member of the medical profession. Or we go out of our way for an old woman because she is a member of our local church community. Or we allocate a kidney to a member of our own nation before considering foreigners. In other words, our special relationships make a difference in our care. We act in part out of and for the sake of these relationships. Thus, we might make an extra effort to stay with one patient during the night through a critical period in her illness, even though we would legitimately pass a new patient on to another competent colleague. We make these distinctions because of the special relationship of trust and concern we have established with the first but not the second patient.

All three foci of care can be present to various degrees in the way a professional relates to a particular patient. Still, one or another form of care likely will be predominant at any particular moment, and one or another may at times be appropriate, inappropriate, or problematic. For example, giving some extra attention to the son of a colleague can be appropriate, but taking charge of our own daughter's hysterectomy is not. Our gravitation toward enjoyable cases becomes problematic to the degree it renders us less ready to deal with bothersome patients.

Thus far, I have described "care" as a complex amalgam of four aspects: beneficence, benevolence, responsibility, and affection. I further qualified care by considering for whose sake we act. I want now to look more closely and at length at the affective quality of care, as the other features of care generally receive ethicists' approval, but the role of emotions is too frequently either neglected or denigrated in medical ethics.

THE AFFECTIVE QUALITY OF CARE

We experience the world within us and beyond us with emotion. Certain parts of the world are hot for us, others are palpably cold, most are tepid. A walk through a hospital is charged with positive and negative importances, as well as with a host of nearly neutral objects. For example, this syringe on the emergency room floor is a temptation for the drug addict, a reminder to the nurse of two nearly simultaneous cardiac arrests, and just one more piece of litter for the night janitor. Or, again, this young child—it pains me to say—almost died last night; that old man—I'm so relieved—will finally die soon; and these people passing through are unknown to me.

Our emotions are "intentional" acts in the phenomenological sense that they put us in touch with the world within and beyond us. Emotions are not just "tingles" down the spine; they are "about" something (Solomon 1980, 250–54). Because of them, we experience objects as having different kinds and degrees of salience (de Sousa 1980, 137–38). A life without emotions is a life without importances. Emotions can put us in contact with what is objectively valuable *qua* valuable.

The language of value is commonly used vaguely and loosely. We are said to give value or to decide what shall be valuable; and outside our bestowal or decision, things are said to be without value. In this relativistic view, health is not itself a value; rather, it is good only if a person (autonomously and ultimately arbitrarily) decides he or she wants to be healthy. Alternatively, "value" is commonly used as a synonym for virtue, as when someone says courage is a value, but greed is not. In this essay, by "value" I mean a quality of a thing whereby it is good in itself or good for another (or bad, in the case of disvalues). All things, both real and ideal, possess value, indeed, many values. As I use the word, then, "value-education" teaches students what is important and how one importance compares with another. It teaches, for example, that Beethoven's music is more profound than that of the Beach Boys, that human beings are more valuable than pet frogs, and that generosity is good whereas greed is bad. Such learning, of course, is a complex cognitive process.

Martha Nussbaum rightly argues that emotions are cognitive acts that complexly interact with intellectual acts, volitional acts, behavior, and so forth (Nussbaum 1999, 256–65). As Diana Fritz Cates notes, "Our best feeling is thoughtful feeling (i.e., passion that has been educated over time to arise and to persist 'in the right way'), and our best thinking is feeling-full thinking (i.e., thinking that takes place fundamentally in the service of love)" (Cates 1997, 171). I cannot here probe deeply the relationship between emotions and these other human acts, but I must give some indication of the complexity of emotions themselves. They have four aspects.

Openness to Value in General and Regions of Value

The first aspect of our emotional life is our openness to the world as valuable. We are essentially beings-who-care. Caring is part of our very humanity. Consider the following scene depicted by the fourth century B.C.E. Chinese philosopher, Mencius:

> Suppose a man were, all of a sudden, to see a young child on the verge of falling into a well. He would certainly be moved to compassion, not because he wanted to get in the good graces of the parents, nor because he wished to win the praise of his fellow villagers or friends, nor yet because he disliked the cry of the child. From this it can be seen that whoever is devoid of the heart of compassion is not human. (Mencius 1970, 82–83)

As this text incidentally indicates, our emotions may often be directed to various collateral values of an event (here: pleasing parents, getting praise, ending an annoyance), but our emotions can and should be directed to the central value (the child's safety) in and for itself.

It is intrinsically human to respond to events of value and disvalue. If nothing makes a difference to us, then we are (nearly) dead. As Bernard Lonergan wrote, without emotion, "our knowing and deciding would be paper thin" (Lonergan 1972, 30–31). Rarely if ever does a human being reach such a state of "apathy." Rather, all of us have a fundamental affective openness to value in general. Just as the eyes open the world of color and the ears open the world of sound, so too our emotions open the world of value.

Within our broad, general sensitivity to value, each of us is more or less sensitive to various delimited regions of value. The same person can be doctor and scientist and wage-earner and mother, and each of these personae has different regions for its concern. These concerns may complement or compete with one another. They may also allow or even promote blindness to other regions. As Lonergan writes, "what lies beyond one's horizon is simply outside the range of one's knowledge and interests: one neither knows nor cares" (Lonergan 1972, 236). Accordingly, Mark Doorley writes, "The first role of feelings in the deliberative process concerns the establishment of a subject's horizon. The horizon of a subject refers to a limit of his concern" (Doorley 1996, 78). For example, the need for data for our research project may blind us to the negative side-effects of an invasive test we order.

Because our emotions reveal some values even as they blind us to other values, because they are often conflicting, and because they both motivate as well as restrain us, our emotions build the stage and set the scenes for our moral life. Whereas some people are highly sensitive to instances of sexism, racism, religious prejudice, dishonesty, suffering, or self-denigration, other people are almost numb to these evils (Blum 1994, 46–47). People are moral, in part, to the degree they have developed appropriate sensitivities to various regions of value. Robert Solomon points in the right direction when he writes: "Caring about the right things—one's friends and family, one's compatriots and neighbors, one's culture and environment, and, ultimately the world—is what defines rationality" (Solomon 1994, 297). Far from being antithetical to our moral life, our emotions are part of its very foundation.

Health professionals are people who care about the specific region of health values. Within this region, they will likely have greater concern for certain kinds of health values than others. One health professional may get excited about surgical breakthroughs, but be nearly indifferent not only to discoveries in, say, architecture, but also in dentistry or cardiac nursing care. She will have developed her care for surgical goods, much as a particular art critic develops a special interest in Rembrandt. As a consequence, where an internist sees medication as the best first step to curing an illness, the surgeon will be equally confident that outpatient surgery is the appropriate course of action.

This openness or sensitivity of professionals for their own special area of health values likely will itself wax and wane over time. Many professionals experience lesser and greater forms of burnout. They may no longer care very much about what they are doing, even if, technically, their skills in healing are greater than ever and even if, paradoxically, they still care about particular patients. A similar rhythm of enthusiasm and aridity pertains to all human experiences of value, including, for example, those related to teaching or praying. Arid periods serve either to deepen one's commitment to a region of value or to displace this region in favor of another region of concern.

Value Perception

The second aspect of emotional experience is the perception of particular values. Emotional experience is an affective perception of value qualities. Particular emotions bring to light particular forms of beauty or good. No one ever sees "color." Rather, we see this red apple and that orange sunset. Similarly, typically we don't just feel; rather, we feel the values of particular "objects." For example, different kinds of pleasure reveal that this apple is tasty, that chapel service is uplifting, this idea is just the solution we have been seeking, and so forth.

Cognitions   Emotions, generally, are cognitions of particular objects. (I leave aside the important class of emotions such as anxiety or awe that may have no particular object.) To have an emotion is to apprehend some object as, in some aspect or another, positively or negatively valuable. Through our emotions, we learn the good or bad, the beautiful or ugly, the harmful or helpful, the enlivening or deadening, the brilliant or dull, the holy or defiling, and so forth. Thus, on the one hand, if we want to learn "what" a thing is, we examine it with our intellect. If we want to discover the solution to a logical problem, we employ our deductive reasoning. On the other hand, if we want to learn the value or values of an event, person, relationship, and so on, we originally do that learning through our emotions (Lonergan 1972, 37). Often in the history of human experimentation, as Tom Beauchamp and James Childress point out, it has not been the "reasonable" scientist who has first protested abusive medical research; rather it has been "persons who were able to feel compassion, disgust, and outrage" (Beauchamp and Childress 1994, 89).

Whenever we do not have our own personal, emotional experience, we can still know objects as valuable in a second-hand way. Second-hand knowledge is not wrong knowledge. In fact, most of our knowledge—both intellectual and affective—in any area of life is largely second-hand, perhaps learned in school or on TV. Yet that knowledge is still true. But second-hand knowledge depends on someone's first-hand perception. When parents have an immediate experience of their newborn baby or of their injured daughter, their emotional experience teaches them human preciousness. They do not reason to this preciousness. But once they or others have had such an experience, then it can be generalized and communicated as second-hand knowledge. It may be formalized into propositions such as: "Persons are infinitely valuable" or "People have a right to basic health care." These propositions can then instruct and guide in other situations. Indeed, recognizing that almost all of us tend to block feelings correlative to the human dignity of strangers, we wisely turn our insight concerning the preciousness of those who are dear to us into laws that protect the dignity of every human being. In short, someone's first-hand, overriding emotional experience of human dignity precedes second-hand rules such as "Do no harm to other human beings, regardless of how you feel." Ethics fundamentally begins not with principles, but with affective experiences of value.

Basic emotions such as love or fear are not, as John Rawls and many other intellectualists suppose, second-order activities that occur only after we have already determined what is good or bad (Rawls 1971, 96; cf. de Sousa 1980 and Greenspan 1980). Rather, they are independent or concomitant first-order activities that disclose what is valuable. We are immediately frightened by a rattlesnake or by a bleeding wound. Our original fright has its own "rationality," that is, its own aptness to its object (de Sousa 1980, 128–29). If we are not afraid of what is dangerous, we fail to appreciate reality. Later, we may mentally judge that we are relatively safe because the snake is separated by a zoo window or the blood is part of routine surgery. Subsequently, we may barely be moved. But our initial encounter revealed a real danger.

In the midst of daily medical practice, we may not be able to feel much emotional movement. This should not be misinterpreted to imply that emotions are only momentary (Solomon 1994, 294). Many emotions have long-standing, "quiet" duration, for example, a fear of death, a love of friends, a passion for justice, and, importantly here, care about health values or compassion for the sick. Far from being momentary, some emotions, such as those behind racial prejudice, may be nearly ineradicable. Similarly, emotions such as a special sensitivity to sick children have a long life, becoming modified and deepened by each new patient. In other words, emotional knowledge, like intellectual knowledge, can be either short-term or long-term and either superficial or profound.

Finally, I should mention one other very important cognitive function of emotions. Through compassion, empathy, and the like, we also grasp what others are emotionally experiencing. We learn emotionally that they are happy or sad or distraught. This emotional co-knowing is very relevant to determining the sort of care that patients need from health professionals. Reason alone is insufficient (Beauchamp and Childress 1994, 89). Care, in this sense, includes within itself emotions such as distress at another's pain, compassion toward another's tragedy, or elation at another's successful recovery. Through this co-feeling, we come to know people not just as bodily beings but also as full human persons.

Diverse Emotions   We often have mixed or rapidly changing emotions because we commonly experience a multiplicity of values (Greenspan 1980). These values may conflict. For example, a colleague's surgical success in a difficult case may evoke both admiration and jealousy; it may make us proud to be a member of the same service, happy for the patient, and disappointed at being passed over in a major case. One task of reflection is to sort through these various emotions so that we can decide which ones we want to act on and which we want to let go. Each emotion, if not distorted or misdirected, reveals valuable or disvaluable features of the event. If, for example, we are disappointed because a patient got well under someone else's care, then this emotion is perverse and needs to be corrected, a point I will discuss below. If, however, our own disappointment points to our inadequacy in the eyes of others, then we may focus our attention on whether we have the requisite surgical abilities or on whether we are being unfairly evaluated.

Our emotions not only reveal values, they also help establish a hierarchy of values. We experience not only the preferability of positive values to negative; but we also experience among positive values gradations of more and less. Thus we feel the preferability not only of sense pleasure to pain or of interpersonal union to alienation, but also of intellectual brilliance to ordinary intelligence and of deep holiness to superficial piety. We feel satisfaction when we act as a good Samaritan, but we feel a certain emptiness or coldness when we needlessly pass by a bloodied man lying in the ditch. Thus, through diverse emotions we are in touch with an order of diverse values. As these examples indicate, our emotions range from bodily to highly spiritual, from the simplest of sense pleasures that we roughly share with other animals to the scientific delight and religious passion that distinguish us from those animals.

Our affections comprehend values not only as they are now, but also in their broader temporality. The past and the future are part of what our emotions limn. We affectively "feel" in the mangled arm not only present pain, but also some sort of horrible accident. Our affections toward our infant daughter open out into a future filled with smiles and laughter. At the other end of life, we may feel in our aging bodies not only that we are presently weary, but also that our lives have run out and will not be restored. Just as the mind can think things that do not actually exist, so too emotions can feel values that are only possible. We can emotionally feel what is at stake in imaginary or ideal situations. We are, for example, drawn toward perfect health of mind and body or toward a world at peace, even though such things do not, never have, and never will exist this side of the grave.

Our emotions not only point to values in the world about us. They may also reveal our own growth or decline in goodness. Thus, a morally sensitive physician may at some point grow uneasy with treating only wealthy patients. She may enjoy working with each rich patient, but her discomfort may suggest a conflict between who she is becoming and what she aspires to become. Her discomfort might point her toward taking on pro bono work in a poor neighborhood clinic because her exclusive practice is changing the physician in ways that are not good for her or not consistent with her religious commitments. Perhaps she is beginning to expect the privileges of the rich or perhaps she is growing insensitive to the poor. In brief, our emotions point not only to the value of objects (events, goals, people, etc.), but they also indicate to us who we are and who we are becoming.

Forms of Learning   As a form of cognition, we learn our emotions in ways similar to how we learn to think. Emotions are no more innate than thoughts. Emotions are also not a matter of insightless, behavioral training any more than thinking is simply a matter of thoughts drilled into us. We are by nature broadly predisposed to think and to feel, and we learn particular thoughts and emotions by interacting with particular objects.

We experience our emotions as social beings. Without social influence, we would be extraordinarily limited in the way that we relate to the world. Our emotional knowledge, no different from our intellectual knowledge, is socially formed. Still, our emotional knowing is not simply a matter of social convention. Our emotions are directed to the world as valuable; when correctly working, they objectively attain the values of the world. In other words, society, at its informative best, teaches us to feel what is really there. What we feel through our socially informed, emotional knowing really refers to the world.

The process of this emotional learning may take several forms. I begin with a contemplative mode. In order to appreciate adequately values such as the beauty of a particular painting we must let the canvas "speak" to us. We "drink in" the beauty of, say, Monet's water lily paintings. Such appreciation is not available to the person who approaches the world as a problem to be solved or who takes the attitude of an inquisitor, trying to uncover the secrets of the world. Rather, we must, so to speak, relax and allow ourselves to receive whatever values a particular object shows us. We may not know those values in advance. We open ourselves and wait. The religious experience of revelation from God often takes this form, as does an appreciation of the sacredness of a sleeping baby lying in a maternity bassinet. Thus it is not the case, as some hold, that truth and value are what one has after exhausting all the questions we might ask. Rather, truth and value are sometimes given only if we cease our interrogation.

Alternatively, we are educated emotionally when certain values grab our attention. For example, we are occupied with filling out a patient's chart, and then a raving, raging mental patient rushes in. For a moment, the chart and every other concern disappears. Or, for example, as we are going about our routine rounds, we see a patient dangling from her bed, throat tangled in IV lines; all our attention becomes concentrated on freeing her. This process is like the previous one in that it presupposes a general openness to a particular region of value. If we were insensitive to life-threatening rage or danger, no change would occur. It is also like the first process in that we are not seeking some value. But unlike the first process, we do not relax, clear our minds, and wait for a revelation. Rather the value, as it were, grabs our attention and, unless we are resistant, crowds out other concerns.

At still other times, we actively seek some value. We are attentive in a heightened way. For example, during diagnosis of a patient we look for symptoms that will confirm our suspicion of diabetes. The attentiveness can also be more general. Medical professionals are sensitized to notice a wide range of signs of illness, for example, jaundice, an unstable walk, or hesitancy in speech. Though we ordinarily describe this sensitivity as an intellectual skill, it is built upon an affective attentiveness to the abnormal in the area of health values. Granted, a diagnosis can at times be almost a purely intellectual exercise: the dermatology textbooks say that this kind of rash is caused by that kind of fungus and is cured by these kinds of ointments. Nevertheless, usually underlying even this intellectual activity are several affective responses. To be sure, the dermatologist may at the moment have no affective reaction, but she once did, and the present attentiveness draws on that past experience. Further, the intellectual knowledge the she draws on derives from previous patients who were bothered by this problem and by previous researchers who were intrigued enough by it to investigate.

Emotional Re-Education   Emotions can be corrected and further educated. Because emotions are a kind of cognition, they can be appropriate or inappropriate, and in varying degrees. Not infrequently, contemporary students say that emotions are neither true nor false, neither mature nor immature, neither right nor wrong. Consequently, they argue, emotions are not open to correction, development, or evaluation. But we rightly speak of "shallow love," "unjustified anger," "misplaced compassion," "excessive fear," or a "juvenile infatuation."

An emotion can be shallow or undeveloped in the sense of only slightly grasping its object. We often "appreciate" something only after, and sometimes long after, we first encounter it. For example, it takes a long time to understand affectively classical music or the marvels of biochemistry. Similarly, we can have a mature or immature "feel for" pastoral care or for children's reactions to needles. Again, as psychotherapy shows, often an interpretation or an intellectual insight into one's self lies inert until we are able to connect it with sufficient emotion (Kramer 1997, 220). Where these forms of immaturity occur, development of the emotions is needed.

As we mature, we become ever more morally responsible for our emotions (Laskey 1987, 308). Both psychological and moral maturity involve learning to deepen, differentiate, correct, and expand our emotions. As Lonergan insists, our "moral feelings have to be cultivated, enlightened, strengthened, refined, criticized and pruned of oddities" (Lonergan 1972, 38). We should, for example, learn to distinguish emotionally the "soar" in spirit that comes while singing a song of praise to God from the "rush" that comes while cheering at a football game. We should also learn to distinguish those feelings that are authentically ours from those that more or less automatically reproduce what others have taught us to feel. For example, a child, confused by the conflict between his parents' racism and his own positive experience of racially different classmates, will have to learn to trust his or her own affective perceptions.

Over time, our emotions should become more refined. Thus, our immediate compassion for people who have lost a spouse should become more complex with each new bereavement. Such refining "education" should be promoted in the classroom. As Lonergan remarks, "no small part of education lies in fostering and developing a climate of discernment and taste, of discriminating praise and carefully worked disapproval, that will conspire with the pupil's or student's own capacities and tendencies, enlarge and deepen his apprehension of values, and help him toward self-transcendence" (Lonergan 1972, 32; see also Nussbaum 1996, 39, 50–51).

Over time, our emotions should, where appropriate, also become more generalized. Thus, our anger at injustice done to ourselves should expand to an activist outrage at injustice done to the poor. But in other cases, we should learn to focus a diffuse emotion on its own proper object. Even our more basic or "primitive" emotions are subject to this focalizing education. We may initially fear all snakes, but over time we fear some less than others and some not at all. Thus, the process of education includes the development of our capacity not only for generalization but also for particularization.

Emotions must not only be developed and refined; they must also be corrected. Just as our senses of hot and cold can be deceived, and just as our intellect can make mistakes, so too our emotions can be disordered or mistaken, thereby missing what is really important or what is truly at stake. Some of us may be tempted to love our dog more than the neighbor's child. And all of us at times make the mistake of misidentifying the object of our emotion. For example, we might attribute the current dullness of our job to the work itself and not to our depression over a friend's death.

Again, just as a chain of "reasoning" or an analysis of the "facts" can go astray, so too an emotion can be irrational in the sense of "inappropriate" or untrue to its object. We may feel contempt for the drunken man on the emergency room gurney chiefly because he reminds us of our alcoholic father. Where these forms of irrationality occur, correction is the appropriate response. Correction, however, is not the same as disregarding. Just as we don't distrust all sense experience because our ice-cold hand feels cold water to be warm, and just as we don't deny all deductions because we added our bank account incorrectly, so too we need not and should not distrust all our emotions (Blum 1980b, 34). Rather, our task is to critique, reform, refine, or redirect our emotions.

Quite frequently our emotions need to be corrected not in the accuracy with which they intend one value, nor because there is disorder among our emotional evaluations, but in the way one set of emotions excludes emotional attention to other sets of values. If, for example, our attention is fixated on the political power of the patient who is lieutenant governor of the state, that attention might distract us from care-fully attending to her pregnancy. Here the first emotion is true to its "object," but it needs to be complemented and transcended by a more appropriate or requisite second set of emotions that refer to her pregnancy. Otherwise, we are being irrational because we miss what is most relevant to the present medical context (de Sousa 1980, 130–31). Morally and psychologically mature people are generally able to shift appropriately from one set of emotions to another set. Each authentic emotional experience, including a direct love for God, has its own proper time and place that must give way when other emotions become more appropriate.

Strategies for Education   In order to educate our emotions, we may use several strategies. We might learn certain emotions by opening ourselves to well-chosen images, such as those that good fiction or theater present to us (Cates 1998). In particular, we can open ourselves to stories of good and bad medical practice. Because emotions are perceptions, given the proper object the appropriate emotion may follow. For example, Christians read together scriptural texts that tend to evoke similar emotions, and they thereby promote shared valuations. Likewise, health personnel may educate one another and create a common ethical ethos when they share their own set of horror and hero stories.

A similar and especially powerful strategy is to compare and contrast our emotional experience with that of others. We usually are very attentive to the experience of those with whom we share communal life. Thus, teenagers learn to value in accord with valued friends. We also compare our experience with the experience of people who seem most affectively in touch with the world (Cates 1997, 217). As we saw above, through emotions such as empathy we can co-feel the emotions of others. In co-feeling their emotional responses, we learn what may be possible for ourselves. In brief, we can educate our emotions through our ability to feel what others feel. Their tears and laughter teach us what is sad and funny, as well as when and how to respond. The deeper our love for others, the more likely we will learn through their emotional perceptions.

We may also use our intellect and imagination to bring a past emotional experience to bear on a present one. For example, most of us likely have fallen in love with another person, say, with an exciting and witty teacher. In loving her, we may have discovered not only how unique a person she is, but also how precious personhood itself is. Then, suppose we meet another teacher who is not so stirring. Indeed, he is a dullard. We definitely are not attracted to him. Still, through our intellect we understand that he, too, is a person. That may lead us to the inference that he, too, is precious, not in the unique way that she is, but precious as a person nonetheless. It can then happen, especially if we apply our imagination, that we come also to appreciate him affectively both for the quality of his personhood and for elements of his unique self.

We can also alter our emotions by changing beliefs that either prevent an emotion from arising or evoke inappropriate emotions. As Paul Lauritzen writes, "If emotions are understood to involve a complex web of moral, scientific, and aesthetic beliefs, then a change in these beliefs has the potential for changing our emotions" (Lauritzen 1992, 60). We might initially feel ill at ease both with arterial bleeding and with menstrual bleeding; but with further experience, reflection, and instruction (e.g., we learn that menstruation is a normal activity of a healthy woman's body), we recognize a difference in their meaning and value. New thoughts lay the basis for altering old emotions. Most if not all emotions depend on several beliefs. To be angry because my car has been stolen is a very complex activity that presupposes a world with automobiles, the institution of private property, my history with this red Porsche, an attitude toward theft, and so forth. Changing those presuppositions likely will alter the emotion.

Lastly, we can and should pay careful attention to the exact correlation between our emotion and the value it "intends." Quite frequently, we make emotional mistakes through associational learning. For example, we dislike a current patient because of a bad past encounter with a similar person. Or we transmute our distaste for the patient's physical ugliness into a dislike for the person as a whole. By paying careful attention to our emotions and their proper objects, we can not only overcome mistaken associational leaps, but also further refine our emotional acuity.

It is not only through thought or reflection that we modify our emotions. Our emotional life has its own developmental tendencies (Lonergan 1972, 32–33). As adults we ordinarily should have grown to respond emotionally not only to the obvious but also to the more complex needs and qualities of others. Further, our openness should also have expanded to include people who bear no special connection with us. This development of our emotions is a natural tendency that does not need to be argued to or forced, but rather to be consented to and fostered. As we mature, we normally deepen, expand, and correct our loves and hates by loving and hating.

Emotional development is essential to moral growth. In particular, over time, the emotions of care should become modes of our being, that is, of the way we relate to the world. Over time we should become the sorts of persons who are disposed to notice and then respond easily and often without much deliberation to others who are in need or who may benefit from our help or interest. When this happens, we experience a certain pleasure or satisfaction in being solicitous, even when this involves us in another's pain. As we grow in the emotions of care, we become "wholeheartedly convinced that this is the best way to be" (Cates 1997, 187–88). In spite of any increased suffering due to sharing in another's troubles, we would not want to be any other way than sensitive and solicitous.

Being Affected

The third aspect of an emotion is its effect on our selves. When we have an emotion, we not only attend to something as good or bad, but we also are affected by what we perceive. The etymological meaning of "passion" suggests that we are moved or changed. Receptivity is an essential feature of the emotions of care (Cates 1997, 134; Noddings 1984, 30–31). We let go of our detached and objectivizing self, and we ourselves become modified.

This third aspect is highlighted by certain common questions such as, "How does that make you feel?" or "How do you feel about this?" Paradoxically, our answer to such questions provides an evaluation of an external event by talking about ourselves. We say we are "not comfortable with" removing a feeding tube or that we are at peace with writing a DNR order. These statements about ourselves are the subjective correlates of our objective evaluation.

Such experiences as "being comfortable with" or "feeling good about" indicate concord or discord with our already established patterns of evaluation. A feeling of discord may indicate that our morally sound patterns of evaluation are rejecting involvement in a particular practice. Discord may also arise when an appropriate emotional change in our self conflicts with a previously distorted pattern of emotional apprehension, thereby providing an occasion of corrective growth. Similarly, a feeling of concord may indicate that our morally good character agrees with an affective perception of a particular object. Or it may be the result of a blind repetition of old affective patterns in a new situation.

Participatory Identification   Through emotion, we are changed in various ways. If our emotions perceive something bad, we are inclined either away from or against it. That is, we are inclined either to flee or to fight. If our emotions perceive something good, we are inclined either to go toward it or to hold on to it. That is, we are inclined either to pursue or to possess it.

These changes occur through our capacity for participation. We at least momentarily identify with and share in the good we perceive. Thus, going to an art museum lifts our spirit; witnessing a generous gesture expands our heart; and being with lively people enlivens us. We also, again at least momentarily, partake of the evil we emotionally perceive. Encountering a sick child upsets us and makes us feel ill at ease; uncovering open sores, for a brief moment, makes us feel wounded; interacting with a mentally delirious patient tends to throw us off our stride. In a word, through identification we share in good and evil.

Participative identification is a unity-in-difference. Both aspects are necessary. On the one hand, there is the experience that Cates describes of watching her daughter skin a knee: "For a moment there, I was so much a part of her . . . that we seemingly ceased to be separate selves!" She adds, "my experience is not that I am a separate person who uses my imagination to bridge the gap between my own and another separate person's experience. My experience is that we are one extended self, skinning our knees together. There is no distance between us to overcome" (Cates 1997, 140, 99–100). Experientially, we are in an emotionally undistinguished unity with the other. That is, we have gone over to the other; we have become at one with the other. Or, as sometimes happens, we experience that the other has "come over" to share in the experience we are having. Thus we can at least momentarily feel (something akin to) the pleasure or pain that another feels and, at other times, we become aware that they have done the same with us.

On the other hand, this participative identification is distinct from the loss of identity that occurs when we lose all sense of difference of ourselves from what we perceive. Cates' reflection on unity should be held in tension with what Martha Nussbaum writes on difference: "even then, in the temporary act of identification, one is always aware of one's own *separateness* from the sufferer—it is for *another*, and not oneself, that one feels; and one is aware both of the bad lot of the sufferer and of the fact that it is, right now, not one's own" (Nussbaum 1996, 35). Joining these two views, we can with Nel Noddings say: "The one-caring assumes a dual perspective and can see things from both her own pole and that of the cared-for" (Noddings 1984, 63; see also Cates 1997, 135). Both unity and difference are experienced, though in the moment we are not distinguishing. Subsequently, we sort out what belongs to a subjective pole and what to an objective pole.

Participative identification is not the same as remembering that we once had the "same" or a similar experience. Usually, of course, we fill out an act of participative identification by imagining what it was like or would be like for us to experience a similar loss (Reeder 1998, 49–51). This process of embellishment frequently is very helpful, but it is not necessary. We can share another's experience even if we never have had and never will have that experience (Blum 1994, 192–95).[3] An elderly, unmarried man can at least somewhat understand affectively what it is like for a friend to give birth to a still-born child. In other words, our affective understanding of others is not just a matter of recalling or imagining our own experience and then projecting it out on others. We are not limited to understanding only our own private past or possible future experiences. Capable of affective self-transcendence, we are not bound within the confines of our own skin. That is, we can to greater and lesser degrees really share in and understand the experience of others in its otherness. Put correlatively and negatively, an inability to participate affectively in the experience of others *as* other indicates a defect in our own character (Blum 1980a, 509–10).

Usually we do little more than momentarily identify with others; then we get on with our own projects. When, however, we allow the emotion to develop into full-fledged sharing in their feelings, we unite more fully with whatever they are experiencing. In other words, care begins with momentary participative identification, but then it can persist and develop further so that, to greater and lesser degrees, we share in others' weal or woe. We become different because of what they experience.

Subjectivism   There are two common mistakes to avoid in discussing emotion's third aspect of being-affected. The first is to reduce emotions simply to a change in ourselves, denying both the first aspect of an emotional openness to regions of value and the second aspect of our emotional perceptivity of particular values. Thus, it is a mistake to reduce emotions to the tingle down the spine or the flushed face we feel. Emotions are not simply bodily changes. It is also a mistake to understand emotions as merely psychological phenomena going on inside us. To be sure, the uplift we feel before the tabernacle and the helplessness we feel before an intractable cancer are important subjective acts, but they are also "intentional." That is, they refer to something beyond themselves. Just as my idea of my mother standing before me really refers to her and is not just brain or mental activity, so too my emotions really refer to objects beyond themselves. At their highest, our emotions have the same sort of spiritual self-transcendence as our intellect. As Noddings writes, "Caring involves stepping out of one's own personal frame of reference into the other's. When we care, we consider the other's point of view, his objective needs, and what he expects of us. Our attention, our mental engrossment is on the cared-for, not on ourselves" (Noddings 1984, 24).

A second and correlative mistake is to understand the word "value" as referring primarily to our choices and not to the world about us. People sometimes speak of values in a subjectivistic way. Value, they say, has no objectivity, but is simply something we "put on" or "place on" or "give to" an object. Values, they suppose, are not discovered by us; rather, for them, the term "our values" means whatever we choose to value (Lauritzen 1992, 38). In these misunderstandings, emotions are sometimes thought to be an independent source of value. For example, something is thought to be offensive because we are angry; it is not considered that we are angry because something offends. Or, again, a newborn is thought to be precious if a mother cherishes it or can't bear to live without it; it is not understood that mothers cherish their babes and are moved to hold them because they are so precious.

We do, at times, arbitrarily attribute value when we feel affective movement in ourselves. Valuing is a socially influenced process and can be more a matter of social construction than objective reality. Consider, for example, the supreme importance to children of getting this year's "must-have Christmas toy." We also misvalue when we are not careful about the "intentionality" of our emotions. For example, we get angry at the night nurse when we are really angry at ourselves for an error that we have made. But each of these is a subjectivistic mistake. When we become aware that our attachments or attributions of blame are disordered or wrong, we should correct ourselves. The fact that we can recognize mistakes implies that there is a correct intentionality of our emotions.

The danger of "subjectivism," however, should not be taken as an invitation to "objectivism." That is, we should not suppose that human beings can affirm the objectivity of values apart from someone's first-hand affective appreciation of them. Put simply, we don't know objects apart from knowing them, and we don't appreciate the value of objects apart from feeling them. This idea is often overlooked by those who reject the relativism of subjectivism. They speak as if values are known apart from our own socially influenced, affective appreciation.

Values are objectively good in either of two ways. First, commonly, they are good in relation to some being, typically our own self, who is helped by them. Second, they are good in themselves. Thus, on the one hand, a carrot is good or bad relative to our need for nourishment, and people are good relative to our need for companionship. On the other hand, values may be called "absolute" in the sense of "good in themselves." For example, telling the truth is good apart from consequences, and human dignity is precious quite apart from any social contribution.

Mode of Response

The fourth aspect of a full emotional experience is our response. We consent to or dissent from the emotional process, adding our Yes or our No to what we have been experiencing. Consider a parallel. When doing specifically intellectual work, we usually affirm a conclusion that has come about through our reasoning. But we can hold in abeyance our affirmation of the conclusion, and we may even refuse assent if the conclusion does not intuitively feel right. So, too, we can affirm or hold in abeyance or resist our emotional perceptions and the way they affect us. We can even affirm, bracket, or resist the development of our first and more basic openness to regions of value. Noddings, for example, encourages us to foster a "readiness to try to care for whoever crosses our path" (Noddings 1984, 18). Others discourage this readiness, for example, through using the term "bleeding hearts" as an accusation. In short, we have some freedom to modify the four aspects of an emotion.

Emotions as Motives   As we have seen, to be affected means to be inclined to flee, to oppose, to pursue, or to abide with a value. When we consent to one of these ways of being affected, we may then allow it to function as a "motive" for action. We act out of love, out of anger, out of fear, and so forth. Pure judgments of reason are not sufficient for action. We might judge intellectually that some evil is present, yet do nothing (Solomon 1994, 292). Bare determination of our will usually is not sufficient. True, we can will ourselves to perform most actions even when we feel nothing or feel only aversion. But aversion is incomplete human action that rarely perdures. Moreover, such willing usually draws its energy from other emotions, such as fear of punishment or longing for approval.

We need the energizing power of the emotions to make or retain changes in ourselves, in our relationships, and in our world (Scheler 1973, 131). We need a passion for justice and for righting what is wrong. If we don't care, no amount of getting our principles right or making proper deductions suffices to move us into action on behalf of a morally good world. If we don't care, sheer willing of what is not also felt to be good does not endure. At the very least, we must have an affection such as a Kantian "respect for duty." But this particular affection is far too thin to account for most of our moral actions, and indeed it is not central to our ordinary moral experience (Blum 1980b, 118–19).

The etymology of "emotion" suggests that emotions incline or move us to act. Many times when we act, we do not cite the emotion as our reason for acting, for example, out of compassion. Instead, but we name the value or disvalue the emotion points to. We say that we acted because the patient was vomiting or was in pain. Both ways of speaking are intelligible as "reasons." We can say either that we acted out of concern or that we acted because the patient was sick. Whenever emotions are held in suspicion or thought to have merely private significance, then the only acceptable "reasons" to give for our action are the object's values that these emotions point to. But where emotions are themselves the focus, as in psychological contexts, often it is acceptable to name only the emotions themselves. For example, we say we feel comfortable with a decision or that a decision "feels right." In psychological therapy it is not enough to say that another's nasty remark is the "reason" for our outburst. Rather, we must also admit our own anger and search for some underlying and perhaps neurotic sensitivity to such remarks. Some psychologically oriented people are distrustful of any claim about objective values. They accept only emotions as "reasons" for action. In subjectivistic fashion, they hold that the other person's nasty remark has only the value we give it. If we have become irate, that is wholly "our issue." On the other hand, in objectivistic fashion, where emotions are denied their relevance, the other's remark is the only thing that can count as a reason. In a courtroom, for example, the judge claims to punish offenders for their misdeeds, not because he or she is annoyed or perturbed by their behavior. In fact, however, emotional perception and value perceived are correlative; hence, we may name either as reason for action. We must be careful, however, because reasons that name emotion are open to subjectivism and reasons that name objective value are open to objectivism.

Emotions do not automatically cause us to act. We can have an emotion and do nothing. We may be emotionally moved, but then we can bracket the inclination to any action that the emotion prompts. Most of us are, I suppose, moved when we read in the newspaper of a famine in the Sudan; many of us then think ourselves compassionate because we can feel the plight of the unfortunate; but for only a few of us does this compassionate response turn into action (Solomon 1994, 301). As a consequence, our feeling of compassion may feed the self-deception that, because we were so moved and "care" so much, we are actively involved on behalf of the poor. Similarly, the expression, "There but for the grace of God go I" can be a humble act of sympathy and of divine praise, but it can also be a cover for self-righteous inaction as we congratulate ourselves for being so good that we avoid the evil that besets others (Solomon 1998, 517, 523).

Self-deception is not the only reason we do not act on our emotions. We simply cannot act on all the emotions we experience. In fact, an impulsive person is one who exhibits an inappropriately small gap between the onset of an emotion and subsequent action. Most of us, for example, properly take with a grain of salt all the emotional appeals that come our way through advertising. Further, there are many other reasons for not acting on our emotions. Real obstacles often stand in the way of realizing particular inclinations. Then the obstacles themselves may become objects of our emotions; for example, we are happy that we don't have to do anything because we can't. When this happens, we must sort through these conflicting emotions and what they reveal as goods-to-be-achieved and difficulties-to-be-overcome or drawbacks-to-be-accepted before we decide to walk one path and not another.

Qualifying Emotions   Emotions not only motivate, but also qualify our acting. As we have seen, it is possible for someone to be beneficent without care-as-benevolence or care-as-affection, but this is incomplete human action (Beauchamp and Childress 1994, 89). If the attending pediatrician is incapable of feeling a mother's loss of her child, he or she might be credited with having done all the appropriate medical procedures, but he should be judged to be an incomplete human being and physician.

Moreover, emotions are often essential to the very meaning of what we are doing. For example, we cannot be coldly or reluctantly generous; to be generous we must give gladly and with desire. Similarly, a chaplain who visits a patient simply out of duty does a different act from one who visits because she cares. Part of the very meaning of the second chaplain's visit is to express concern and thereby to boost the patient's spirits (Noddings 1984, 59). Accordingly, care is part of the very meaning of her act (Blum 1980b, 144–46). If a third chaplain visits out of an aggressive love for winning converts, he likely victimizes patients rather than offering them God's care. In other words, as Lawrence Blum notes, "the emotion itself is often part of what makes the act the morally right or appropriate one in a given situation" (Blum 1980b, 142).

Accordingly, the emotions of care are usually very important to the recipient of health care. All of us want to make a difference in another person's life. We don't want to be the object of emotional indifference, even if care-as-benefit is just what our bodies need. When, as a patient, we make a difference to our care givers, we know that we do not suffer alone, and we know that we are valuable.

Emotions may be integral to the very manner of giving health care. Beauchamp and Childress well observe, "it is not only important what the physician does ... but also how actions are performed" (Beauchamp and Childress 1994, 85–86; see also Carse 1996, 92). A surgeon might be truly sad about the loss of a patient on the operating table, but if he communicates the bad news to the family with a smile, he fails in communication (Beauchamp and Childress 1994, 467). A gynecologist who goes about a pelvic exam in a cold, uncaring manner can do harm, no matter how accurate his medical diagnosis. By contrast, Noddings observes of the one who cares: "If she tends the sick her hands are gentle with the anticipation of pain and discomfort. . . . She feels the excitement, pain, terror, or embarrassment of the other and commits herself to act accordingly" (Noddings 1984, 59).

Lastly, emotions affect which medical benefits will be offered. As we have seen, a caring professional will act carefully, that is, with attention to all that is relevant (Cates 1998, 412). The emotionally sensitive nurse is far more likely to observe and take care of the hospital patient than an equally well-trained but uncaring nurse. Without the appropriate emotions, care givers are less likely to notice either the physical or the psychological condition of their patient. Thus, they may fail to give the appropriate treatment.

Emotions and Freedom   Many ethicists mistakenly hold that we have no freedom in regard to our emotions and that thus our emotional life is outside of the sphere of morality. To the contrary, I have claimed that we have some freedom in cultivating particular desirable emotions and in correcting errant emotions. We also have some freedom in restraining or bracketing emotions that are accurate but lead us in directions we do not want to go. Thus our anger at a particularly uncooperative patient may be justified, but we can still decide not to let anger dominate our affections, and we can decide to treat him well out of respect for his dignity.

Admittedly, we do not have complete control over our emotions. We also do not have complete control over our thoughts or even over our own will. We cannot simply decide faultlessly to solve a complex mathematics problem. We cannot simply decide to will only the good, as the Christian doctrine of sin constantly reminds us. Similarly, we are not free to feel anger at what is innocently fun, and sometimes we cannot even feel the humor in a good joke. But we have enough freedom to cultivate our emotional life in a variety of ways, and we should do so. Fernando Flores and Robert Solomon rightly propose a " 'cultivation thesis' [that] attempts to develop a middle ground ... insisting that we are responsible for our emotions but, nevertheless, they cannot be understood as 'willed.' ... Indeed, the realm of the mental has too long been forcefully partitioned by a philosophical 'green line' between straightforwardly 'willable' deliberate intentional actions and purely victim-status passive experiences" (Flores and Solomon 1998, 227).

We can help in the genesis of particular emotions. To be sure, emotions ordinarily have a spontaneous quality. We cannot simply choose to have a particular emotion. For example, if, without further impetus, a man decides to be sympathetic, his concern likely will both be and appear to be forced and hardly heartfelt; in other words, it won't be sympathetic. Still, just as we human beings have an innate capacity to begin thinking, so we have a capacity to feel. Given the right object, as the text from Mencius cited earlier indicates, the appropriate emotion likely will follow. Thus, as we have seen, one strategy for generating emotions is willfully to present ourselves with objects of value and then freely foster the emotions that may arise. Over the course of our lives we should expose ourselves to a rich array of different kinds of objects. We can and should freely encourage the emotions that then occur, as long as they are appropriate both to these objects and to the course of our lives.

In addition to the limited freedom we have in the genesis of emotions, we also have some freedom to affirm or deny their development. It is a common mistake to imagine that emotions are inner forces that have an independent life of their own, controlling us but unable to be controlled by us. Again, it is sometimes said that an emotion will, if stifled and not expressed, necessarily pop out uncontrollably at another moment. This mistake imagines that emotions are forces or fluids obeying the laws of physics. Solomon calls this approach the hydraulic theory of emotion. Simple reflection, as well as sophisticated research, has demonstrated its falsity. In extreme form, this sort of mistake leads to the claim that all emotions are "irrational" forces (Blum 1980b, 125). Rather, we have the freedom to bracket, reject, or confirm the development of an emotion. We can dissociate ourselves from our emotions, in effect saying, "This is what I am feeling, but this is not how I want to be" (Blum 1980b, 181–82). We can resist our emotions, saying, "I feel this, but I will do what I can to change my feeling this way." We can consent to what we are feeling, saying, "This is the very feeling I want to feel."

We can also expand a particular kind of feeling, looking for ways that will extend its range of objects or that will increase its depth and subtlety. Emotions are not restricted to material objects. They extend to groups and spiritual objects. Further, if we reflect on emotions such as racial prejudice or hatred, we can readily see that emotions generalize themselves. As Solomon points out, "It is not reason (as opposed to emotion) that allows us to extend our reach to the universal, but rather the expansive scope of the emotions themselves" (Solomon 1994, 297). We also can freely promote greater depth of our emotions, for example, from a superficial love to a profound love or from a passing anger to a pervasive anger. We can become ever more supple and subtle in our emotions. An undifferentiated "I want to help people" can become a free desire to care for Jack and Jill, and for each in an appropriately different way. At a more profound level, we can consent to the very way we are becoming when we have a particular feeling, saying, "I want to be an angry (or loving, etc.) person."

Character Formation   Our emotions are not valuable simply because they are motives for action or because they qualify our actions. The emotions involved in care are also valuable in themselves (Blum 1980b, 153–57). They help constitute our humanity. Through caring we fulfill our nature as relational, valuing, self-transcending beings able to be involved with others. Even if there is no external act that we can do for patients, it is still a basic human good to feel care for them (Noddings 1984, 49). In short, in order to flourish as human beings we must care. To be caring is a central part of what it means to have a morally good character.

Speaking more broadly, the development of an *ordo amoris*, of an appropriate set of emotions, is constitutive of our moral life. Particular affections, when freely consented to, gradually (or sometimes suddenly as in a "first experience" or in a traumatic situation) become character traits. For example, fostering an emotional reaction to the poverty of others can gradually expand our sensitivity and become a passion for justice. Through our freedom we can habituate a series of emotional acts into an affective virtue that is part of our character. As Cates writes, "whether or not we are habitually disposed toward passionate perception ... depends on whether or not we want to be the sorts of persons who are deeply, complexly, and sometimes painfully affected by others in our moral encounters with them" (Cates 1997, 10).

Our character-building freedom is especially apparent when we experience "mixed emotions." In fact, every situation potentially presents us with many different values and thus with the possibility of many different emotions. In making a decision, we follow one set of emotions and often must set aside another set. There are, by contrast, necessary interconnections among certain emotion-based virtues. We need not despise the second (or third or fourth) set of emotions; we simply decline to act out of those emotions. In other words, we may honor each emotion as a correct value-perception, yet we may act on only one emotion and in favor of its correlative value. In so doing, we affirm that we want our character to remain attuned to a great variety of values, even when we can realize in practice only one set. For example, courage and self-sacrificial altruism are not possible if we do not also feel the goodness of our own selves. If we hate ourselves we will not experience danger as a threat to our own good and thus cannot be courageous; similarly if we hate ourselves, we do not give up any great good in giving ourselves. Thus, courage or self-sacrifice requires self-love, even though courageous or self-sacrificial actions may harm the self. In short, our freedom allows us both to honor the truth of all our emotional sets as well as to act in accord with only one or other among them (Greenspan 1980, 238–44).

A moral analysis that looked only to the actions we perform would fail to note how our character can remain richly diversified even as it focuses on particular tasks. Indeed, it is possible genuinely to value certain activities even though we never perform them. We might always have more important matters to attend to. For example, we can value dentistry even when we are a podiatrist; and we can value pro bono work even when we are too worried about our own family's welfare to help the poor. It should be obvious that the possibilities for self-deception in this regard are large. But the absence of action does not mean we have a morally deficient character. Indeed, one aspect of a strong character is its ability to deny one desire when that desire conflicts with another more important or more pressing desire.

We have not only the freedom to realize good, we can also bring about evil. When we freely consent to emotional identification with evil, we likely will experience some debilitation. Free participation in evil will weaken our character if, as is likely, it eviscerates our normal, contrasting sense of beauty, goodness, healthiness, holiness, and so forth. Still, emotional experiences of evil need not harm our character. Because we are free and have the power of self-transcendence, we can usually turn any encounter with evil into some good. For example, we may momentarily be disturbed by encountering the derangement of a psychiatric inmate, but we can turn this emotional upset into compassion for the patient and then into a desire to bring about some relief for that patient. In the face of someone's illness, we have the freedom to shift from "I must protect myself" to "I am strong enough to do something for the other" (Noddings 1984, 81). In so doing we develop our character. We become good persons.

This virtuous character, however, should normally be developed out of the corner of our eye, so to speak. When we care for another, the other is the focus of our attention, not ourselves. In caring for another, we are concerned not for our own development of virtue, but with the other's well-being. Other-love should not be reduced, as is so often done, to an act of prudential self-love. Steven Hendley rightly observes that "it does not, therefore, appear descriptively adequate to characterize care for the other as merely an extension of my care for myself. It is, rather, a matter of being called to attend to the needs of the other in their own right" (Hendley 1996, 512–14).

EMOTIONS AND PROFESSIONALISM

If it is true that emotions are essential to the moral practice of medicine, what are we to make of the common claim that emotions interfere with medical practice? We hear stories praising the professional who, rather than getting emotional, remains cool and calm as the key to doing what needs to be done. On the other hand, we hear stories of people who get so emotionally involved in their work that they suffer "burnout." And we read some feminists who claim that the emotions of care lead to excessive self-sacrifice (Carse 1996, 104).

To the contrary, I have argued that the emotions involved in care, like all emotions, help us to see and do what needs to be done. They are acts of evaluation and participation. As a consequence, emotions should make us more, rather than less effectively attentive to patients' needs. It is a mistake to think that the "cool, calm, competent professional" lacks emotion. A lack of emotion in the value-rich medical context would border on the pathological. Rather, the emotions of such a professional likely are very focused on the deed that needs to be done (Cates 1997, 196). Emotional focus or control is not the absence of emotions.

What about "burnout" or "over-involvement"? We should not succumb to the stereotype of emotion as a state of being out of control. Basic emotions such as love for medicine or peace with our vocation can and should give us a sense of direction, as well as the stability to deal with medical problems and crises (Lonergan 1972, 32–33). Furthermore, compassion and other emotions of care should give us the strength to persist in the pursuit of health values (Blum 1980a, 512–15). These are not emotions that are the source of the problem of burnout. We never really "love too much," but only love the wrong things or love in an unbalanced or disordered way.

To be sure, emotions can interfere with our professional lives. If we lose "control" of our emotions, we thereby add stress to an already complicated life. Because emotions contain an aspect of being affected, we can be so strongly affected that we are unable to act. We can become overly involved, to the exclusion of other balancing emotions. For example, the oncology nurse who has few outside sources of "life" will be prone to burnout because, as we have seen, his emotional identification does, at least momentarily, unite him with the disvalues of his patients' disease, dying, and death (Beauchamp and Childress 1994, 467). Or the oncology nurse might so focus on "failures" that he cannot see the good done in offering comfort measures to all patients and, additionally, in providing cures for some. Or burnout may occur when the nurse affectively experiences things that diminish his own sense of self-worth, such as dismissive doctors, overly demanding supervisors, or abusive patients. Again, the nurse may have allowed himself to slip into unfulfilling activities, for example, winning the pyrrhic victory of water-cooler gossip. As a last example, he may be full of unresolved, conflicting emotions, such as when racial prejudice clashes with a desire to help all people in need.

We need not, however, be controlled by our emotions. Some emotions, such as anger over an insult, have a tendency to grab hold of consciousness like a pitbull terrier. Such emotions tend to dominate consciousness, thereby excluding other emotions that may be appropriate and necessary in a particular medical context. Still, we have at least some freedom vis à vis even these tenacious emotions. Usually, we can modify our emotions through various mental moves such as thinking of different objects or considering an object under a different formality, for example, we reconsider the rich, tempting dessert as the source of a future heart attack. Similarly, we can set aside our over-involvement in one patient's illness and replace it with care for another patient who needs our prompt attention. Just as scientists who are not able to consider evidence contrary to their pet theory fail an intellectual challenge, so health professionals who are unable to make the transition from one kind of emotional involvement to another fail in their professional responsibilities.

Health care professionals should be able to retain the emotional flexibility to respond to an ever-changing reality within the medical context, but also outside that context. All human beings have this requisite ability some of the time; a mark of moral perfection is the ability to remain flexible most of the time. Without denying or suppressing one emotion, such as grief over the death of a patient, a doctor should be able to leave the hospital looking forward to her own children. Her sense of loss may continue, but it need not exclude other emotions.

In brief, professionals need to practice emotional hygiene. They should do so not solely for the sake of being able properly to care for others, but also as a form of self-care. All human beings need a healthy rhythm of different emotion-laden activities, from raising children to sports activities. Health care professionals should enjoy life not only in their work, but also beyond their work.

One last worry deserves comment. Feminists quite regularly warn against the dangers to women of the practice of self-sacrifice (Andolsen 1996, 356; Beauchamp and Childress 1994, 91). They fear that women in medicine will lose themselves if they get emotionally involved with caring for people in great need. Although such warnings were and are in order, they should not be taken to exclude affective care in medicine, for at least two reasons. First, as Solomon notes, "Caring about others is not necessarily putting their interests before one's own much less sacrificing oneself on their behalf" (Solomon 1998, 527). Rather, as social beings, our care often unites us with others in a way that enriches us. Although self-sacrifice cannot be a focal object of self-care, such sacrifices often do, paradoxically, achieve the ultimate goals of self-care. There is evidence—which should not be surprising to Christians—that professionals who selflessly care for their patients achieve the greatest fulfillment (Scudder and Bishop 1986, 149). Still, in order for self-sacrificial activities to redound to the good of the care taker, it is usually necessary that the care taker have already developed a rather strong sense of self-love, so that the giving flows from an already rich self. Those who sacrifice generously are often, although not always, those who grow the most as persons.

Second, history hails as heroes and heroines many who have sacrificed themselves greatly for others. In fact, it would be a rare hero or saint who did not make great acts of self-sacrifice. Christianity is, for example, founded on a man who gave his life for others. His self-sacrificing greatness continues in Christian saints, some of whom have been lustrous stars in world history.

Thus, genuine self-sacrifice out of care for others is, at times, not only acceptable but also praiseworthy or even mandatory. Indeed, in cases of epidemics such as the AIDS crisis, society often criticizes health professionals who abandon their patients out of fear for themselves.

BROADER SPHERES OF CARE

Patients have overlapping memberships in various groups. So do professionals. These groups also elicit and deserve affective care. Thus, professionals should care for more than just individuals. Professionals do worry about the practice of medicine in their hospital, city, country, and world. They know how deeply various cultural, economic, and religious forces influence the health of patients, as well as their own practice of medicine. Hence, they should be affectively concerned about the groups that influence these forces, wanting to promote their good qualities and diminish their failings.

An individualist ideology, of course, denies that groups exist. Though this position is false, I need not here claim that groups have a metaphysical status. Rather, I point only to the common experience that we do develop emotional relationships with groups. We admire the work of a particular hospital; we get disappointed when scandal hurts our alma mater; we feel tarnished when a fellow psychiatrist is convicted of sexual abuse. In short, professionals and their clients belong to groups that affect the practice of medicine, and professionals should care about such groups.

Patients and professionals are related not only to one another and not only to a variety of groups. By God's grace they are related to God and interrelated among themselves in God (Vacek 1996). This supreme relationship and these religiously dependent relationships evoke and deserve our affections of care. The Christian life is first and foremost a relationship with God. Having been touched by the God of life and love, we want to become more involved with this God. Forming something of a partnership or covenant with this God, we want to do our part to uphold and develop that partnership (Vacek 1994, 133–40). We also want to become involved in the activity of God, wherever this is possible. We especially desire to contribute our distinctive talents to this enterprise.

As God desires not only the salvation of souls but also, as is evident in Jesus' ministry, the salvation of bodies and psyches, Christians will want to assist in God's work of healing. Health care professionals contribute directly to this saving work. Indeed, whether by God's choice or by metaphysical necessity, healing bodies and psyches (ordinarily) occurs only through a human contribution. In other words, God does God's work through humans. Thus, because of the covenant Christians have with God, this work is not theirs alone, but also God's.

A direct relationship with God is manifest in worship and prayer, and care for human beings should never replace this direct relationship. God is not humanity, but the creator and redeemer of humanity; and so care for humanity is not a substitute for our care for God. Nonetheless, our God is not simply transcendent to creation. God is also with us, healing and uplifting us. Christians rightly praise God whenever and wherever the blind see and the lame walk again. However much such healing events are humanly mediated, in them God's own healing activity is realized. In Jesus' healing miracles, the reign of God was at hand. His ministry of healing continues in the work of his disciples down the ages. In our care for healing and health, the reign of God is still at hand.

Endnotes

1 I have worked these three out in greater detail and nuance in Vacek 1994.

2 For some of the dangers of a purely agapic view of the moral life, see Davenport 1998.

3 Hence I disagree with the portrait given in Nussbaum 1996, 34–36, 48. Nussbaum insists on similar possibilities as a necessary condition for compassion.

References

Andolsen, Barbara Hilkert. 1996. Elements of a Feminist Approach to Bioethics. In *Feminist Ethics and the Catholic Moral Tradition: Readings in Moral Theology*, no 9, ed. Charles Curran, Richard McCormick, and Margaret Farley, 341–82. New York: Paulist Press.

Beauchamp, Tom, and James Childress. 1994. *Principles of Biomedical Ethics*, 4th ed. New York: Oxford University Press.

Blum, Lawrence. 1980a. Compassion. In *Explaining Emotions*, ed. Amélie Oksenberg Rorty, 507–18. Berkeley: University of California Press.

———. 1980b. *Friendship, Altruism and Morality*. Boston: Routledge & Kegan Paul.

———. 1994. *Moral Perception and Particularity*. New York: Cambridge University Press.

Carse, Alisa. 1996. Facing Up to Moral Perils: The Virtues of Care in Bioethics. In *Caregiving*, ed. Suzanne Gordon, Patricia Benner, and Nel Noddings, 83–110. Philadelphia: University of Pennsylvania Press.

Cates, Diana Fritz. 1997. *Choosing to Feel*. Notre Dame, Ind.: University of Notre Dame Press.

————. 1998. Ethics, Literature, and the Emotional Dimension of Moral Understanding. *Journal of Religious Ethics* 26/2 (fall): 409–31.

Davenport, John. 1998. Levinas's Agapeistic Metaphysics of Morals: Absolute Pas-
sivity and the Other as Eschatological Hierophany. *Journal of Religious Ethics*
26/2 (fall): 331–66.

de Sousa, Ronald. 1980. The Rationality of Emotions. In *Explaining Emotions*,
ed. Amélie Oksenberg Rorty, 127–52. Berkeley: University of California
Press.

Doorley, Mark. 1996. *Place of the Heart in Lonergan's Ethics*. New York: University Press of America.

Flores, Fernando, and Robert Solomon. 1998. Creating Trust. *Business Ethics
Quarterly* 8/2 (April): 205–32.

Gordon, Suzanne. 1996. Feminism and Caring. In *Caregiving*, ed. Suzanne Gordon, Patricia Benner, and Nel Noddings, 256–77. Philadelphia: University of
Pennsylvania Press.

Greenspan, Patricia. 1980. A Case of Mixed Feelings: Ambivalence and the
Logic of Emotion. In *Explaining Emotions*, ed. Amélie Oksenberg Rorty,
223–50. Berkeley: University of California Press.

Gunderman, Richard. 1998. Medicine and the Pursuit of Wealth. *Hastings Center Report* 28/1 (January-February): 8–13.

Hendley, Steven. 1996. From Communicative Action to the Face of the Other.
Philosophy Today 40/4 (winter): 504–30.

Kramer, Peter. 1997. *Listening to Prozac*. New York: Penguin.

Laskey, Dallas. 1987. Empathy and the Moral Point of View. In *Morality Within
the Life and Social World*, ed. Anna-Teresa Tymieniecka, 299–311. Boston:
Dordrecht.

Lauritzen, Paul. 1992. *Religious Belief and Emotional Transformation*. Lewisburg,
Penn.: Bucknell University Press.

Lonergan, Bernard, S.J. 1972. *Method in Theology*. New York: Herder and
Herder.

McCormick, Richard. 1998. The End of Catholic Hospitals? *America* 179/1:
5–12.

Mencius. 1970. In *Mencius*, trans. D. C. Lau. New York: Penguin.

Noddings, Nel. 1984. *Caring*. Berkeley: University of California Press.

Nussbaum, Martha. 1996. Compassion: The Basic Social Emotion. In *Social Philosophy and Policy* 13: 27–58.

————. 1999. *Sex and Social Justice*. New York: Oxford University Press.

Rawls, John. 1971. *A Theory of Justice*. Cambridge, Mass.: Harvard University
Press.

Reeder, John, Jr. 1998. Extensive Benevolence. *The Journal of Religious Ethics* 26/
1 (spring): 47–70.

Scheler, Max. 1973. *Selected Philosophical Essays*. Evanston, Ill.: Northwestern University Press.

Scudder, John, and Anne Bishop. 1986. The Moral Sense and Health Care. In *The Moral Sense in the Communal Significance of Life*, ed. Anna-Teresa Tymieniecka, 125–58. Boston: Dordrecht.

Solomon, Robert. 1980. Emotions and Choice. In *Explaining Emotions*, ed. Amélie Oksenberg Rorty, 251–82. Berkeley: University of California Press.

———. 1994. Sympathy and Vengeance: The Role of the Emotions in Justice. In *Emotions*, ed. Stephanie H. M. van Goozen, 291–311. Hillsdale, N.J.: Lawrence Erlbaum.

Vacek, Edward Collins, S.J. 1994. *Love, Human and Divine*. Washington, D.C.: Georgetown University Press.

———. 1996. Love for God—Is It Obligatory? *The Annual of the Society of Christian Ethics* 221–47.

Waerness, Kari. 1996. The Rationality of Caring. In *Caregiving*, ed. Suzanne Gordon, Patricia Benner, and Nel Noddings, 231–55. Philadelphia: University of Pennsylvania Press.

5

The Psychology of Emotion and the Ethics of Care

Sidney Callahan

The theory and practice of ethics have been transformed in recent decades. Twenty-five years ago I co-led bioethical workshops with a philosopher colleague who would hold up two flow charts displaying formulas for making ethical decisions. One chart laid out the steps in a decision tree to reach a deontological solution and the other demonstrated how to reach a utilitarian answer. "Can it really be so simple?" I would protest.

Today, overly abstract methods of ethical decision making have been found wanting. Consequently, many new approaches to ethics have emerged or re-emerged, such as casuistry and virtue ethics, feminist ethics, narrative ethics, relational ethics, discourse ethics, ecological ethics, and care ethics. All of these theories react against standard abstract methods by agreeing that turning to human experience is necessary. Persons cannot engage in effective moral deliberation without activating their subjective responses of emotion, intuition, and imagination, all of which operate within the implicit assumptions and narratives of their communities.

However, it is far easier to assert that moral deliberation is always shaped by intuitive and emotional processes that initiate, direct, shape, challenge, and sustain a person's thinking than it is to understand *how* this happens. Although there has been a recent upsurge in the study of consciousness in psychology, no one yet fully understands how self-consciousness operates (Damasio 1999; Flanagan 1992; Rychlak 1997). This chapter explores the process of subjective consciousness that operates in moral decision making. In particular, I focus on the nature of emotions and their significance in the moral life, especially as understood within an ethic of care. When focusing upon care ethics, it is important to understand the psychology of care, and to appreciate that care is an emotion that can be cultivated and thus, to some degree, controlled. Care can also promote effective moral reasoning.

THE PSYCHOLOGY OF EMOTION

To understand care as an emotion, one needs to know what emotions are and how they operate. Defining what counts as an emotion is not easy, despite the fact that in recent decades, there has been a remarkable amount of research done on human emotions. The new sub-discipline of the psychology of emotion is part of what I call the "emotion explosion." It followed psychology's "cognitive revolution," which rehabilitated the study of thinking (Gardner 1985).

If an ongoing stream of human thought and consciousness shapes and affects behavior, then clearly some conscious experiences are more personally arousing, qualitatively colored, and vividly "hot" than others (Frijda 1986, 1988; Izard 1993). Thinking about one's cancer operation tomorrow morning is different from planning how to rearrange one's bookshelves. Affect and emotion (I will use these terms interchangeably) are embodied responses that signal intense personal interest, self-focus, and self-investment.

The boundaries of an emotion are difficult to delimit because the emotion system is so complex (Griffiths 1997). Having an emotion consists of feeling an internal private experience while exhibiting differentiated facial displays, postural and physiological responses, and predispositions to action (Izard 1993). I am angry and want to attack; I love and seek to approach the valued object. The different brain and bodily components of the emotion system consist of conscious and nonconscious elements that usually, but not always, work together. It is possible to have an embodied emotional response that remains below the threshold of experiential self-awareness. No one as yet understands exactly why or how this happens, although everyone has observed an obviously angry person who does not recognize his own anger. Other bodily functions such as heartbeat or respiration can also remain unnoticed, so perhaps the occurrence of nonconscious emotion is much the same. Emotions differ from moods, which are states that are more diffuse and longer lasting than emotions. Emotions, as compared to moods or other kinds of generalized background states that reflect internal bodily conditions, emerge more acutely into consciousness and display different patterns of onset and dissipation (Damasio 1999; Katz 1999).

Another puzzle in the psychology of emotion involves the number of different basic emotions. Most lists of basic emotions include joy, fear, anger, disgust, contempt, shame, guilt, and for some theorists, interest and surprise (Izard 1992). Love is considered a combination of joy and preferential interest that emerges very early in infancy (Hatfield and Rapson 1993). By contrast, shame and guilt appear only after a young child has the intellectual equipment to know that certain social standards exist and that he or she has violated them (Saarni 1993).

Cognitively elaborated emotions are shaped by experience and learning and are sometimes called the social or secondary emotions. Yet the stimuli that induce an emotion may not be consciously perceived. All emotion is induced by the perception of an internal or external stimulus. The secondary social emotions are induced by stimuli given meaning by previous associations. Very early in the course of each individual's experience his or her emotions become associated with thoughts and images, forming cognitive-affective associative structures. These associations are stored in an individual's memory where they can be easily accessed by either the cognitive meaning or the affective feeling. If I feel sad, I will tend to think of other sad things; thinking of sad things will make me feel sad. These learned cognitive-affective structures and stored emotional prototypes, scenarios, or scripts can change over time. Associations and combinations of emotions can also become stable and habitual. An individual's cognitive-affective structures and patterns of emotional response make up a great deal of the uniqueness of a personality (Izard 1993).

Every unimpaired individual while awake and conscious has a private ongoing stream of consciousness that includes thoughts, emotions, sensory signals, and behavioral responses that interact in alternating or complementary ways (Damasio 1999; James 1950). Consciousness operates in different intensities, ranging from hyper-alert awareness to near-sleep. Musical images of a fugue or a symphony have been used to describe how emotions emerge, fade, and join with ongoing thinking, sensations, and behavioral responses within a person's stream of consciousness (Damasio 1999). When the emotional themes in the symphony of consciousness come to the fore, they signal qualitative states of self-investment, arousing the emotion system. Other themes in consciousness can, in turn, become salient and absorbing, as when a person engages in problem solving or abstract information manipulation. Insistent sensations from physiological drives can also become dominant. These are neither thoughts nor emotions, but can stimulate or fuse with both. When hungry, I focus on food and become anxious if none is available. Pain is a physiological signal that can be interpreted as a threat to the integrity of the self and thereby become amplified into the emotion of suffering (Cassell 1991). Many stimuli can induce emotions that are experienced in many different intensities, combinations, and associations with thought and behavior. The human organism has many parallel functions that operate simultaneously and ordinarily as a unity.

Emotional experiences can be positive or negative. In the context of psychological research on the emotions, the terms "positive" and "negative" do not reflect normative evaluations. Positive emotions are defined as those that are experienced as innately rewarding and pleasing to the individual. They induce approach and satisfaction. Negative emotions are defined as innately aversive, punishing states that usually induce avoidance or unpleasant feeling. One can experience combinations or mixtures of positive and negative emotions at the same time because positive and negative emotions exist as independent subsystems in the brain, arise from different sources, and follow different functional rules (LeDoux 1999). For example, some kinds of suffering can be experienced at the same time as joy, as in a bittersweet encounter or a blend of love and sorrow while caring for an ill person.

In the dynamic process of human functioning, the individual's cognitive, emotional, and behavioral systems respond to each stimulus to the organism from the constantly changing internal and external environment (Greenberg and Safran 1987; Katz 1999; LeDoux 1999). Mutually determining interactions and feedback loops continue the nonlinear processing, which takes place so fast that, when emotions emerge into conscious awareness, they appear to come out of the blue, seeming to arise automatically and without effort, just as sensory perceptions do. In the same way that we see and hear, or feel pain, we seem to feel most emotions without freely choosing to do so. Automatic, nonconscious responses are necessary for human life, as no one could consciously will and intelligently direct all of the bodily and mental functions that an organism requires to operate.

Following in Darwin's footsteps, most psychologists today consider emotions to be very old products of evolutionary pressures for survival (Buss 1995; Tooby and Cosmides 1990; Wright 1994). Human emotions are adaptive because they make up core consciousness, amplify physiological drives, enable human communication, and are primary motivators for human action, including sustained acts of problem solving (Izard 1993). Emotions, like the capacity for language and logical thinking, are pan-specific, genetically inherited human programs that develop from birth and operate always and everywhere throughout the life span in every known culture (Ekman and Friesen 1971).

The universality of basic emotions and their embodied expressions enable interpersonal communication. Human beings are innately equipped to display and read other people's nonverbal emotional signals in their facial and other bodily responses. Emotions convey information about an individual's inner state and personal reactions to environmental conditions. Individual emotions are "vital signs" or read-outs of the self's relationship to self and environment, particularly the interpersonal environment. The psychologists Greenberg and Safran affirm that "emotion is a type of information processing about the self in interaction with the environment"; in fact, "emotion can be thought of as a form of tacit knowing" (Greenberg and Safran 1987, 147). When the tone of voice, face, and posture differ from the verbal content of a message directed to us, we tend to trust the nonverbal signals. All health care workers have had the experience of reading nonverbal emotional signals of their patients that differed from what the patient said. Patients, too, try to read their physicians' emotional responses in order to gain information. Moreover, when emotions are displayed and seen by another they tend to elicit an instantaneous corresponding response. Your tears and grief bring tears to my eyes; your panic makes me afraid. Emotions communicate so well that they seem to be contagious.

It has often been noted that negative emotions appear to be more numerous and occur more frequently and intensely than positive emotions (Frijda 1988). Evolutionary psychologists attribute this asymmetry to the need to ensure human survival in a dangerous environment. Vulnerable individuals must be on the defensive and hyper-vigilant to any threat. Fear of a predator must be an instantaneous reaction, induced even by ambiguous stimuli, if an organism is to escape quickly enough to live another day (LeDoux 1999). Better to flee from what may be a snake across the path than to wait to identify it as a harmless vine. Instantaneous fear motivates flight or freezing, and bursts of anger motivate an attack upon any threatening danger or frustrating obstacle. More complex negative emotions of grief and disgust, along with shame, guilt, and contempt, also work to ensure human survival. Human beings are a social species dependent upon group support; interpersonal relationships and commitments must be kept in good repair. Negative emotional responses are punishing and initiate a change in behavior. Social punishments serve to ensure an individual's conformity to prescribed group norms.

The positive emotions, which give pleasure and induce approach, tend to receive less attention in research, perhaps because they do not present the disturbing problems that maladaptive and excessive negative emotions do. Much human misery arises from phobias, depressions, and hostile outbursts of aggression, but love, joy, and interest, the primary positive emotions, make life worth living and enhance human flourishing. Recently, scientific research has begun to focus on positive emotions and optimal experiences, with inquiries into love, happiness, joy, and altruism (Diener and Larsen 1993; Sober and Wilson 1998). Here, too, evolutionary psychologists would claim that positive emotions evolved because they strengthen social bonds, restrain aggression, and produce the altruism and cooperation that ensure the survival of the group. As positive emotions induce relaxation and reduce defensive vigilance against predators, they also induce group protection and thereby promote survival. Altruistic sacrifices of self-interest for the sake of offspring, kin, and other group members become more likely when affectionate bonds and a sense of positive identification with others exist. Human families and communities are held together by mutual love and collective celebrations of joy. The familiar tends to be liked, and positive affection for one's own people and one's own territory keeps people and groups together.

The positive emotional responses of interest also motivate people to explore the new. From infancy, individuals display a fascination and delight in the novel. Curiosity induces human beings to investigate, learn, invent, and create culture. Intense interest in carrying out goals produces pleasure. Children love to play games, and when play turns into adult work, interest and enjoyment remain. Being intensely interested and absorbed in an appropriately stimulating task produces a kind of optimal experience described by psychologists as "flow" (Csikszentimihalyi 1990). Absorption in goal-oriented projects produces material achievements, but interest also motivates and sustains thinking and problem solving. Goal-oriented thinking and other creative work are motivated by delight found in the desire to explore, to know, and to solve problems—even ethical and moral problems.

CARE IS AN EMOTION THAT CAN BE CULTIVATED

Love is a blend of interest and joy that motivates approach, sustained attentiveness, and a positive valuing of its object. Love, like all emotions, can come in many varieties, intensities, and blends. Sexual love fuses with the physiological drive for sexual consummation. Care, by contrast, is a nonpossessive, nonsexual, cognitively elaborated, altruistic love. Care can be identified with the Christian concept of charity; it is a love that seeks to benefit the valued other for his or her own sake. The person who cares for another focuses attention and invests interest and energy in bringing about his or her welfare. Because it takes thought to discern what is actually good for another, care usually becomes blended with cognitive content and functioning. One intuitive cognitive capacity that relates to care is empathy, which is an intuitive intelligence concerning what another is feeling. It is empathy that makes emotional contagion or communication possible. When empathy is consciously elaborated by intelligent thinking and fused with the emotion of care, care givers can take the role of others and imagine what will best serve their interests from their own point of view.

When actively caring for another, a care taker can become self-forgetful, especially when engaged in a face to face mutual relationship. The give and take can become engrossing and produce flow (Noddings 1984). A mother nursing her child can become absorbed in the interaction. Parents and children can become emotionally attuned to one another while carrying out a joint activity (Stern 1985). Emotional attunement arises when each person reads the other's emotion and demonstrates that understanding through an appropriate emotional response. Such attunement brings the sense that one is understood and cared for. All caring resembles the giving and receiving of attentive presence and response found in nurturing families. Happily, although care is altruistic and may include suffering as well as intense effort, it can also produce joy for the care giver. A parent may suffer while donating an organ to save his or her child's life, but at the same time feel joy in being able to do it. Nurses or physicians may make sacrifices in order to care for their patients, but also be happy in their ability to relieve suffering (Sulmasy 1997). The human ability to care for one another is an intrinsically good emotional capacity. Nothing contributes more to human flourishing.

Although emotions usually arise in consciousness as involuntary responses, they are not completely removed from the influence of the self-regulating will. As emotions are intense embodied responses, it is not easy to suppress or mask their presence once they arise, but with practice it is possible to control their expression, as well as the actions that they motivate. Indeed, because emotions can be so disturbing and contagious, every culture strives to regulate emotions for the sake of the community. In the course of socialization, every child tries to learn self-control and the display rules that apply to various emotions (Saarni 1993). Different cultures, or social groups within them, approve and encourage the expression of certain emotions and proscribe others. Our culture is no exception, as psychological research on emotional regulation reveals (Gross 1998).

People attempt to mask and suppress emotional displays by controlling facial muscles and motor behavior, and especially by employing mental strategies. Detaching attention from disturbing stimuli by acts of will is an ancient method of emotional control, recognized at least from the time of the

Stoics. Other strategies to control the emotions were devised and practiced in spiritual disciplines long before the development of modern psychology. Although many psychologists still resist the idea of free will and claim that unconscious psychological mechanisms always determine behavior, more researchers and theorists have come to explore the power and freedom of self-conscious acts. Recent research on cognition and consciousness explores the power that an aware and awake self has to freely and self-consciously make plans and choose between alternatives (Cantor and Blanton 1996; Rychlak 1997). Following the work of William James, many psychologists believe that the self is dipolar and consists of an "I" who is an observer within the stream of consciousness and who can observe the "me" or the self's material, social, and spiritual dimensions (James 1950). I can observe my body, my social role playing, and my mind working out a problem. I can also alter aspects of who I observe myself to be. The power to change oneself resides in the power to set a goal, and to fix attention upon that goal and the steps needed to obtain it. Once one grants that the conscious self has the power to observe and alter its own responses to itself and its environment, then the stage is set to affirm that it is possible to regulate emotions.

A person can spontaneously experience an emotion while ignoring it and refusing to respond to its action tendencies. Or one can welcome, attend to, cognitively elaborate, and act in order to sustain and amplify an emotion. As a person develops what used to be called strength of character and is now often called ego strength or emotional intelligence, he or she learns to govern the stream of consciousness and the behavioral responses of the emotion system. I do not bare my teeth, howl with anger, or strike an infuriating opponent. "Emotional intelligence" has become a new watchword in popular psychology. The term refers to a person's ability to attend to his or her own emotions, regulate them, and understand and respond appropriately to the emotional responses of others (Goleman 1995). Feeling one's emotions or allowing emotions to emerge into consciousness is important to receiving the tacit information or vital signs that emotions provide. A person who lacks emotional intelligence may engage, for example, in denial or suppression. These are handicapping and can have negative effects on physical health (Gross and Levenson 1997). Self-knowledge is necessary for self-care and self-direction (Higgins 1996). A person who lacks emotional intelligence may also become "emotionally hijacked," and lose self-control as consciousness is flooded by intense emotional responses (Goleman 1995; LeDoux 1999). Destructive episodes of unregulated rage, fear, jealousy, and suicidal depression produce many of the tragedies that fill the daily news reports. Such pathologies obscure the fact that most normal people regulate their negative emotions most of the time, and that morally appropriate positive emotions play a significant part in most people's lives.

Although one may grant that spontaneous emotions can be controlled, there remains the intriguing issue of whether emotions can be voluntarily engendered. There has been little psychological research on this question. Experimenters have studied actors who have been instructed to display emotions, and they have also devised experimental mood induction procedures to put people into happy or unhappy moods before testing their memory or some other capacity. Mood induction procedures may ask people to remember happy or sad memories or to listen to favorite music or annoying noises. Inducing frustration or failure reliably creates negative feelings in experiments. Tests show that beautiful and ugly rooms induce, respectively, positive and negative emotional effects. Experimenters providing direct and immediate stimuli can induce emotions, but can people voluntarily make themselves feel an emotion? Apparently so, at least to a certain extent. Humans have the ability to create imaginative constructions in consciousness, call up memories at will, and provide vicarious experiences for themselves. Many actors report that they create imaginative stories and recall personal memories in order to engender the emotions they wish to display in a role. Role playing is an ability that actors refine and elaborate, but other people also possess it. When people recount stories, they reenact the emotions that accompany the events of the narrative.

There are many entry points in the complex emotion system in which to intervene and exert influence. Because emotions are constituted by physiological responses, behavioral dispositions, facial displays, and conscious feelings infused with cognitive meaning, the conscious self can act in many ways to bring about desired emotional responses (Gross 1998). Engaging in deep breathing, relaxation techniques, eating, sleeping, and exercising can change emotional responses, as can the intake of psychoactive drugs. Voluntarily assuming the facial expressions of an emotion can give a person feedback and thus help create the feelings associated with those expressions. Pollyanna, the glad girl of the children's books, always put a smile upon her face in order to make herself feel happy. Experimenters have tricked subjects into producing smiling expressions by gradually taping their lips upward; these subjects have reported themselves to be happier than subjects of a control group (Ekman 1993; Ekman, Levenson, and Friesen 1983). Other behavioral strategies include adopting the postures and bodily movements associated with a desired emotional response. If I stand up straight, smile, and march to work whistling a happy tune, I may soon feel cheerful.

Another related way to engender desired emotions is to move into a different environment, whether internal or external. Once we know that certain environments affect us by eliciting certain emotional responses, we can move into the environment that encourages the responses we desire. Walking outdoors beside still waters may induce happy calming responses, and entry into a bustling, crowded social environment may induce interest and alertness. Listening to music or going to the theater or a movie can change emotions. Socially, we can seek out friends or those supportive groups that give us a lift. Group celebrations, artistic performances, and worship services can also induce positive emotions. Seeking the company of like-minded others can increase emotional energy and synergy. Just as problem drinkers seek places where they can be surrounded by other heavy drinkers, so other people go to AA meetings to avoid alcohol abuse. Groups exert powerful influences upon individual emotions and behavior. In battle, soldiers endure harrowing fire and advance into great danger moved by their emotional attachments to their units, as well as by the desire to avoid being shamed as cowards.

A more direct way to engender, shape, or control an emotion is to employ self-directed thoughts and commands. The suppression of negative emotions can often be achieved by a self-instruction like "Stop!" Sometimes we can muster reasons to induce positive feelings. The self can direct rational arguments to the self, and as in the case of actors, consciousness can call upon specific memories, images and narratives in order to induce an emotion. Attention makes a remembered feeling more vivid and real. Often, a person can voluntarily recall past moments of shame, guilt, or pride and re-experience the flood of feeling, although it may be all but impossible to induce the automatic, built-in fear that responds to a sudden environmental threat unless there is an external signal of danger. Emotions that are fused with particular physiological states may also be less subject to imaginative maneuverings. I cannot experience suffering over physical pain without experiencing some sensation of physical pain. But altruistic care can be engendered because it includes imaginative cognitive constructions of the other, the other's needs, and the self's commitment to respond with interest.

We can thus evoke care for others in the ways that we can evoke other emotions. We can welcome, attend to, and amplify care when it occurs spontaneously. We can induce care by acting in a caring manner and by placing ourselves in the presence of other caring people within nurturing environments. Just as groups of soldiers can function together to conquer fear on the battlefield, so communities of care, such as churches and health care teams, can induce and model care giving in difficult situations. If momentarily irritated or disgusted by a sick and irascible patient, a person can consciously dissipate the irritation by imagining the other's neediness and discomfort. A person can remember his or her commitment to care giving, and he or she can enlist the help of others who share that commitment simply by calling to mind past feelings of caring and being cared for. Gratitude and memories of having been cared for in the past help generate care. Religious people can think of God's care for them while remembering the command to love others as God loves us.

Emotion-laden behavioral responses are shaped by conscious control efforts, as in "boys don't cry" or "don't hit back." From an early age people engage in "character planning," which involves the shaping of emotional and behavioral responses (Elster 1999). Timid, shy children can aspire to be braver or extroverted, bumptious children to become more self-controlled (Kagan 1999). Human selves who live into an imagined future from a remembered past can in the present aspire to self-transformations, seeking an ideal self (Allport 1955; James 1950). Often a beloved, admired model is remembered and imitated. Christians seek to imitate Christ, the great saints, and other exemplars. Caring for one's own ideal self and future helps generate care for others.

Emotional responses and associated thoughts that are repeated become internalized. Each response strengthens and builds up a pattern of behavior. Habitual emotional responses become part of one's identity. Those who choose over and over again to care for others and act benevolently will find themselves doing so more and more automatically (Bargh and Barndollar 1996). After choosing to be attentive and receptive to spontaneous feelings of care and repeatedly making the effort to induce the emotion of care for others, caring becomes part of a person's second nature. The habitual disposition to feel care and enact caring behavior has important implications for care ethics.

CARE CONTRIBUTES TO GOOD DECISION MAKING

If it is true that emotions are an essential part of all thought and behavior, emotions will necessarily be a part of moral reflection—whether acknowledged or not. Thus, people who aspire to suppress emotional responses as much as they can in order to be as rational and objective as possible are engaging in a futile and self-handicapping strategy. Theorists who stress the adaptive moral role of emotions cite evidence that involuntary emotional responses are not generated solely by the more primitive parts of the brain that we share with other animals. The higher cortex plays a crucial role in the emotion system, especially in those more cognitively elaborated emotions that are elicited through social experience. When certain specific parts of the higher cortex are injured, an individual's social and moral functioning become seriously impaired. Antonio R. Damasio, the noted neurologist, reports on brain injured people who can achieve high scores on I.Q. tests but cannot make other kinds of socially appropriate judgments that enable them to take care of themselves or hold a job (Damasio 1994, 1999). Damasio thinks that emotions not only accompany all states of consciousness, but furnish individuals with personal and social values that give direction and purpose to rational thinking. The emotional contribution to value assessment is automatic, but vital. Emotional responses may be mostly involuntary, but they are not alien to the person; they reflect internalized past choices and deployments of attention.

Surely good moral decision makers need emotional intelligence or the ability to read the signals and listen to the emotions of everyone involved in any individual or group situation. Negative emotions can be as important as positive ones, especially one's own negative emotions. Knowing, for instance, that one is disgusted, bored, angry, or afraid in a situation can prevent morally evasive strategies of thought and behavior. Even our most instinctual defensive emotions of fear may give us valuable information about the environment. So, too, sensing another's fear, sadness, or anger makes it easier to understand them. It is also important to realize that when humans are under stress or tempted to regress morally, the higher cognitively developed emotions of love and loyalty can provide strength and sustain commitments to morality. Positive emotions of care give direction to thinking and strengthen the value priorities built up by past decisions.

Feeling the emotion of care as a matter of habit tends to increase the adequacy of moral functioning in additional ways. As noted above, when a person is unimpaired and awake, there is a constant interaction of cognitive, emotional, and behavioral responses. Different themes in the musical fugue become salient and influence each other. A person can direct attention to different elements of consciousness. Feeling the emotion of care can induce preferred behavioral approaches to others, increase communication, and sustain cognitive attention and interest in them. Those things or people that are loved, desired, and cared for capture interest because they are experienced as rewarding and valuable objects. Focusing caring attention produces increased information about a person, his or her environment, and the relationships between the two. Increased understanding of a situation from different points of view can improve ongoing thinking and induce more positive emotional responses. Care for others not only directs attentive personal interest toward them, but sharpens the cognitive focus upon their situation (Isen 1993). Care also contributes to moral creativity, for it allows one to engage many concerns and many dimensions of ongoing events. The positive emotion of care arouses and focuses reasoning and enlarges problem-solving goals beyond simple efficiency.

Care also motivates perseverance in ethical thinking. In time-scarce and distracting health care environments it becomes tempting to cut short difficult ethical problem solving and save energy and effort by deciding on the first available solution that is minimally acceptable. Carelessness encourages sloppy thinking and mindless routine performance. But emotionally caring for persons will not allow shortcuts. The investment of care gives a care taker energy to return again and again to the person's needs and continue seeking the best outcome for the other.

Indeed, when analyzing the accepted midlevel principles widely used in ethical reasoning, one can discern within each principle a crystallized emotional scenario or emotional prototype of care. Ethical principles and guidelines can be seen as condensed prescriptions to act upon the caring emotions that one should have for others, despite distractions, provocations, or countervailing personal desires. In the principle of beneficence we see the implicit prescription to care for the well-being of others. In the principle of nonmaleficence we see the command to care enough about others to avoid harming them when possible. Respect for autonomy implies caring for another by taking his or her point of view and valuing it for the other's own sake. In seeking to follow the principle of justice a person embraces the importance of caring, not only for some, but for all. Thus the emotion of care motivates, infuses, and informs abstract processes of ethical reasoning.

The process of ethical decision making is always dynamic. A person must try to synthesize principles or decide which principles and which reasons apply in specific cases. The directed active reasoning process takes place within a stream of consciousness that includes emotional responses, intuitions, and imaginative scenarios. Spontaneously emerging or enacted emotions can change or direct reasoning, but reasons and reasoning can also inform and change emotional responses (Callahan 1988, 1991). Abstract reasoning can operate in a flexible, far-ranging manner and produce novel ideas that do not come from past embodied experiences, implicit intuitive knowledge, or immediate reactions to the present environment. Yet reasoning, like emotional responses or instant intuitions, can be misleading. Mutual testing and a measure of skepticism seem to be the safest strategies during ethical inquiry.

A caring decision maker feels his or her attention shifting back and forth in consciousness, moving through different responses while at the same time reflecting upon those responses and their outward effects. A person's internal subjective commitment to pursue the good can be questioned and his or her performance scrutinized. Consulting with others and tapping into the resources of wisdom in one's professional and moral traditions while attending to the objective external problem to be solved can inform the mutual testing and circular processes of deliberation. Dialogue with others produces information, but it is even more critical for helping one avoid self-deception, bias, or personal lacunae in either reasoned or emotional responses. Religious people seek guidance and critique from their faith commitments, their religious communities, and holy exemplars. Believers may also pray to God in an effort to seek rational insight and to energize their emotional commitments to care. Insights obtained from prayer may arise into consciousness from implicit intuitive knowledge garnered from past religious practice, or from creative syntheses of old and new ideas.

When a person reflects upon a given ethical decision, it becomes invested with internal personal authority and produces an ethical pull or obligation to act. A truth seeker may remain open to more information or better insights, but in the real world ethical decisions have to be made and acted upon. If one later becomes convinced of better arguments or has different emotional experiences and responses that impel new insights, then a person will change. Every person and every institution experiences moral change over time. Moral progress is always possible, as is moral regression. Self-correction is built into a caring commitment to the good because care for self and others motivates a constant effort to grow in moral discernment. Sometimes new experiences of care for some group, such as slaves or the mentally ill, have inspired reassessments of the accepted ethical reasoning supported by current authorities. Sometimes new reasons and new information have produced new ethical standards of care, for instance, in decisions concerning definitions of brain death and the treatment of the dying.

One can employ reason to judge and correct instances when the emotion of care itself becomes distorted or deformed. Emotions rightly cause concern in ethics when they are distorted and hijack consciousness. At times, emotional distortions of thinking may be due to some physiological clinical disorder such as mania, depression, or schizophrenia, but even in unimpaired but immature people, emotional wildfires can incite thoughts that produce disordered emotions, which prompt impulsive actions that cause harm. Often emotional wildfires involve defensive episodes of rage, but love and care can themselves be consuming. They can become obsessive desires to control events and to relieve suffering in the receiver, as well as the giver of care, instantly and at any cost. Many cases of mercy killings seem to follow this pattern. The emotion of care loses its nonpossessive, altruistic quality and becomes distorted by a rage against life's circumstances. Under stress the cognitive elaborations that usually fuse with care break down and a passionate desire to cut off the sufferings of patient and observer engulfs consciousness. A person who is emotionally overcome no longer possesses the free and flexible play of attention that can take the point of view of others or attend to what is best for the common good. Such distortions and narrowing of attention have given rise to the maxims that love is blind and that emotion clouds the mind.

Care becomes distorted when one fails to attend to the moral claims of everyone involved in a situation. Altruistic care fails when one forgets that care givers and other members of an individual's family and community also need to be cared for. Everyone's needs count. Because women have been the principal care givers in our society, their own needs have often been sacrificed. Even if a person desires to lose him or herself in a caring relationship, others may be rightly concerned for the care giver's well-being and try to intervene. Altruism is consistent with an ethic of care; self-destruction generally is not.

JUST CARE AND THE EDUCATION OF EMOTION

Feminists have advocated an ethic of "just care" (Farley 1991; Young 1991). Care should not ignore the wider claims of justice, even as justice is initiated, informed, and sustained by the ability to care. "Justice is love's absolute minimum," as Pope Paul VI said. Justice and loving care should not be seen as polar opposites or even as complementary. Rather, they are points on a reflexive, mutually interacting round of continuing thought and emotional response. Justice in its many forms can be thought of as a rational principle of equality, but it can also be defined as meeting everyone's need for compassionate care now and in the future. Demands for empathy and care at one point in time have to be enlarged by the individual's imagining and taking seriously future caring, as well as the emotional needs of the whole community. If, for instance, today a mother shrinks from having her child hurt by an inoculation, she must imagine the emotions she would feel if in the future her child became ill with polio. And how would the other families feel whose children might be infected by her child? Caring emotions extended into the future and toward others in the community transmute the feelings and behaviors of the moment.

Acts of imaginative projection into the future are necessary in the practice of care ethics. Nurses in a burn unit cannot let their present empathy for their patients' pain keep them from carrying out the painful treatments that can save lives and bring future recovery. A professor may be empathetically engrossed with a medical student's learning process, but still should not shrink from giving the painful negative evaluations without which the student will not exhibit competence in the future. Almost every claim of justice and the common good can be seen as a need to care for others within an enlarged, communal, and long-term perspective. Ethical decisions are not decided by contrasting the claims of reason versus emotion, but by comparing one cognitive-emotional scenario with a more adequate and comprehensive cognitive-emotional narrative.

Ethical thinking is not simply a matter of individual responses and private behavior. As bioethics has matured, it has become clear that acute clinical dilemmas faced by individuals are not the only matters that need to be addressed; the scope of moral attention has to be enlarged to focus upon groups and social environments. Ethical analyses should focus upon corporate actors and institutionalized policies and practices—especially upon the operating moral assumptions that rarely get noticed or examined. Here, too, caring enough to find out the emotional responses of everyone involved in the system can give vital information about the moral environment. Care givers must take the point of view of everyone involved in an institution and invest in everyone's flourishing.

Throughout the course of history strong defensive emotions have resisted moral progress and fueled ethical regressions. Primal defensive emotions of fear, often automatically and unconsciously triggered, can exert powerful obstacles to ethical behavior because embodied emotions are experienced more intimately and vividly than abstract thoughts (LeDoux 1999). After all, emotions gain their usefulness and power by signaling passionate investments of the embodied self in the environment. Emotional reality seems convincingly real because the unique bodily self is reacting. Thus habitual emotions or emotional landscapes may change more slowly than a person's cognitive beliefs. To believe that one should care for others will not instantly produce caring. Notional assent to a new concept must become a real assent marked by emotional conviction. This explains why new emotional experiences are the most potent ways to effect personal changes in mind and behavior (Greenberg and Safran 1987). Psychotherapy and religious conversions induce changes by providing new emotional responses and new personal relationships. Emotional changes accompany moral and ethical growth—or moral regressions. Nazi medical selections and experimentations done by physicians upon concentration camp inmates were carried out by people who had numbed their emotions of care. The Holocaust murders and other recent instances of genocide and ethnic cleansing were fueled by hatred, contempt, and disgust for the victims. Often the hatred that enables people to act cruelly is incited and magnified by demagogues and evilly manipulative propaganda. Hate-mongers who arouse hatred in the mob may themselves be filled with hatred and contempt. The fact that negative emotions can be used to fuel destruction, even among medical professionals, means that an ethic of care must constantly be valued and encouraged.

Care inhibits aggression. Care can overcome fear and disgust toward the ill. Caring can be stronger than fear because, as the Gospel says, "Love casts out fear." The early Christian martyrs impressed their pagan countrymen by their steadfastness and fearlessness in meeting death. According to some observers, the spread of Christianity in the ancient world was facilitated not only by the example of courageous martyrdoms, but by the fact that Christians committed to love of neighbor did not flee the cities during plagues, but rather stayed to nurse the ill (Stark 1996). Feelings of disgust and contempt for the weak and ill can be overcome by feelings of compassion and care for the needy. In the history of Christianity there appears a huge body of spiritual writing specifically devoted to transforming selfish emotions of fear, greed, contempt, disgust, sloth, and pride into altruistic care. Acute psychological insights into the workings of emotion exist in spiritual exercises, such as those of Ignatius Loyola, which work toward the personal transformation of the believer.

Modern psychotherapy is also devoted to personal change by the re-education of the emotions. The main way people change in therapy is through corrective emotional experiences of care. New personal relationships take the place of harmful early socialization into distorted "emotional prototypes." Families or peers who may have inculcated maladaptive cognitive and emotional responses lose their influence as new positive experiences take place with a therapist or supportive group. One can bring distorted cognitive-affective structures and negative personal relationships that have in the past or present produced malfunctioning into full awareness within a safe and caring setting. Becoming fully conscious of the ways that one's thinking and feeling interact can give one the freedom to change. New emotional experiences support reflection and new patterns of action, changing ongoing mindless responses. Care ethics should emphasize the importance of tutoring and encouraging emotional responsiveness and caring behavior in professional care givers. Technical competence is necessary, but not sufficient.

Health care givers constantly face the challenge of flexibly enacting and sustaining appropriate emotions in the difficult challenges of their practice. Obviously they should not give in to fear, disgust, anger, or contempt, and they should work continually to engender and sustain the positive emotions of care. But at the same time, care givers such as emergency room teams need to remain calm and controlled enough to carry out the upsetting procedures that are needed. William Osler, the great pioneering physician, recommended that his medical students cultivate equanimity, composure, imperturbability, presence of mind, or "a judicious measure of obtuseness" in order to care for their patients well (Carr 1999). To dissolve into tears or collapse emotionally in response to a patient's pain and suffering will not help those in dire need. Emotional contagions or collapses should be resisted in the hospital. But the emotional control that is necessary to steel oneself against incapacitating responses must never become so dominant in the person that it results in emotional numbing. Osler himself could be the most compassionate of physicians at the bedside. Heartfelt compassion and attentive care should be the habitual and dominant emotional response cultivated by care givers. When we speak of innately healing personalities or gifted healers we are speaking about those persons who are fully present in each personal encounter because they deeply care for others.

CONCLUSION

Caring infuses ethical reflection with heartfelt emotional knowledge and produces the interpersonal relationships that enable good communication and good decisions. Wisdom differs from narrow and abstract intellectual skill because it combines emotional investment and emotional intelligence with acute reasoning. A narrowly abstract analysis will often miss the depth, the subtleties, the nuance, and the interpersonal dimensions of an ethical challenge. Care ethics emphasizes the emotional responses and maturity of the persons who as agents must make moral decisions and act. When we judge the moral character of persons, we are judging the quality and appropriateness of their emotions as well as their behavior. Unless a person is mentally ill or impaired, we hold him or her responsible for the emotions he or she has, or fails to have. We understand that present emotions and behavior are partly the result of innate temperament and contingent environmental experiences, but they are also the fruit of past choices and willed conduct.

Practicing an ethic of care, although arduous, increases positive emotional responses such as interest, joy, and flow. Besides serving the individual and common good, caring produces its own experiential validation in an inherent sense of being good and doing the right thing. Traditional spiritual counselors recognized the role of joy and care in authenticating one's moral decisions and practices. Care expands our attentiveness, opens us to the world, and makes us free and willing to engage and serve others. Care and happiness can be a sign that our lives are going well. Care ethics encourages the most positive of all emotions and sustains the bonds of community that undergird the moral enterprise. With practice and good will spontaneous feelings of just care can become habitual. Care ethics is an enterprise whose time has come.

References

Allport, G. 1955. *Becoming*. New Haven, Conn.: Yale University Press.

Bargh, J. A., and K. Barndollar. 1996. Automaticity in Action: The Unconscious as Repository of Chronic Goals and Motives. In *The Psychology of Action: Linking Cognition and Motivation to Behavior*, ed. J. A. Bargh and P. M. Gollwitzer, 457–81. New York: The Guilford Press.

Buss, D. M. 1995. Evolutionary Psychology: A New Paradigm for Psychological Science. *Psychological Inquiry* 6: 1–30.

Callahan, S. 1988. The Role of Emotion in Ethical Decision Making. *Hastings Center Report* June/July: 9–14.

———. 1991. *In Good Conscience: Reason and Emotion in Moral Decision Making*. San Francisco: Harper San Francisco.

Cantor, N., and H. Blanton. 1996. Effortful Pursuit of Personal Goals in Daily Life. In *The Psychology of Action: Linking Cognition and Motivation to Behavior*, ed. J. A. Bargh and P. M. Gollwitzer, 338–59. New York: The Guilford Press.

Carr, M. 1999. A Tale of Two Physicians. *Update* 15 (June): 3–6.

Cassell, E. J. 1991. *The Nature of Suffering and the Goals of Medicine*. New York: Oxford University Press.

Csikszentimihalyi, M. 1990. *Flow: The Psychology of Optimal Experience*. New York: Harper & Row.

Damasio, A. R. 1994. *Descartes' Error: Emotion, Reason, and the Human Brain*. New York: Putnam.

————. 1999. *The Feeling of What Happens: Body and Emotion in the Making of Consciousness*. New York: Harcourt Brace.

Diener, E., and R. J. Larsen. 1993. The Experience of Emotional Well-Being. In *Handbook of Emotions*, ed. M. Lewis and J. M. Haviland, 405–15. New York: The Guilford Press.

Ekman, P. 1993. Facial Expression and Emotion. *American Psychologist* 48: 384–92.

Ekman, P., R. W. Levenson, and W. V. Friesen. 1983. Autonomic Nervous System Activity Distinguishes between Emotions. *Science* 221: 1208–10.

Ekman, P., and W. V. Friesen. 1971. Constants across Cultures in the Face and Emotion. *Journal of Personality and Social Psychology* 17: 124–29.

Elster, J. 1999. *Alchemies of the Mind: Rationality and the Emotions*. Cambridge, U.K.: Cambridge University Press.

Farley, M. 1991. Love, Justice, and Discernment. *Second Opinion* 17: 80–91.

Flanagan, O. 1992. *Consciousness Reconsidered*. Cambridge, Mass.: MIT Press.

Frijda, N. H. 1986. *The Emotions*. Cambridge, U.K.: Cambridge University Press.

————. 1988. The Laws of Emotion. *American Psychologist* 43: 349–58.

Gardner, H. 1985. *The Mind's New Science: A History of the Cognitive Revolution*. New York: Basic Books.

Goleman, D. 1995. *Emotional Intelligence*. New York: Bantam Books.

Greenberg, L. S., and J. D. Safran. 1987. *Emotion In Psychotherapy: Affect, Cognition, and the Process of Change*. New York: The Guilford Press.

Griffiths, P. E. 1997. *What Emotions Really Are*. Chicago: The University of Chicago Press.

Gross, J. J. 1998. The Emerging Field of Emotion Regulation: An Integrative Review. *Review of General Psychology* 2: 271–99.

Gross, J. J., and R. W. Levenson. 1997. Hiding Feelings: The Acute Effects of Inhibiting Negative and Positive Emotion. *Journal of Abnormal Psychology* 106: 95–103.

Hatfield, E., and R. Rapson. 1993. Love and Attachment Processes. In *Handbook of Emotions*, ed. M. Lewis and J. M. Haviland, 595–604. New York: The Guilford Press.

Higgins, E. T. 1996. The Self-Digest: Self-Knowledge Serving Self-Regulatory Functions. *Journal of Personality and Social Psychology* 71: 30–40.

Isen, A. M. Positive Affect and Decision Making. In *Handbook of Emotions*, ed. M. Lewis and J. M. Haviland, 261–77. New York: The Guilford Press.

Izard, C. E. 1990. Facial Expressions and the Regulation of Emotions. *Journal of Personality and Social Psychology* 58: 481-98.

————. 1992. Basic Emotions, Relations Amongst Emotions, and Emotion-Cognition Relations. *Psychological Review* 99: 561–65.

————. 1993. Four Systems for Emotion Activation: Cognitive and Non-Cognitive Processes. *Psychological Review* 100: 68–90.

James, W. 1950 [1890]. *The Principles of Psychology*. New York: Dover Publications.

Kagan, J. 1999. Born to Be Shy? In *States of Mind: New Discoveries About How Our Brains Make Us Who We Are,* ed. R. Conlan, 29–51. New York: John Wiley & Sons, Inc.

Katz, J. 1999. *How Emotions Work*. Chicago: University of Chicago Press.

LeDoux, J. 1999. The Power of Emotions. In *States of Mind: New Discoveries About How Our Brains Make Us Who We Are*, ed. R. Conlan, 123–49. New York: John Wiley & Sons.

Noddings, N. 1984. *Caring: A Feminine Approach to Ethics and Moral Education*. Berkeley: University of California Press.

Pinker, S. 1997. *How the Mind Works*. New York: W.W. Norton.

Rychlak, J. F. 1997. *In Defense of Human Consciousness*. Washington, D. C.: American Psychological Association.

Saarni, C. 1993. Socialization of Emotion. In *Handbook of Emotions*, ed. M. Lewis and J. M. Haviland, 435–46. New York: The Guilford Press.

Sober, E., and D. S. Wilson. 1998. *Unto Others: The Evolution and Psychology of Unselfish Behavior*. Cambridge, Mass.: Harvard University Press.

Stark, R. 1996. *The Rise of Christianity: A Sociologist Reconsiders History*. Princeton, N.J.: Princeton University Press.

Stern, D. N. 1985. *The Interpersonal World of the Infant*. New York: Basic Books.

Sulmasy, D. P., O. F. M., M. D. 1997. *The Healer's Calling: A Spirituality for Physicians and Other Health Care Professionals*. New York: Paulist.

Tooby, J. and L. Cosmides. 1990. The Past Explains the Present: Emotional Adaptations and the Structure of Ancestral Environments. *Ethology and Sociobiology* 11: 375–424.

Wright, R. 1994. *The Moral Animal: Evolutionary Psychology and Everyday Life*. New York: Vintage Books.

Young, I. M. 1991. *Justice and the Politics of Difference*. Princeton, N.J.: Princeton University Press.

6

Caring for Girls and Women Who Are Considering Abortion: Rethinking Informed Consent

Diana Fritz Cates

It was an evening that I would carry with me for many years. When I arrived at Laura's, Judy was already there. The two of them had been sitting in the dimly lit living room, talking. The room seemed thick with apprehension, as if momentous words had already been spoken or were lying in wait, about to be spilled.

I had not seen Judy for a long time, so we played catch-up while Laura got some snacks and checked on the baby. As Judy and I exchanged the usual Midwestern niceties, I began instinctively to brace myself for a coming storm. When Laura returned, the niceties soon gave way to a probing emotional intensity.

Laura's eyes pulled me in. "Judy was just telling me about a difficult decision she has to make."

"I've already made the decision. There's no way that I can have a baby now." Judy hesitated and drew a difficult breath. "When I told Don that I was pregnant, he got really quiet. I was hoping that he'd be happy—that he'd be excited about starting a family—but he wasn't. He kept mumbling something about a baby not being such a good idea for us. It took a couple of days, but I managed to get him to tell me what was wrong. We've been married for a year, but this is the first time he's ever opened up to me about his family. He told me about his father—about the years of physical and emotional abuse. It was like he was trying to communicate the horror of his childhood, but without having to unleash the dreadful pain of it. I can see that he still has wounds from that abuse. And the idea of being a father himself fills him with terror. He doesn't want to be a father. He doesn't trust his instincts on this. He's not ready."

"Can't Don get some counseling to deal with his fear?" Laura pressed. "I don't see why you and he can't talk with someone about this. I mean, few people ever really feel ready to become parents. There's almost always a sense of risk and worry that you won't be strong enough or smart enough or good enough. Besides, it seems important to Don and to your marriage that Don come to terms with his past."

"I've already talked to him about that. He's willing to at least think about getting some help, but let's face it—given where he's at right now, and how deep the roots of his problem lie, and the fact that he's never had counseling before, there's little chance that he could adjust to the idea of fatherhood by the time a baby would arrive. In any case, he doesn't want to take that chance. I'm afraid that, if I were to go through with this pregnancy, I would lose Don, I mean really lose him. Our marriage would come undone, and I'd be left to raise a kid on my own. I don't want that. I can't handle it."

Laura was quick to respond. "But Judy, you told me a couple of months ago, after your dad died, that you wanted a baby more than anything else in the world. You laughed and cried about how you wanted a new life to hold, to shower with love, to fill that void in your life. You wanted a little one, and you got what you wanted. And now you want to destroy it?" It wasn't really a question.

Judy shifted in her chair. "It's not like I'm going to destroy a developed human life. The fetus is only a potential life at this point. It won't feel any pain; it'll never know the difference between being born or not being born."

The tension between Judy and Laura continued to build. "You talk about potential life as if it's just a blob of tissue. It's a potential baby, Judy. If you give it the rest of its nine months, it will be a baby, just the kind of baby that you were hoping and praying for." Tears began to stream down Laura's face. She went on and on about how much Judy had wanted a baby, how it made no sense that she could now be so sure that she didn't want this baby, how she needed to acknowledge that she got pregnant on purpose, how it didn't seem right that Don had so much influence over her choice.

Judy was becoming tearful herself and increasingly defensive. I wanted to rein Laura in somehow. I didn't know the whole story, but it was clear that Judy had wanted to see us, her friends, in order to get some support. What Laura was giving her didn't feel like support. When I suggested this to Laura, she said, "I'm sorry, but . . ." She went on, clarifying that she loved Judy and wanted to be supportive, but she had this horrible feeling that Judy hadn't really worked through her decision, and because of this, Judy was about to do something that she might regret for the rest of her life.

"Look, I'm sharing this with you because I need your support. I don't need the third degree. I've thought it through as much as I care to, and I've made my decision."

Knowing these women as well as I did, and caring for them, I could feel the power of both of their perspectives. Judy is an idealistic and sentimental person who weeps openly over beautiful and fragile things. I could imagine her gushing tearfully about having a baby. I could also hear Laura saying how wonderful it would be if Judy had a baby soon; then their children would be relatively close together in age, and Judy and Laura could share in the adventures of parenting. I could see that Laura was already grieving—and also resisting—the loss of this possibility.

At the same time, I could imagine how crushed Judy was when Don did not respond to her news as she had hoped. I felt the pull of her desperate desire to do what she could to minimize the psychological risk to Don, who was much more frail than I had realized. I knew that Judy was herself rather vulnerable, as she was still mourning her father's untimely death. I could see that she needed for us to be with her on this—to trust that she was capable of making a good choice. I imagine that she also wanted us to agree with her choice.

Yet Laura was not willing to grant that Judy had made a good choice. At least, not yet. I slowly began to figure out why. It was not simply that Laura wanted to hang on to certain possibilities for herself and her relationship with Judy; it was also that Laura was concerned about Judy's decision-making process—and the way that process reflected on Judy morally. That is to say, she was concerned about Judy's moral well-being. Laura is strikingly honest and brave when it comes to facing the most painful aspects of life. She notices when people are hiding or running from something, and she commonly wants to talk about these fears until they become workable. It seemed strange to Laura that, although Judy was upset over how the conversation was going, she did not appear to be very upset at the prospect of the abortion itself. Judy seemed to be deflecting a discussion of how it felt to conceive new life within her body, to experience the power of pregnancy, to imagine her fetus as a baby and to see herself nurturing that baby, only to have her hopes dashed. Laura suspected that Judy was deceiving herself about how much loss she was already suffering and how much more she would suffer in getting an abortion. Laura hoped that Judy would face the truth of her situation partly by acknowledging this loss.

Judy was not entirely disengaged emotionally. She was very concerned about Don's well-being. Actually, it is a mistake to speak of Judy's well-being and Don's as though the two were straightforwardly separate, as though Judy could promote or diminish Don's well-being without at the same time indirectly promoting or diminishing parts of her own well-being. When Don suffered, Judy tended spontaneously to suffer with him. When Don experienced terror at the prospect of being a father, Judy felt his terror extend into her own body, causing her own muscles to tense up and her own palms to sweat. For Laura, this was not in itself troubling. She knew this sort of intimacy in her own marriage. What *was* troubling to Laura was that Judy's co-suffering of Don's terror—her impulse to save Don and by extension herself from disaster—seemed to be dominating Judy's deliberations. There were other important goods and evils at stake. Judy needed to experience and reflect upon the relative attractiveness and repulsiveness of these other possibilities, especially the ones that affected Judy apart from Don, before she could reach a sound decision. Or so Laura thought.

To Judy, it seemed that Laura was trying to make her feel grief-stricken or guilty for destroying her fetus and her dreams for herself and that fetus, whereas Judy had decided early on, after receiving Don's reaction, to disengage emotionally from her fetus. In my view, there was something disrespectful and even violent about the way that Laura was trying to make Judy feel the way that Laura thought she should feel. It seemed cruel to insist that Judy open up a can of worms that she would probably not be able to sort through in the limited time that was available. Yet Laura's insight (quite apart from its mode of presentation) would not let go of me. I wondered whether it was a good idea for Judy to make a decision of this magnitude in what appeared to be a state of selective emotional numbness. I was gripped by the possibility that she was making a decision in the absence of relevant information that could be gleaned only by feeling (and at the same time reflecting upon) certain painful emotions.

Regarding Don's influence on her decision-making process, Judy thought that Laura underestimated the moral weight of Don's fragile psychological state. Judy agreed that she had needs of her own that deserved to be weighed in the balance, but it was clear to her that Don's need to be protected from emotional injury—and her own need to be a wife who respected her husband's limits and honored him in his acknowledged weakness—tipped the scale toward terminating the pregnancy. This made sense, but again, Laura's perspective tugged at me. Judy had always wanted to have children, and it was an immense sacrifice for her to abort this potential child; yet it appeared that she did not feel the full weight of this sacrifice. I shared Laura's worry that a part of who Judy was apart from Don (a part of her that Laura and I had known for years) had been lost in the shuffle—not deliberately sacrificed, but simply neglected.

Judy got the abortion. I never talked to her about it. I went back to school, and we gradually lost contact. Laura never talked to her about it, either. Judy never invited her to. Laura's reaction to Judy's announcement had caused a rift in their friendship. They tried for some time to mend the relationship, but they eventually drifted apart.

To this day, I am troubled by this encounter, by the question of what friendship required of Laura and me in responding to Judy. More specifically for the purposes of this essay, I remain captivated by Laura's insights into possible problems with Judy's decision-making process. Was Judy in a good position to provide an informed consent to abortion? Was she well-informed? Was she doing well in exercising her autonomy? In order to pursue these questions it is necessary to introduce the concept of informed consent as it functions within medical ethics.

INFORMED CONSENT

When Judy arrived at Planned Parenthood a few days after our conversation, she probably met with a pregnancy counselor just prior to obtaining her abortion. Such a meeting may last from 10 to 45 minutes; given institutional time constraints, it usually lasts less than 20 minutes (Brien and Fairbairn 1996, 77–78; Simonds 1996, 6; Winn 1988, 44). In that time, the counselor would record Judy's medical history and her vital signs. She would explain the procedure that Judy was about to undergo, its medical risks, the physical pain that she could expect to feel during and after it, her options for anesthesia, and so on. She would answer any questions that Judy had, and then she would ask Judy to confirm that she wanted to end her pregnancy. In sum, the counselor would have an exchange with Judy that culminated in Judy's signing one or more consent forms authorizing clinic personnel to perform an abortion (Simonds 1996, 12).

The practice of securing signatures on consent forms reflects one prominent way of thinking about informed consent. As Ruth Faden and Tom Beauchamp explain, informed consent can be construed as a "legally or institutionally *effective* . . . authorization from a patient or a subject. Such an authorization is 'effective' because it has been obtained through procedures that satisfy the rules and requirements defining a specific institutional practice in health care or in research" (Faden and Beauchamp 1986, 280). According to this understanding of the concept, Judy's signature amounted to an informed consent, not so much because it documented a particular state of mind on her part, but because it was the result of a standard disclosure procedure on the part of the clinic that most likely was adopted on the advice of counsel primarily in order to avoid legal liability (Appelbaum, Lidz, and Meisel 1987, 176–80).

It is possible that, in the process of taking her medical history and disclosing relevant medical information, the counselor also spoke with Judy about some of her social and sexual history. She may have asked whether Judy or her partner used birth control and in what form, why she was seeking an abortion, whether she had considered other options like adoption, what financial constraints she was under, who else was involved in the choice, how these other people felt or would likely feel about her decision, whether she had any special needs that the clinic could address through referral, and so on (Joffee 1986; Simonds 1991). Then again, her counselor may have chosen to avoid such questioning. At a clinic researched by Wendy Simonds, "health workers and medical staff usually did not question a client's decision to abort her pregnancy unless she took the initiative to speak of her ambivalence. Health workers saw this *lack* of interrogation as feminist; they believed that conventional abortion-clinic practice forced women to justify their decisions and placed clinic staff in the role of judgmental, and potentially condescending, authorities" (Simonds 1996, 36–37; see also Kushner 1997, 58). Nevertheless, if Judy's counselor did take the opportunity to explore Judy's state of mind, she may have done so not simply because she wanted to dot her institutional "*i*'s" or because she distrusted the authority of Judy's decision-making powers, but because she hoped to enhance Judy's experience of her own authority, as well as her sense of being cared for.

Exploring a woman's understanding of herself, her situation, the choice that she is about to make, and its possible consequences for her life can help medical care providers confirm that her signature on a consent form represents not only proper procedure, but also a specific sort of act. A second way to think about informed consent is to construe it as "an autonomous action by a subject or a patient that authorizes a professional either to involve the subject in research or to initiate a medical plan for the patient (or both)" (Faden and Beauchamp 1986, 278). An authorization constitutes an informed consent in this sense "if a patient or subject with (1) substantial understanding and (2) in substantial absence of control by others (3) intentionally (4) authorizes a professional (to do [an intervention])" (278). An interest in obtaining such an authorization typically reflects not simply a pragmatic concern to avoid litigation, but also a respect for persons' autonomy, their capacity for reflective self-governance.

This second definition of informed consent provides an excellent framework for the rest of our inquiry. It allows us to make more explicit two of the issues raised by Judy's story. First, respecting persons' autonomy requires providing them with information that is relevant and material to their decisions to undergo proposed medical interventions. It also requires taking steps to ensure that persons understand the information provided. The provision and discussion of factual information is crucial, but for many girls and women who face the intervention of abortion, moral considerations are also material to their decisions. A "substantial understanding" of an abortion and its consequences (#1 above) may include an understanding of the moral dimensions of both. Moreover, moral understanding commonly has an emotional component. For many women, feeling certain moral emotions can be partly constitutive of a substantial understanding of an abortion and its possible effects on their well-being. Making an abortion decision on the basis of this understanding can both express and enhance autonomy.

Second, most medical ethical reflection presents autonomy as a capacity whose exercise ought to be promoted by allowing and encouraging people to make their own decisions, "in substantial absence of control by others" (#2 above). The typical model of the autonomous moral agent is of the individual who has the right and the responsibility to be self-determining and thus free from coercion and manipulation by others, including those who would treat him or her merely as a means to their own ends (e.g., as a source of income) and those who, in exercising their professional authority or in caring personally for the agent, think that they know better than the agent what is in his or her best interest (Faden and Beauchamp 1986, 8). This model of autonomy is valuable in that it accounts for the need to protect individuals from abuse on the part of more powerful people and institutions. It also accounts for something that many of us (despite postmodern criticisms) are unwilling to relinquish, namely, the notion of personal moral responsibility. However, this model of autonomy does not capture the experiences that many girls and women (and, I expect, many others as well) have of being selves-in-relation whose moral agencies are properly bound up with the agencies of others. There is no doubt that girls and women can be controlled and manipulated in considering abortion. We must consider carefully, however, the sense of self that we wish to promote as we seek to protect and enhance their moral authority.

In what follows, then, I investigate first what it is to have a substantial understanding of the act of aborting one's own fetus and, accordingly, what it is to make an abortion decision partly on the basis of this understanding. The emphasis here is on the relationship between autonomy and moral understanding. I consider second what it is to deliberate and decide about abortion in the substantial absence of control by others. The emphasis in that section is on the relationship between autonomy and relationality. In each of the two main sections, I follow the same pattern of inquiry. I introduce the issue and begin an analysis of it with regard to Judy in particular. I then analyze the issue further with regard to a few other women who have shared their abortion experiences. Finally, I try to remain close to my understanding of these experiences as I extend the analysis in light of some literature of medical ethics. Attending to the experiences of a few women (and we can perforce attend to only a few) makes manifest the need to reformulate some standard theoretical insights of medical ethics that purport to apply to all people, but have not been examined with due regard to particular women.[1]

This analysis is governed by a conviction that attempting to be respectful and compassionate is a necessary condition for understanding the moral dimensions of abortion and making appropriate evaluations of particular abortion decisions. No one possesses the virtues of respect and compassion in their perfect form; and most of us are probably mistaken about the degree to which we possess them; but all who wish to render moral judgments about girls' and women's choices in the matter of abortion—and this includes girls and women themselves—are morally required to cultivate these virtues and bring them to bear, as much as possible, in their reflections. Because the following analysis seeks to draw both author and reader into the work of respect and compassion, and also because I argue that respect and compassion require certain things on the part of persons who stand in relationship to those who are considering abortion, it is necessary to indicate what I mean by respect and compassion before proceeding.

Traditionally, philosophers have thought of respect as a rational attitude of reverence regarding the power that persons have to act according to universalizable maxims and in obedience to the rational moral law (Kant 1990). Recent research has done much to correct for hyper-intellectual/hypo-emotional interpretations of this attitude (Engstrom and Whiting 1996). Still, I find it more helpful to construe the reverence that is properly felt toward persons as the expression of a virtue—a moral virtue in the Aristotelian-Thomistic sense (Cates 1997). Respect is a habit of perceiving persons as having profound moral and spiritual value, and experiencing this value on an emotional level. It is a habit of approaching people with caution, standing at moral attention before them and perhaps also at a certain moral distance from them, giving them some privacy and leeway in the exercise of their moral agencies, and thereby honoring the separate and inviolable moral space that they occupy as personal subjects. It is a habit of being stopped short in our impulses to ignore persons, dispose of them, control them, or in other ways use them as mere means to our own ends. Respect is, at the same time, a habit of receiving and responding to persons as beings who are fundamentally like us and therefore stand with us on the same moral ground. It is a habit of approaching others with a passionate interest in protecting the basic rights and responsibilities that belong to all of us simply because we are persons.

Conceived as such, the virtue of respect is closely related to the virtue of compassion. Whereas respect disposes us to perceive every person we encounter as a being who is of immeasurable and irreplaceable value, compassion disposes us to perceive every person we encounter as a being who is vulnerable, who suffers, and whose suffering ought ordinarily to be alleviated. Compassion is a habit of noticing people who are suffering and approaching them with such openness and attentiveness that we are able to experience elements of their suffering as partly our own. It is a habit of responding, partly out of the experience of co-suffering, in a way that is likely to ease the suffering. Compassion is, at the same time, a habit of discerning how not to become so engrossed in the suffering of others that we are overwhelmed and thus incapacitated in our efforts to provide help. It is a disposition to help others partly from a position of leverage outside the immediacy of the other's experience.

In what follows, I take a virtue ethics approach that considers the requirements of respect and compassion taken together. "Care," as I use the term in this chapter, refers to a synthetic unity of respect and compassion. I assume that persons do best as moral agents, and that they relate best to other persons, when they exercise both virtues. One virtue may appear to be more important than the other in a given circumstance, but both are always or almost always relevant. Persons always possess basic dignity, and they are always or almost always undergoing some form of suffering. A virtuous person consistently registers these truths (in appropriate ways) in her or his relations with other persons.[2]

AUTONOMY AND MORAL UNDERSTANDING

It was early in high school that Judy and I first became friends. Many things about her character drew me into her company and held me there. Most remarkable, perhaps, were her perceptual acuteness, her attentiveness to the details of experience, her intellectual curiosity and clarity, and the way that all of these gifts were infused with a palpable emotional intensity and honesty. Judy was someone who came across as being fully alive. She had a penchant for following fascinating but ultimately unanswerable questions. She sought to understand human beings and their relationships in all of their complexity, brokenness, and dignity. She was relentless, though not desperate, in her effort to discern what is most valuable in life, and what would make *her* life, in particular, most satisfying and worthwhile.

For Judy, to understand something of moral significance was, in part, to be moved. It was to receive an impression of how things are—and ought to be—with humans, partly in feeling and reflecting upon dull and inchoate or more vibrant and focused emotions. For Judy, and for those of us who learned so much from being with her, to understand the dignity of a person, for example, was partly to stand in awe before an unspeakable abyss that was not—and would never be—within our grasp or at our disposal. To understand the evil of murder was partly to be shaken and sickened by an unfathomable loss and by a human spirit so crushed that it could not feel this loss. To understand the good of friendship was partly to delight in pursuing with each other open-ended, character-forming inquiries into the meanings of life and love. Although Judy's emotional responses were not always on target (no one's are), I encountered in them a touchstone to moral value (see C. Taylor 1985, chaps. 1 and 2).[3]

J. Giles Milhaven identifies a way of knowing good and evil that he provocatively calls "bodily knowing" (Milhaven 1991; see also Milhaven 1993). This mode of moral knowing includes making truthful evaluative judgments, but for Milhaven, making such judgments properly involves being moved by the goods or evils at issue and thus experiencing pleasant or painful bodily reverberations. In Milhaven's view, a moral judgment tends to be incomplete, overly abstract, and untrue to human reality when it lacks an embodied emotional dimension. For example, Milhaven, who is white, explains that he long regarded racism as a serious moral evil. He sought to undermine it through personal acts and the exercise of institutional responsibilities. It was only in feeling compassion for a particular black person, however, who addressed him through the words of Martin Luther King, Jr. and whose suffering caused his stomach to sink, that Milhaven began to realize how weakly he had previously known the evil of racism. It was only in co-feeling the "horror, repulsion, longing, anger, despair, hope" of someone who, as Audre Lorde puts it, "[metabolized] hatred like a daily bread," that Milhaven began to grasp as a whole person what is evil about racism and how evil it is (Milhaven 1991, 241; see also Lorde 1984, 152).

Milhaven pursues with another example of what it is to know the good or evil of abortion. He explains that for many years he was unconditionally and vocally pro-choice:

> I thought long on the issue, discussed it with fellow ethicists, and arrived at what I believed was a sound, sensitive, moral position on abortion. However, on this issue I never listened attentively to the experience of women who had chosen to have abortions. Neither did I listen to the experience of women who, despite motives against having another child, chose not to have an abortion but to give birth. I knew nothing of the experience of women who were at peace with their choice, whichever it was. Of women who regretted their choice. Of women faced with the choice and struggling to make it. (Milhaven 1991, 239)

It was only when he listened and, as I interpret him, listened *with compassion* that he was able to let go of the security of his considered intellectual position and feel the heart-rending difficulty and ambiguity of many women's reproductive and moral lives. Only in the exercise of compassion did it dawn on him that, for many women who sought abortions, abortion was in their own judgment "a serious evil." Only in being moved by particular women who were caught up in unique and complex predicaments of pregnancy did he understand, intellectually and viscerally, that abortion can nevertheless be the best choice for many women. It was partly in sharing pain that he grasped that "there are other bad things, worse evils, that the continuation of the pregnancy can bring" (Milhaven 1991, 239).

Ordinarily, Judy's understanding of moral value was deeply and reflectively emotional. It included a bodily component that typically manifested itself in Judy's own verbal descriptions of her feeling states, as well as in altered physical movements and facial expressions, altered speech, sweating, crying, and the like. But as Laura saw things, Judy was not experiencing in a full-bodied way that the fetal life within her body was of value. She was not feeling in her flesh and bone the loss of the prospect of preserving and nurturing that life. Had Judy experienced an emotional acknowledgment of these features of the situation, she would have suffered more pain in her decision making. That in itself would have been sad, but in Laura's view, it would have been sad in a good way. Judy's decision would have been more truthful, it would have honored more of the different and competing goods at stake, had it been made partly in sadness.

Digging deeper into what was only implicit at the time, I believe that from Laura's perspective, making the abortion decision with emotional eyes wide open would have helped Judy to avoid self-deception and thereby exhibit courage; it would have allowed her to experience more respect and compassion for herself and for other women who are troubled by their abortions; it would have allowed her to cultivate many other moral virtues that grow only when one slogs through the pain of life, rather than skirting around it. One could judge Laura's perspective to be judgmental, moralistic, paternalistic, and even subtly sadistic. Indeed, on the face of it, Laura seemed to want Judy to suffer, to pay an emotional price for what she was about to do, so that the abortion would not be too simple or easy. I grant that Laura's motivations were probably mixed. The rather aggressive way in which she presented her concerns to Judy suggests that she wanted, for whatever reason, to exercise some control over Judy's emotional state. Still, I trust that compassionate motives predominated. Laura believed, on good evidence, that Judy had previously ascribed considerable value to the fetus and to the prospect of mothering the fetus, yet she was not presently admitting this value into her conscious awareness. Judy was suppressing relevant emotional information and sensation in order to make her decision more bearable. Laura could appreciate this, but she thought that it would be better for Judy to struggle with the pain up front than to make a decision that did not serve her well as a moral agent.

To anticipate subsequent formulations of this concern in terms of the discourse of medical ethics (even though Judy and Laura did not think in these terms), Laura wanted to help Judy make an informed choice, and she intuited that for Judy this would have to be an emotionally informed choice. She also wanted to help Judy make an autonomous choice, and she intuited that if Judy's choice was to be truly her own—if it was to express her capacity for reflective self-governance—then it would have to be based on a full or deep understanding of what she was about to do. An overly intellectual and emotionally flat understanding would not suffice. Laura believed that if Judy were to go through an abortion experience in the mode of a disembodied mind, Judy's ability to identify with her decision and thus take responsibility for it would be diminished.

Listening to Other Women

When one listens to other women's abortion stories, one hears many of the women raising similar concerns, after the fact, about their own decision-making processes. In particular, one encounters many women who seem to have engaged in forms of denial and self-deception. One woman, Fritzi, when questioned about her abortion experience, can hardly recall it. Eve Kushner narrates her story: " 'I don't remember,' she answers, and then laughs, 'It must have been awful.' Fritzi continues, 'I just blanked out a lot of it. It's scary,' she says of this unfamiliar behavior. She likens it to another experience: 'Sometimes if I told a little white lie, it's the same. I try to ignore it. It's something I put behind me and I don't look back at it. I separate it from myself' " (Kushner 1997, 102). Another woman, Irene, kept so busy before and after her abortion that she did not have time to think or feel about it. " 'I didn't feel it the whole time beforehand. I just laughed it off.' As the abortion occurred, however, she 'didn't feel that disconnected.' During the procedure and directly afterward, she had 'a moment of hysteria.' . . . Now, she says, thinking about 'the actual procedure' is 'the only thing that really upsets me. I don't know if it's because that's the only part I couldn't really deny,' she muses. Otherwise, Irene notes, 'I just don't feel it. I don't let myself get like that' " (Kushner 1997, 103). Similarly, Janet, who obtained an illegal abortion in a motel off of the highway recalls, "I think also that the three of us [she and her two sisters] were in a way—well, we were scared and my boyfriend was sad—I think that we were kind of afraid to really acknowledge what was going on, because I think it would have been too hard to deal with" (Hoshiko 1993, 34). Many other women feel, as they move through their abortion experiences, like they are on "automatic pilot" or "hot and numb, lost in space" (Kushner 1997, 29–30; Winn 1988, 60).

Different women experience emotions differently. Some are characteristically less inclined than others to register events on an emotional level. Moreover, different women experience the value of human fetuses differently, and for apparently good reasons (Hoshiko 1993, 82, 138; see also Kushner 1997, 82). Nevertheless, it appears to be the case that some women who go through abortions feeling very little or no emotion do so because they are unable or unwilling to acknowledge, as whole persons, the implications of what they themselves take to be true, which is that even if a human fetus is merely a *potential* person, still it is a potential *person*, who if nurtured will likely eventuate in a thinking, feeling being just like them, with a moral standing equivalent to their own.

One woman who had an abortion proclaims, " 'I think you're a cold person if it doesn't hit you. You've got a screw loose if you can do it and have no problem with it at all' " (Kushner 1997, 17). Respect and compassion require, however, recognizing that self-deception and denial are terribly common human phenomena. Few of us even notice the painful moral ambiguity that characterizes most of our actions and interactions, and few are strong enough to feel the full force of what we see. Respect and compassion also require trying to understand women's motives for shutting down emotionally. Some women are afraid to admit how much they care about the competing goods at stake because they want to make a decision that is as straightforward as possible. They want to make a "tight" choice that will not leave any loose ends dangling, undermining their peace of mind (they fear) for the rest of their lives. Especially in environments where people do not talk about their abortions, or in religious contexts where the voice of judgment and punishment predominates over that of forgiveness and mercy, or more specifically where women do not have a relationship with a divine power that helps them to shoulder the weight of their burden, it is hard for women to trust that they will find adequate emotional and spiritual support from others if they turn off the "auto-pilot" and attempt to navigate.

I take it that most women who choose abortion experience their fetuses to have *some* moral value and their abortions to have *some* moral significance. Some women who have abortions believe that their fetuses have the same status as a baby or a full grown person. But most women who have abortions believe that their fetuses have more limited moral value—a value that increases with fetal growth and development, but remains, at least for the first trimester, less or even much less than that of a baby or an adult person.

One would expect women who ascribe a significant amount of value to their fetuses, and who acknowledge this value on an emotional level, to experience *some* pain as they choose to destroy or withdraw support from this value (McDonnell 1984, chap. 2). Within the moral domain one would expect different women to experience this pain differently, depending partly on how they conceive of morality—whether in terms of human flourishing or a personal ideal, a standard of common human decency, a conception of virtue, a set of values, a sense of responsibility, a system of principles and rules, or convictions about religious or spiritual obligations or goals. In general terms, one would expect—and one finds—that women commonly experience pain in the form of grief and guilt (among other feelings) (Gardner 1986, 87–88; McDonnell 1984, chaps. 2 and 3). They experience grief and guilt as modes of registering their own (and other people's) judgments that their abortions and, in some cases, their broader life circumstances, are morally problematic.

Grief and Guilt   One woman, Wanda, has had two abortions. For years after her first one, she continued to feel occasional grief about it. She said to her partner, " 'Honey, I'm really upset about this.' He did not understand, so Wanda insisted, 'I miss it. I miss that child. I lost something.' Wanda remembers panicking and yelling, 'You don't understand. There's something gone!' She adds, 'It's like I went into the room, they gave me the anesthetic, and all of a sudden something's gone that I will never, ever get back' " (Kushner 1997, 61). Wanda coped with her grief by leading a support group for men with HIV. Kushner narrates more of Wanda's story:

> She told the members her reason for joining: "I had an abortion and I feel like there's a little part of me missing or that I took a little something away from the world." By running the group, she gave something back. In the group, Wanda came face to face with people's grief and loss, as well as her own. Although her abortion losses caused her great pain, she did not shy away from experiencing those feelings again. . . . She believes that her grief may indeed ebb someday. But, she notes, "That's not what I'm looking for." Wanda is more interested in accepting her abortions and feeling the grief they have brought than in dulling her pain. (Kushner 1997, 63)

Another woman, Dana, began to work through her grief even before she got her abortion, by establishing a relationship with her fetus. "I thought it was a girl, I had named her, and . . . I talked to her all the time. The night before [the abortion] I kind of started this process of talking to her and telling her what was going on. And telling her, asking her how she felt about it. This may sound a little strange. And she understood, and she's at peace with it, she wasn't angry. She said to me that we would meet again, and that she will come back in my life someday." During her abortion, Dana said goodbye to her fetus and then started sobbing. "And when I cried, I've never cried as deep before. It was like, the core of my being.

And it felt really good to be screaming, to cry, and just be there with all the pain" (Hoshiko 1993, 109). For Wanda and Dana, grief appears as an embodied realization that they have lost something, not only of private, personal significance, but of broader human significance. Grief provides them with access to a moral truth that they desire to know, and in light of which they desire to live—the truth about how precious or vulnerable or difficult or tragic human life is. Grief contributes to their understanding of the moral dimension of their abortions.

In addition to grief, many women feel guilt about their abortions.[4] Some feel guilt because they believe that they are killing or have killed a "child." One Catholic woman, Annika, felt guilt because, " 'There was this little life that depended on me to grow. And I was just going to toss it. The fragility and helplessness and dependency really were making it problematic for me.' " After her abortion Annika was convinced that she had violated God's will and deserved to be punished. She could not bring herself to return to church. Then one evening, "she heard 'a gentle voice.' She explains, 'It was clear to me that it was Jesus. All it said was, "Come to me." I started crying.' She fell asleep and woke up Sunday morning to find the same thing again." So she went back to church. The entire service spoke to her with the voice of forgiveness, and she was released from a lot of her guilt (Kushner 1997, 153).

Other women feel guilt because, even though they disagree with their church's stance on the morality of abortion, they cannot eradicate church teachings from their minds. Some feel brainwashed by the churches in which they were raised, and they believe that part of their spiritual task is to arrive at more autonomous judgments about their abortions. Kushner narrates the story of Abigail. After a second abortion, Abigail was overcome by the thought that God was going to punish her.

> Shocked to find herself having such thoughts, Abigail says she "had to reconsider my beliefs." She adds that she "evaluated how much I wanted to buy into a fear-driven religious system that seemed to have invaded my mind without my being conscious of it." She eventually succeeded in removing these ideas from her mind and says, "I now do not consider abortion a sin and feel sorry for those who torment themselves by that thought. I think the whole punishment ideology professed by a religious right is so manipulative and unneeded, considering everything else stressful that is caused by abortion." (Kushner 1997, 145)

Stories like these help us to realize that thoughtful, decent people disagree about the morality of abortion. People will disagree accordingly about whether guilt feelings can contribute to a sound moral understanding of one's abortion or whether, instead, they embody inauthentic, imposed-from-the-outside moral misunderstandings.

Guilt and Moral Understanding   An ad for a feminist health care clinic reads, "NO WOMAN SHOULD EVER HAVE TO FEEL GUILTY FOR HAVING AN ABORTION." Some women who have their abortions at feminist clinics do so because they believe that abortion is an act of little or no moral significance, and they want to go to a health care facility where they can count on people to agree with them. Bernice was perturbed by what she took to be pressure to feel guilty about her abortion. Workers at the clinic that she went to " 'wanted me to talk to a counselor. I was like, "No, I just need the operation. I don't have any doubts or questions. I don't need whatever you're trying to give me.' " Bernice adds, 'People at times made me feel strange because I wasn't questioning myself, because I wasn't saying, "Is it a life? Should I do this?" I was just, "I'm pregnant. I need an abortion." ' Bernice says slowly, 'I think I'm supposed to feel guilty and horrified, like I'm bad. But I don't feel that way, because what was right for me was having an abortion' " (Kushner 1997, 143).

Other women, including feminists, resent it when staff appear to white-wash the moral seriousness of abortion. Kushner presents Brittany: " 'I didn't like the way they were talking to me.' They told her, 'It's a fetus' and 'a tissue,' not 'a baby,' the term Brittany prefers. ... Smacking her hands together, she imitates how the clinic workers implied, 'There's nothing wrong with what you're doing.' She did not find their method reassuring and says, 'There wasn't really an opening for me to have an opinion. It was like, "This is the way it is." ... 'I think they were used to having to reassure people about it' " (Kushner 1997, 58). Some women report feeling chastised by feminist abortion providers for thinking that their fetuses are more than "just a collection of cells and da-da-da-da-da" (Kushner 1997, 148; see also McDonnell 1984, 34, 47). In a sense that we could finesse if we were so inclined, it may be true that no woman should ever *have* to feel guilty for having an abortion. But what if a woman already feels this way? It is more respectful and compassionate to help women who feel ambiguous or partly at fault over their abortions to explore their moral emotions with an appropriate person than to imply that they should feel stupid, immature, or even guilty (unfeminist) for feeling guilty.

Still, the matter is never simple, for there are many ways that one can go wrong in feeling guilt.[5] It is difficult to sort these out, and beyond the scope of this chapter to try. I would argue, in general terms, that it is not morally good to feel guilt over an act that is not, in one's soul-searching moral judgment, wrong. One ought not simply to dismiss communal moral standards as bogus, but neither ought one to be dominated by authorities with whom one has good reason to disagree. One ought not to feel guilt for acting in a way that one community judges to be wrong, when one has determined, through a discernment process involving members of other communities, that acting in that way is right. It should be noted, however, that most often when we do things that are right, we do things that are only *on balance* right or best. We do things that uphold one good while at the same time neglecting other goods. Feeling guilt may be a way of acknowledging the goods neglected or the morally mixed nature of a given choice; however, nearly all of our moral choices are impure in this way, and there are limits to the human ability to deal with impurity and ambiguity.

One can go wrong in feeling guilt by feeling it too often, too destructively, or for too long. We could perhaps identify a virtue that orders feelings of guilt—to use Aristotle's language, a disposition to feel it at the right times, with respect to the right acts, for the right end, in the right way, and so on (Aristotle 1985, 1106b, 17–24). Determining what constitutes the right kind and amount of guilt in a given situation is the work of practical wisdom. For religious believers it is also the work of prayer, the reception of grace, and the practice of religious virtue. All I can do here is to suggest that we ought not to dismiss feelings of guilt as always inauthentic, slavish, obsessively self-lacerating, or unproductive. Guilt feelings *can* be an indication that we have violated our own moral standards or those of a community that matters to us. We may upon reflection wish to repudiate these standards, or we may judge that it was necessary to violate one standard in order to uphold another. But the fact that we appear to have violated a standard is important information for those who seek to avoid self-deception (see G. Taylor 1985).

Many women who obtain abortions experience grief and guilt (in addition to other emotions). These are painful emotions, and most people are inclined to avoid pain. Yet many women like Wanda, Dana, Annika, and Brittany choose to face this pain. They choose to undergo the grief and guilt that arise within them, rather than trying to distract themselves from these feelings. They do so, I believe, because they intuit that something good might come of this encounter. It appears that well-formed feelings of grief and guilt can register features of an abortion event and its consequences that might otherwise be missed. Grief and guilt help some women to acknowledge what they themselves, on some level of awareness, regard as the moral import of the deliberate destruction of fetal life. Feeling these and other feelings throughout the deliberative process, and reflecting as lucidly as possible upon them, helps some women to become more transparent to themselves, more fully present to themselves in their decision making. It helps them to understand what they are doing—or have already done—on every relevant level, and thus to make decisions that are powerfully their own.

The Literature of Medical Ethics

No one that I know of has probed in their scholarship the importance that moral emotions can have for understanding one's own abortion and thus for consenting to it in a well-informed and autonomous way,[6] but my argument receives indirect support from Faden and Beauchamp. On the matter of being well-informed, they contend that "A person has a *full* or *complete* understanding of an action if there is a fully adequate apprehension of all the relevant propositions or statements (those that contribute in any way to obtaining an appreciation of the situation) that correctly describe (1) the nature of the action, and (2) the foreseeable consequences and possible outcomes that might follow as a result of performing and not performing the action" (Faden and Beauchamp 1986, 252). The authors recommend that medical professionals seek substantial, rather than complete understanding with their patients, but even substantial understanding can have a moral dimension. They refer to a patient whose understanding of a blood transfusion includes the judgment that, "If I consent to this blood transfusion I will burn in hell" (254). To extend the example, such a person's understanding of the morality of receiving another's blood may have an emotional dimension; it may include, say, a desire to honor God as the source of eternal life and a fear of being forever separated from God. To connect with the broader issue of autonomy, it seems that for such a person to make an autonomous choice about a transfusion, he or she would have to make the choice partly on the basis of his or her religious beliefs and their emotional pull, rather than irrespective of them—at least to the extent that these have been formed by rational reflection (which is admittedly a sticky issue). Otherwise the decision would be based on an incomplete grasp of what the decision means *for that person.*[7]

Becky Cox White explores further the element of "affect" as it bears on the making of informed and autonomous decisions. She argues that "Decision-making data usually include not merely facts, but how one *feels* about those facts; not merely the variety of possible outcomes, but which of those one would most prefer. One's preferences commonly count as reasons for choices, and these preferences do not come from reason alone" (White 1994, 71). White admits that emotions can be epistemologically off target, but she holds that they can also steer our attention toward what is important. They can promote "an understanding of the overall nature of one's current situation" (128). More specifically, emotions can promote understanding by signaling the extent to which a proposed intervention will likely promote one's well-being. "Persons relate present and preferred states of affairs to their well-being by paying attention to felt emotions and identifying whether or not those are preferred. If present felt emotions are not desired, they motivate persons to change their circumstances so as to acquire preferred felt emotions" (129).

It is a mistake to reduce the emotions that contribute to good human functioning to those that are "preferred," for people commonly prefer pleasant to painful emotions, even when painful emotions are the most appropriate to a situation. Moreover, White's explanation does not illuminate situations of serious moral ambiguity in which we struggle with many different emotions, on different levels, at the same time. But she is right that painful emotions *can* warn us that a proposed action may threaten our well-being. She is also right to suggest, within an academic and professional world "that demands unadulterated rationality as the basis for choices," that attending to such warnings is likely to enhance, rather than inhibit, the exercise of our autonomy (72). There is a growing consensus among philosophers, psychologists, and even scientists of the brain and of consciousness that there is no such thing as "unadulterated rationality" in humans with healthy brains, and that, even if there were, such a state would be dangerous and disabling (see Damasio 1994).

Once we admit that emotions can sometimes enhance understanding and autonomy, we are led to ask whether girls and women *ought* therefore to experience certain emotions in choosing for or against abortion. An ethic of virtue seems to require delineating the feelings that girls and women who are considering abortion ought to experience, and in what manner, in order to do well at being human and at being the particular people they are.[8] Given that most implanted human fetuses have the potential to become persons, and persons have considerable moral standing, it is prima facie morally fitting to regard developing fetuses with a degree of *something like* the respect and compassion that we extend toward persons. It is thus prima facie an indication of good human functioning to experience *some* emotional pain in choosing to end the life of a fetus. However, it is not appropriate to say categorically that a woman who feels emotionally unmoved at the thought of aborting her fetus must be in poor working order as a moral agent. Nor is it possible to specify categorically in any detail what she or any other woman ought to feel in deciding whether or not to abort. Making such judgments requires knowing a great deal about who a particular woman is, how she regards herself and the goods that are at stake for her, how she values her fetus and how she arrived at this evaluation, how she understands the responsibilities of her other relationships, and so on.

Those of us who seek answers to the problem of abortion are well-advised to start by listening to some of the people who have faced this decision. As soon as I began to ponder women's abortion stories, I found myself caring for these women to a surprising extent. I felt affection for them, and I drew close to them in my imagination, as one does with certain characters in a good novel. I extended myself into a fragment of their lives and began to glimpse their worlds partly from their perspectives, informed by their emotion-laden memories, dreams, longings, and fears. I felt their vulnerability, their need to be loved, the horror of their abusive relationships, the seductive power of their addictions and their temptations to self-hatred and suicide, the devastation of their poverty, and the constraints posed by so many other features of their lives—features that are almost never noticed, let along discussed when scholars scrutinize the morality of abortion. As I experienced all of these things, abstract ethical questions about the requirements of moral goodness slipped quietly from my mind. These questions did not cease to be of import, but their import began to re-appear in particular, personal ways, against the horizon of particular women's relational lives. It was only then, when these questions arose in relation to a whole range of other questions about the well-being of these strong and wise and fragile and injured women and the other people in their worlds, that I was in a position to reach meaningful moral insight (see Lauritzen 1994, 1998).

Some people who are duly sensitive to the painful predicaments of girls and women may nevertheless insist that there is a need to specify a principled limit beyond which it would be impossible for *anyone* to justify an abortion. I have not yet encountered a proposal for such a limit that does justice to the powerful moral claims that girls and women make on us. Some ethicists try to establish moral boundaries by reasoning about cases, beginning with those that seem the least controversial. Many scholars have appealed, for example, to Judith Jarvis Thomson's reference to a case in which abortion would be "positively indecent," namely, one in which a woman in her seventh month of pregnancy wants an abortion "just to avoid the nuisance of postponing a trip abroad" (Thomson 1997, 87). The use of such a case, however, is highly problematic. It misrepresents the kinds of moral struggles that most girls and women must undergo in order to make sense of and finally justify a course of action that will remain part of them for the rest of their lives. This is not the place to discuss the use of cases in ethics. Instead, I wish to indicate how important it is to learn the meanings that abortion can take on within particular women's lives, and to consider the ways that abortion decisions can emerge within these lives as consistent with women's own (imperfect) exercise of virtue.

To conclude this section, we ought in our reflections on the morality of abortion to be governed by, among other things, respect and compassion for girls and women. To focus on the matter of informed consent, respect and compassion require that we ponder what it is for a given woman to understand an act of abortion and its possible consequences for her life. Understanding the act may include understanding its moral dimensions, and reaching moral understanding may include feeling and reflecting upon certain moral emotions like grief and guilt. If we care about girls and women as moral agents—if we want them to have the experience of functioning well—we will care that they have the opportunity to engage such emotions in productive ways, in the company of wise and gentle people. Where women believe that fetal life has some moral value, we might help them to acknowledge this value, along with the other values that are at stake in their particular decisions, in a bodily-resonant way, in order that they might sort through these values with honesty, integrity, and growing clarity. Such sorting can both reflect and contribute to autonomy.[9]

Yet psychology and common sense provide ethics with a "reality check," for when one listens to girls and women, one finds that many are not ready or able to introduce so much emotional complexity and weight into their deliberations. Respect and compassion may sometimes require honoring the present depth—and content—of a woman's moral understanding, even if it appears to us to embody some moral misunderstanding. I propose this specifically with regard to abortion partly on account of the fact that people of good will harbor serious moral disagreements about the moral status/es of human fetuses; I would not grant the same amount of discretion to women who are considering killing a child or a grown person. In most circumstances, a commitment to moral goodness requires that appropriate people invite girls and women into shared reflection aimed at increased truthfulness. One must acknowledge, however, that the lines between helping people clarify their own beliefs and feelings, offering comments to provide perspective, seeking to persuade, and manipulating are notoriously fine.

What this means for those who work in abortion clinics is that the role of moral emotion in constituting an adequate understanding of one's abortion and, thus, in providing informed consent, ought to be taken seriously. Caring for girls and women requires attending to them as persons whose future self-understandings may depend to a significant extent on how they work through the issues surrounding their abortions. This does not mean that women who are in denial, who are laughing off their abortions in order to do what they must do but cannot bear to do—or those who still feel torn and unsettled—ought to be denied abortions because they appear unable to consent to them in a substantially informed way. It may, however, mean asking some women to meet with an additional counselor or to wait a few days. It may mean talking with them long enough to observe at least some increasing clarity and transparency in their understandings of themselves and their proposed action. Girls and women are beings with awesome moral and spiritual power and responsibility. Abortion providers ought to furnish health care that avoids, as much as possible, committing violence against girls' and women's personhood (either by denying them appropriate abortions or by providing them with inappropriate ones). Providers ought also to furnish health care that is likely to enhance girls and women's overall well-being.

AUTONOMY AND RELATIONALITY

The Judy that I knew at 25 was like a lot of people whose senses of self are fundamentally relational. She lived most of the unfolding moments of her life in more or less vague awareness of the imagined or real perspectives, thoughts, desires, and feelings of others, and she experienced the world partly as these contributions led her to experience it. Her mental-emotional life comprised a kind of community, the many members of which existed both as individuals outside of her and as resonant voices within her memory and imagination. Generally they remained at the periphery of her consciousness until their contribution became relevant. Then they would enter into her perceiving, thinking, or feeling, sometimes gently, sometimes naggingly, sometimes as strangers or well-known enemies, and sometimes as welcome familiars. Contributors to this conversation offered opinions, gave advice, moved Judy, delighted and saddened her, reminded, reprimanded, and sought to shame her, engaged in serious dialogue, and provoked heated debate. Judy's own voice, the one that seemed to her to be the dominant and organizing voice at the center of the conversation, sometimes made itself known as a voice of suspicion or resistance. Sometimes it came into prominence as a desire to quiet the chatter. Sometimes Judy's voice emerged as a lavish assemblage of relevant insights from her own and others' experiences, so that this assemblage just was, for Judy, her way of encountering the world (Cates 1991, 1997; Keller 1986; C. Taylor 1989, 35–40).

Mary Midgley offers a memorable description of the sort of internal dialogue that can characterize someone's decision-making process and, indeed, can partly compose the decision maker him or herself.

> Some of us have to hold a meeting every time we want to do something only slightly difficult, in order to find the self who is capable of undertaking it. We often fail, and have to make do with an understudy who is plainly not up to the job. We spend a lot of time and ingenuity on developing ways of organizing the inner crowd, securing consent among it, and arranging for it to act as a whole. (Midgley 1986, 122–23)

Midgley anticipates that some readers will think that people who live within this sort of inner conversation are "dotty." She insists, however, that "When real difficulties arise, everybody becomes conscious of [some such dialogue], and has what is recognizably the same sort of trouble. There are then actually advantages in being used to it" (Midgley 1986, 123).

Judy's inner life appeared to me to be well-organized. She was a series of shifting relational connections, but she was a reasonably coherent and stable series. Her life was full of affect, spontaneity, and creativity, yet it was focused and effective in the world. It had a great deal of narrative unity, even though Judy, like the rest of us, had to compose this unity day by day, especially in accounting for major challenges and disappointments. The apparent unity to Judy's character and story enticed those who loved her into an encounter with the secret behind or beneath the unity. To stand in relation to Judy was to encounter within her a mysterious, unfathomable depth, and a capacity hidden in that depth that enabled her to determine, to some extent, how the various contributions to her perceiving, thinking, and feeling assembled into her unique engagements with the world. As a Christian, Judy might have related this capacity to the workings of God's grace. It remains a mystery, in any case, how the exercise of this capacity of self-determination, this personal power, related to the causal forces that were exercised on every aspect of her moral agency by the persons and events of her past. Judy's power to be uniquely Judy presented itself as a result of, and in terms of, these contributions, yet also as something that caused these contributions to coalesce in certain ways rather than others.

There were a few people who were so important to Judy that she allowed them to play a substantial role in the constitution of her experience and, thus, in the exercise of her moral agency. (There were no doubt many others who entered more surreptitiously into her ways of perceiving, thinking, and feeling.) Her way of construing events, for example, was affected by a usually vague but sometimes acute awareness of how her parents would construe them. Judy slipped in and out of (what she imagined to be) her mother's perspective, her father's perspective, her perspective on their perspectives, and her own, separate perspective on the events themselves. Her thinking about what was going on in her encounters with other people gave weight to what her friend, Sara, had said about various relationships in the past. As Judy continued to update her opinions and evaluations, she listened to internal assertions, questions, and criticisms that seemed sometimes to be attached to Sara's voice or face but seemed, at other times, to arise and persist independently of any awareness of Sara. Judy's ways of being moved emotionally were shaped by the ways that she had observed Don being moved. She found herself wanting not only what she wanted before she fell in love with Don, but also what Don wanted, precisely because he wanted it—although it also occurred to her that Don sometimes wanted things that she did not experience to be good for her or for him, which is to say that her own, separate desires created resistance. It is artificial to divide things up like this, as if each person influenced only one aspect of Judy's agency, but this provides an initial glimpse into what it is to function as an extended self (see Cates 1991, 1997).

Judy was remarkably receptive and attuned to others, yet there was something more to her, an irreducible remainder, a power capable of noticing and altering at least some of the influences that others had on her. I wonder, looking back, if it was this unspeakable power that Laura was looking for in our conversation with Judy. Laura had the impression that Judy's way of construing the prospect of bringing her fetus to term had been virtually consumed by Don's view of the matter, as if Judy's agency had been overpowered by Don's. It was doubtful that Don had manipulated Judy into feeling that his perspective was the only one worth considering, that his needs would automatically take priority, and that Judy was confused and could not trust her own feelings about the situation; Don is too humble for that. I imagine that, from Laura's point of view, it was more likely that Judy had wanted so much to please Don and protect him from injury that, after receiving his reaction to her news, all she could see were red flags. All she could feel was Don's desire to stop this racing train (the pregnancy) or jump off as soon as possible.

It is appropriate in exercising the virtue of compassion to allow oneself to be drawn into an encounter with some of the powers that constitute another's moral agency. It is fitting to experience those powers as partly one's own. When one allows oneself to see with a common set of eyes, one perceives what the other perceives with such force that one cannot easily look away. When one reasons with a common mind, one is inclined to give the other's reasoning as much of a hearing as one ordinarily gives one's own. Some of the other's reasoning may turn out to be confused, but because it comes to mind initially through a participation in the thinking of another, it is nevertheless taken seriously and not simply dismissed. When one experiences emotions within the frame of a common body, the other's terror can cause one's own heart to pound, and one can begin to understand partly in this pounding the meaning that the terror holds for the other. Yet this is only one moment in the work of virtuous compassion. Even as one participates in the perceiving, thinking, and feeling of another, one must have access to perceptions, thoughts, and feelings that one experiences as distinctively one's own, for these are what keep the self from collapsing into the other and thus becoming ineffectual in providing perspective, comfort, and aid.

In my view, Judy retained a sense of her own separateness. She was not simply a sponge for Don's terror. She had not become, like Don, incapacitated by that terror. Rather, what she experienced in co-suffering caused her to reform the desires that were previously distinctively her own. What she originally regarded as desirable, she could no longer regard as such, knowing what would likely happen to Don, and thus by extension to her, if she were to carry her fetus to term. Here we begin to see, however, how difficult it is to understand what autonomy amounts to for selves that are constituted through reciprocal movements in and out of other selves. Judy seemed to be "free from controlling interferences by others and from personal limitations that prevent choice" (Faden and Beauchamp 1986, 8). She seemed to be free to enter into a state of co-suffering with Don in the hope of showing him compassion. Yet in her co-suffering, she shared Don's desire to flee the prospect of parenthood, and this shared desire was so compelling that one wonders if any other desire could have pulled strongly enough in any other direction to make a difference in her deliberations. At what point does the beloved's desire become a controlling influence for the lover? Many women habitually put others' needs before their own, so that they make it their business to intuit the needs of others and seek above all else to meet them. At what point does sensitivity to other people's desires compromise a person's autonomy?

What, exactly, is the capacity or the power that we are looking for when we ask someone to make an autonomous choice? One author who seeks to articulate a new paradigm for informed consent puts forward an old and familiar conception of autonomy as involving "independence," "self-direction," "rationality," and "a developed sense of self" (Switankowsky 1998, 11). When one attends to the reflections of girls and women who are pondering abortion, one finds in many of them—or perhaps one finds oneself looking for—a power that cannot quite be captured by these terms. This is a power that sets them apart from others, but reveals itself especially in the ways that they negotiate the responsibilities of their relationships. This is a power that provides direction, but mainly by functioning like a rudder through the waves of ongoing relational exchanges. This is a power to reason through what goodness requires, but in a way that is always duly impassioned, informed by emotion. This may be a power that makes it possible for someone to "decide for him/herself precisely what s/he will endure based on his/her inner self" or "core" (Switankowsky 1998, 13), but it is also a power that comes into its own through increasingly reflective interactions with others.

The power that I am pointing to is decidedly not a power to escape the influence that others have on who we are. It appears, however, that most of us have a capacity to become increasingly aware of at least some of these influences. We have a capacity to become more deliberate about how these influences shape our character and our actions. Yet even our caring about the sorts of persons that we are—even our efforts to become more aware of the factors that are forming us, and our efforts to transform ourselves in light of this awareness—occur or fail to occur to us on account of the influences of others that have accumulated since our earliest days of consciousness (Taylor 1989, 35). It is only in being with others who regard us as persons that we become persons. It is only in choosing to spend our time with persons who share our commitment to being good that we find much success in becoming more deliberately ourselves (Cates 1997). The roots of our social formation lie much deeper than is ordinarily assumed.

I must, however, leave the development of a theory of relational autonomy (and the mysteries of freedom and determination) for another occasion. In what follows, I move beyond the way that Judy's self presented itself to me—as autonomous and yet at the same time relationally constituted. I present some other women's ways of being selves-in-relation. Paying attention to the experiences of ordinary women and trying to imagine how they could become more self-governing without ceasing to share their selves intimately with others promises to help medical ethics move beyond overly simple, individualistic conceptions of autonomy.

Listening to Other Women

When one listens to a woman's abortion story, it is common to encounter a self that is composed of actual or imagined contributions from the hidden and more visible past of the woman herself, from the histories of her relationships with parents, friends, partners, and other intimates, from the anticipated looks of neighbors and strangers, from the teachings of religious figures or the convictions of religious communities, from popular media images and arguments, cultural ideologies, and more. It is common to encounter a self that gets a lot of the inspiration and direction it needs in listening and responding to this crowd, whether in feeling a surge of resistance to what is said or in recognizing an opinion as expressive of its own deepest insights. Yet one also encounters a self that struggles to establish or defend boundaries, to keep the crowd from overrunning its inmost desires and thoughts. Or one encounters a self that already has a power to engage the inner and outer crowd, at least to some extent, with a critical ear and a commanding voice.

Consider the reflections of 25-year-old Sarah, who feels "like a walking slaughter-house" as she decides in favor of a second abortion.

> Well, the pros for having the baby are all the admiration that you would get from being a single woman, alone, martyr, struggling, having the adoring love of this beautiful Gerber baby. Just more of a home life than I have had in a long time, and that basically was it, which is pretty fantasyland.

It is not very realistic. Cons against having the baby: it was going to hasten what is looking to be the inevitable end of the relationship with the man I am presently with. I was going to have to go on welfare. My parents were going to hate me for the rest of my life. I was going to lose a really good job that I have. I would lose a lot of independence. Solitude. And I would have to be put in a position of asking help from a lot of people a lot of the time. Con against having the abortion is having to face up to the guilt. And pros for having the abortion are I would be able to handle my deteriorating relation with [the father] with a lot more capability and a lot more responsibility for him and for myself. I would not have to go through the realization that for the next twenty-five years of my life I would be punishing myself for being foolish enough to get pregnant again and forcing myself to bring up a kid just because I did this. Having to face the guilt of a second abortion seemed like not exactly—well, exactly the lesser of the two evils, but also the one that would pay off for me personally in the long run because, by looking at why I am pregnant again and subsequently have decided to have a second abortion, I have to face up to some things about myself. (Gilligan 1982, 91–92)

There are many fascinating features of Sarah's description. What I wish to highlight here are the multiple, competing perspectives that eventually converge into a particular way of looking at herself and her situation that Sarah experiences to be *her* way. Sarah's perspective is relationally composed, yet there is a part of her that is beginning to make more reflective contributions to this composition. The center of her moral agency comes partially into view as a power that assesses capabilities, confronts limits—including moral limits—experiences guilt and the inclination to probe its meaning, feels a growing sense of responsibility, and makes connections between these things.

Sumi Hoshiko records a story of another woman whose mature moral agency begins to emerge only after years of painful struggle. Donna "was around a lot of drinking and fighting and arguing" from the day she was born (Hoshiko 1993, 113). Living with her mother and her mother's many boyfriends had a profound impact on Donna's power to imagine, desire, and seek a good life. "She [Donna's mother] had two other kids. I call them illegitimate, because one man, he was married, and she had a child. And the other man, he would just come by drunk and take her money and leave. But I always said I was not going to do this. And everything I said I wasn't going to do, I did it" (114). She tells of her first serious relationship:

Somehow we started living together. We had a real heavy sexual relationship. Eventually it started getting to the point where I was losing myself. I thought he was so real. . . . So then he started throwing abusive words at me and everything. But I was past the line, I was in love or whatever, because he seemed to show some consideration or compassion that I never felt before. . . . Every other weekend I was moving out. He was putting me out, we was fighting. Because he made me leave because he wanted to see another woman. And he would mess with my girlfriends and everything. And nothing never clicked, you know, why don't you leave him alone? . . . It was a destructive relationship. . . . Because the home I came from, all I know was fighting, fucking, making up. You can scratch that out. But that's what it was like. You fight this minute, you do the thing, and then you make up. I would go stay with him, so then when he would get tired of me, would send me back home to my mother. So it was just back and forth, living out of bags. (115)

Donna married this man, and the relationship continued to deteriorate. She details her spiral into drug and alcohol addiction, murderous thoughts, prostitution, and crack houses. In the midst of this horror, she discovered an unwanted pregnancy. In a way, the decision was simple for her because the pregnancy presented itself as nothing more than an inconvenience. "Insanity told me I couldn't get pregnant. But when I did get caught, it's like: Well, that's what the abortion clinic is for" (121). Yet the decision to end the pregnancy was not fully hers because at that time she was compelled in all that she did by multiple, interlocking addictions to various people, processes, and substances, and she could not quiet these controlling voices enough to consider how she, Donna, really felt about being pregnant or getting an abortion.

Donna began to turn the corner, after her abortion, when she went to live with her aunt, who introduced a different voice into Donna's self-awareness. "She was a positive woman. She said, 'Donna, go on. You can go on. You don't have to stay on at this. Set your mind.' She wouldn't down me, like my mother did. She wouldn't put her feet on me and keep washing me in it. She said, 'Today, start anew. You don't have to look back, just start now.' I really appreciate that woman today" (125). With the help of this aunt and other people who were committed to recovery, Donna began to experience within herself a power to submit to certain influences more than others, and to grow stronger in self-affirmation under these influences. She began to feel like "a real woman" who was capable of making her own decisions, most notably the decision to seek the right sort of support (126).

Drug and alcohol addiction complicate questions about autonomy, but it is important to see that this does not set Donna's story utterly apart from the stories of other women. As Donna's story reveals, addictions to abusive relationships can be part of the same tangled web. Moreover, many women who are not addicted to the men in their lives—and have relatively violence-free relationships—are nonetheless in the habit of turning to these men to tell them what to think, want, and do. Many women feel unable to say "no" to their lovers' demands for spontaneous and constraint-free sexual contact, fearing that if they refuse, these men will seek this pleasure elsewhere. The power we are looking and hoping for in those who are pondering abortion includes the power to experience the relational self as more than its relationship with one man. As Donna's story shows, however, the power to imagine one's life taking alternative relational forms may arise only under the preferred influence of yet other relationships.

A third woman, Dana, was "clear as a bell" about wanting a baby, but when she became pregnant, this clarity gave way to a kind of inner cacophany. To read her detailed account of how she arrived at her decision is to read the way that her thoughts, perceptions, and desires were formed and repeatedly reformed by reading and rereading the reactions of several people, focusing especially on her partner Jim. "That first week it was like, 'My god, first, we're not ready to have it, and Jim probably doesn't want to have it, so I'm going to have to go through an abortion. But I don't want to!' And that thought would make me ill, physically ill" (Hoshiko 1993, 104). Then Dana met with some other friends and encountered another set of perspectives. "My best friend was pregnant at the time. And she had her two-year-old. And I remember it was that day that I got support from a few people ... to not only think about not having it, but to open my mind to think about having it. I remember that day very distinctly, my thoughts shifting, opening to more possibilities" (104). After extended joint counseling, Jim and Dana decided to have the baby. "We agreed after weeks of thinking and planning, and questioning and crying, and going through our stuff. It's like I felt like we both agreed to do it, so I felt it was clean. We both believed in it, and that's the only way I would have felt good about it. Because it felt like we were doing what we wanted to be doing" (107).

But then Jim changed his mind, which was devastating for Dana. She made a decision, in anger, to have an abortion. It is as if the anger was necessary to push Jim far enough away from her to give her the moral space to make her own decision—even though her decision rested largely on the realization that Jim did not want to have a baby and she did not want to "do anything with anyone that they [didn't] want to do" (108). Dana's anger softened as she arrived at the clinic and her feelings of loss asserted themselves; it subsided further during the procedure when Jim began to cry.

> I've seen him cry before, but he was choking and gasping and sobbing. And it made me feel so good, that he was feeling some pain over it. So we were there crying together for a little while. Because we did, once, [feel] we were going to have it. So I was hoping some depth of feeling about it was there. So it was nice to see him letting himself feel it. He was also probably crying about the pain that he saw me in. I was just really glad he was crying like that; then I felt like I wasn't alone with it. (109)

It seems that Jim had considerable influence over Dana's feelings. Dana shifted from anger to grief to a sense of comfort and even satisfaction at least partly in response to what she perceived Jim to be doing and feeling. I would argue, however, that Dana's unique moral agency reveals itself, to some extent, in the form of insistent, mostly painful feelings that register within her what is really important to her, and in her desire to pay attention to these feelings. Dana appears to be most comfortable with her painful feelings when she perceives that Jim feels the same way, but she does not wait for Jim to share her feelings before feeling and attending to them herself.

Dana's relationship with Jim eventually came to an end. It is instructive to hear her final words concerning what she is discovering in her new relationship:

> You know something I'm noticing in this relationship, and comparing it? It's like I started to realize in the last couple months as we're together, how really special I am. I don't need to be with a man where I need to either convince him of anything or be tugging at . . . there's things I want, and either I'm going to be able to get them or not. Everything's a process, but being in this relationship now, I'm getting everything I want, without having to . . . it's not like I'm pulling teeth. I'm just in the relationship, enjoying it. (112)

As I interpret her, Dana is coming into the exercise of an increasingly autonomous moral agency, not only by attending to her own feelings and the moral lessons of those feelings, but also by attending more fundamentally to what she wants—apart from what the main man in her life wants. This separate, intentional desiring enables her to imagine and choose to be in a relationship in which her most important needs are affirmed and met with relative ease. She will probably still make many of the choices in her life in a way that depends on first reading the reactions of her partner and her other friends; yet she will be able to bring something more—something that is uniquely her/s—to that reading.

Every woman, indeed every person, is different in the way that she composes and understands what she calls her self. But Judy and the other women to whom we have listened have a few things in common. Their selves appear at the interstices of relationships, yet the way in which their selves appear is determined to some degree by a power (however inchoate) that is, in the final analysis, distinctly and irreducibly their own. In my view, these women and many others who have shared their stories are in the process of discovering and beginning to affirm within themselves a depth dimension that is both more and less than a power of independence. It is a power to become uniquely themselves by becoming more attentive to and careful about their ways of being in relation. These women and others are developing a power of self-direction, but this power does not present itself, as Switankowsky and others suggest, as a power to formulate and stick to "a solid, clearly known set of life plans and goals" (Switankowsky 1998, 3), if the implication is that such plans are set and adhered to independently, without also undergoing re-consideration and reformulation within the dynamics of ongoing relational exchanges. The power of self-direction presents itself more as a power to move with growing trust and confidence down a life path that unfolds day by day, in sometimes surprising ways. These women and others are discovering a power to hold relatively loosely to their selves and their plans, especially in times of crisis. Finally, these women and others are beginning to realize a practical rationality that makes them discerning decision makers and effective actors, but their reasoning is consistently informed by the insights of desire and emotion.

The Literature of Medical Ethics

Reading these women in this way, trying to envision what a mature relational autonomy would look like (on the part of men, as well as women), helps us to notice how much work has yet to be done within medical ethics to overcome individualistic conceptions of autonomy and, thus, informed consent. These conceptions have served an important function in protecting vulnerable individuals from institutional abuse, but we need a more nuanced account. The literature is beginning to move in the right direction, but it would be beneficial to pick up the pace.

Recall that an authorization amounts to an informed consent, in Faden and Beauchamp's view, "if a patient or subject with (1) substantial under-standing and (2) in substantial absence of control by others (3) intentionally (4) authorizes a professional (to do [an intervention])" (Faden and Beau-champ 1986, 278). We are presently considering what it is for a woman or a girl who experiences herself to be a relational self, with a more or less open and extensible moral agency, to make an autonomous abortion decision. In their discussion of condition (2), Faden and Beachamp focus on the absence of control by others. Autonomous acts are substantially "noncon-trolled" in the sense that they are "free of—that is, independent of, not governed by—controls on the person, especially controls presented by others that rob the person of self-directedness" (Faden and Beauchamp 1985, 256). The authors have in mind acts on the part of others that go beyond rational persuasion (which is never, in their view, substantially controlling), and take the form of coercion (which is always substantially controlling) or manipulation (which can be, but is not always substantially controlling). In an act of coercion, "one party intentionally and successfully influences an-other by presenting a credible threat of unwanted and avoidable harm so severe that the person is unable to resist acting to avoid it" (339). In an act of manipulation, one party intentionally and successfully influences another "by noncoercively altering the actual choices available to the person or by nonpersuasively altering the other's perception of those choices" (354).

We cannot explore these definitions or their implications in depth, but it is important to note that the authors' conception of "controlled" decision making reflects a picture of the other as one who is clearly separate from the self and who exercises an intentional influence on the self from a position outside of the self (256). Substantially controlled decision making proceeds on the basis of what an external "influence agent" wills for the self, rather than on the basis of what the self wills for itself, from within itself. Typical means of control are irresistible threat, intimidation, and deceit (258). Al-though this sort of controlling behavior is common and can injure women who are considering abortion, what we are concerned with in this chapter are situations in which the other may have no intention to coerce or manipu-late, yet his or her voice sounds so loudly within a woman's own thinking—his or her desires have so much pull within the frame of her extended self—that they threaten nonetheless to become substantially controlling influences. A lot more work needs to be done to clarify what it is to be partly constituted as a self by the reception of another without being controlled by the other's presence.[10]

Some authors have sought to shift the discussion of informed consent from a focus on the self *qua* separate individual to a consideration of the self *qua* relational by attending to patients as family members (Blustein 1993; Hardwig 1990; Kuczewski 1996; Nelson 1992). Much of this discussion concerns the influence that members of a patient's family can and ought to have on medical professionals and patients as treatment options are considered and decisions are made. Most helpful, I think, is the way that Mark Kuczewski shifts the question about families from that of what to do when the wishes of families and patients conflict to the more basic question of how to understand the role that families can productively have in patient decision making.

Kuczewski offers two complementary models of informed consent in which the voices of family members figure prominently. Both models construe informed consent as a process, rather than an event. The first he calls the interpretive model. According to it, "the physician and family assist the patient in interpreting her values and translating them into treatment preferences. This process model allows that the patient has relatively well-developed and stable values but stresses that they may not only be opaque to others, but can also be unclear to the patient" (Kuczewski 1996, 33). When family members help a patient to clarify his or her most important interests and values, they promote his or her self-understanding, and the greater the self-understanding, the greater the likelihood that the patient will understand substantially what a given intervention means *to him or her* (34). The second model is called the deliberative model. According to it, "the physician assists the patient by elucidating the values embodied in the different treatment options. Because the patient's values are [in this case] not fixed, the physician is free, even obligated to advocate certain values. He is helping to shape the patient's values through his recommendations" (34). The family assists the patient by helping the patient not only to clarify his or her values, but also to form new values and set new priorities in response to new possibilities that he or she could not have imagined before. "Because we discover our values in dialogue with those closest to us, the family is naturally an integral part of this process" (34). Once we recognize that medical professionals and patients' family members can play a significant role in patient decision making, and once we begin to encourage this role, we must face the dangers of coercion and manipulation, but it is not Kuczewski's intention to explore these problems (35).

The pendular swing in focus from the patient as singular individual to the patient as family member can profitably be construed as part of a dialectic in our thinking about the self in which we try to appreciate both the social nature of the self, in all of its power and intricacy, and the gripping perception that the self is more than the sum of its social relationships. I am urging, as another moment within this dialectic, that we consider patients as moral agents who may also be partly constituted in and through their engagements with sexual partner/s and friends.

When it comes to making an abortion decision, many girls and women deliberate within the tension of multiple relational bonds. Because they value the experience of mutual belonging, they commonly allow their loved ones to exercise a formative influence on their ways of construing options, imagining scenarios, considering interests, and sorting through feelings that pull in different directions. To help some women make autonomous choices, one may need primarily to help them become more aware of the shape of their relational self-constitution—and more aware of what they want these selves to look like (even though they are not ultimately "in control" of the product). It can be helpful to ask them if they have discussed their decisions with the people who are most important to them and thereby to invite them to reflect on whether and why they may be privileging one perspective over another and giving more weight to certain desires than others. Where it is not possible or advisable for women to have actual discussions with relevant parties, imagined discussions can be beneficial. Being encouraged, for example, to converse with their fetuses before and after aborting them has helped many women toward greater self-awareness and autonomy (Gardner 1986).[11]

In sum, caring for girls and women who are considering abortion may involve encouraging some of them to become more conscious and discerning about the (welcome and unwelcome) ways that the people in their lives are at work inside their hearts and minds, shaping the exercise of their moral agencies. It may be impossible for certain women not to be swayed above all else by the desires of friends, lovers, or husbands. What is important, in my view, is that women be encouraged to make decisions that reflect a growing understanding of this influence and its power.

What this means for abortion providers is that there is no substitute for respect, compassion, and practical wisdom when it comes to treating girls and women in ways that are likely to enhance their autonomy and their overall well-being. Each woman is in a unique situation, the complexities of which we can only begin to appreciate, and each woman emerges out of the thick of these complexities as a unique agent. As Aristotle says, the decision regarding what, finally, to say and do rests with the perception of a fine moral agent (Aristotle 1985, 1109b22, 1126b2, 1143b5). Thinking of the cultivation of virtue as part of the point of one's work is more of a gift than a burden, in my view, but that does not mean that the work is easy.

CONCLUSION

It is not my intent to give specific treatment recommendations to abortion providers, beyond urging some clinics to spend more time with the patients in their care and to improve their abortion counseling (see Brien and Fairbairn 1996). It is my intent, rather, to ask providers, their community supporters, and the rest of us to consider carefully what it would be to provide not only technically competent abortion procedures, but sound health *care* for girls and women. Caring for a girl's or a woman's health includes caring for her as someone who must make decisions about her health. It includes caring for her as a moral agent whose health care decisions can have a profound impact on her ability to fare well as a human being. This much is implied in the growing recognition among health care providers that informed consent is more of a process than a single act. Caring for girls and women who are considering abortion includes providing them with the freedom and the opportunity to seek, not only before, but also during and after their abortions, a substantial understanding of what their abortions mean to them. It includes helping them to reach an understanding that has moral, spiritual, and emotional dimensions. Caring for girls and women also includes helping them in their decision making to emerge from the outer and inner crowd as increasingly aware, confident, deliberate, and responsible.

I am not sure, at this point, whether Judy was able to offer a substantially informed consent to her abortion, although I trust, when all is said and done, that she was. Perhaps I extend this trust as a gesture of care toward someone whose explanation of her decision was not obviously confused or deceitful, and whose complex inner life could not possibly be made transparent to me within a single evening's conversation, even though the conversation was situated within a history of friendship. Judy probably had a substantial understanding of the abortion and its likely consequences, even though her understanding was hindered by a reluctance to confront certain of the moral and emotional meanings of her abortion. And she probably made her decision in a way that was substantially uncontrolled, even though the power that Don's emotions had on her deliberations was considerable. I take it that Judy chose to allow Don's feelings to become partly her own so that she could make a decision partly out of compassion for him. It may be that in their case, within the hiddenness of their marital relationship, Don's vulnerability to psychological debilitation and even collapse really was the most significant moral consideration. In any case, I continue to find Judy's story provocative and the act of attending to it instructive. Her experience raises profound questions for all who wish to promote women's well-being.[12]

Endnotes

1 It was in reflecting on Judy's story, and then turning my attention to the stories of other women, which turned out to be in important respects like Judy's, that I first began to realize that something was lacking in traditional concepts of informed consent. To some extent, I had to employ familiar formulations of this concept from the start in order to interpret the relationship between actual women's experiences and medical ethics; yet I sought to hold on to these formulations loosely, regarding them as provisional, so that I would be able to alter aspects of them that distorted, rather than illuminated, women's experiences. My method of presentation reflects my method of inquiry.

2 I use "care" as a synthetic concept that refers to both respect and compassion much as John P. Reeder, Jr. uses "agape" as a synthetic concept that refers to both justice and care. See his essay in this volume (3–38). I am grateful to Prof. Reeder for helping me, in conversation, to shift from a deontological framework for thinking about respect to a eudemonistic one.

3 I cannot develop here an account of what it is for an emotion to be "on target," but Cates (1997) addresses the issue, primarily with respect to the emotional dimension of the virtue of compassion. Cates (1996) addresses the issue with respect to the emotion of anger. Cates (forthcoming) also offers a descriptive analysis of Thomas Aquinas's view of this issue with respect to desires for food, drink, and sexual contact (many parts of which I do not endorse). For the purpose of this chapter, I simply assume an Aristotelian-Thomistic theory of virtue and emotion, according to which determining whether or not an emotion is appropriate in a given situation is a matter of perception or discernment, and is to be arrived at through the exercise of (among other things) practical wisdom or prudence, within the context of truth-seeking and character-forming friendships and communities.

4 For a philosophical analysis of the relation between guilt and shame, see G. Taylor (1985).

5 There are also many ways that one can go wrong in trying to address another person's feelings of guilt, but I cannot discuss these.

6 John (1984) and Hursthouse (1997) are nonetheless relevant reading on this issue.

7 It is not so much authenticity that I am emphasizing here (see Faden and Beauchamp 1986, 262–68), but more the phenomenon of acting as whole person who is aware of the whole and its parts.

8 I assume that it is possible, at least some of the time, to summon the emotional dimensions of respect and compassion, and feelings of grief and guilt, when they do not arise spontaneously. This assumption rests on a theory of the emotions that I develop elsewhere (Cates 1997). I argue that emotions are best understood as intentional (object-directed) desires that are accompanied by feelings of pleasure or pain, and that emotions can often be evoked or changed by forming or re-forming the intentions that partly constitute them.

9 In my view, acknowledging significant fetal value and feeling some measure of guilt over the destruction of this value does not settle the question of whether abortion is, all things considered, morally the best course of action in a particular situation.

10 The issue of guilt, treated earlier, reappears at this point because emotions can be modes of registering other people' attitudes toward us. The goal of relational autonomy must include the achievement of emotion-laden understandings of moral matters, but *as* persons who are always more than what we take others' moral attitudes toward us to be.

11 William LaFleur, who presented a week-long seminar in 1999 at the University of Iowa on "Religion and Biomedical Ethics in Japan," has written extensively on Japanese rituals that concern the relation between women with their aborted fetuses. His work and that of several others, including Helen Hardacre, have stimulated intense debate. See LaFleur (1992), Hardacre (1997), and the several essays on this topic in the *Journal of the American Academy of Religion* 67/4 (December 1999).

12 I want to thank Thomas A. Lewis, John P. Reeder, Jr., Paul Lauritzen, Gene Outka, Ruth L. Smith, and Joan Henriksen Hellyer for helpful comments on earlier drafts of this chapter. I want also to thank Gene Outka for a 1999 seminar that he presented at the University of Iowa on "The Ethics of Love and the Problem of Abortion," as well as for the discussion surrounding that seminar.

References

Appelbaum, Paul S., Charles W. Lidz, and Alan Meisel. 1987. *Informed Consent: Legal Theory and Clinical Practice*. New York: Oxford University Press.

Aristotle. 1985. *Nicomachean Ethics*, trans. Terence Irwin. Indianapolis, Ind.: Hackett Publishing Company.

Blustein, Jeffrey. 1993. The Family in Medical Decisionmaking. *Hastings Center Report* 23/3: 6–13.

Brien, Joanna, and Ida Fairbairn. 1996. *Pregnancy and Abortion Counselling*. London: Routledge.

Cates, Diana Fritz. 1991. Toward an Ethic of Shared Selfhood. *The Annual of the Society of Christian Ethics*, ed. Diane Yeager, 249–57. Washington, D.C.: Georgetown University Press.

———. 1996. Taking Women's Experience Seriously: Thomas Aquinas and Audre Lorde on Anger. In *Aquinas and Empowerment: Classical Ethics for Ordinary Lives*, ed. G. Simon Harak, S.J., 47–88. Washington, D.C.: Georgetown University Press.

———. 1997. *Choosing to Feel: Virtue, Friendship, and Compassion for Friends.* Notre Dame, Ind.: University of Notre Dame Press.

———. forthcoming. The Virtue of Temperance. In *Essays on the Ethics of St. Thomas Aquinas*, ed. Stephen J. Pope. Washington, D.C.: Georgetown University Press.

Damasio, Antonio R. 1994. *Descartes' Error: Emotion, Reason, and the Human Brain.* New York: G. P. Putnam.

Engstrom, Stephen, and Jennifer Whiting, eds. 1996. *Aristotle, Kant, and the Stoics: Rethinking Happiness and Duty.* Cambridge, U.K.: Cambridge University Press.

Faden, Ruth R., and Tom L. Beauchamp, with Nancy M. P. King. 1986. *A History and Theory of Informed Consent.* New York: Oxford University Press.

Gardner, Joy. 1986. *A Difficult Decision: A Compassionate Book About Abortion.* Trumansburg, N.Y.: The Crossing Press.

Gilligan, Carol. 1982. *In a Different Voice: Psychological Theory and Women's Development.* Cambridge, Mass.: Harvard University Press.

Hardacre, Helen. 1997. *Marketing the Menacing Fetus in Japan.* Berkeley: University of California Press.

Hardwig, John. 1990. What About the Family? *Hastings Center Report* 20/2: 5–10.

Hoshiko, Sumi. 1993. *Our Choices: Women's Personal Decisions About Abortion.* New York: The Haworth Press.

Hursthouse, Rosalind. 1997. Virtue Theory and Abortion. In *Virtue Ethics,* ed. Daniel Statman, 227–44. Washington, D.C.: Georgetown University Press.

Joffee, Carole. 1986. *The Regulation of Sexuality: Experiences of Family Planning Workers.* Philadelphia, Penn.: Temple University Press.

John, Helen J., S.N.D. 1984. Reflections on Autonomy and Abortion. In *Respect and Care in Medical Ethics,* ed. David H. Smith, 277–300. Lanham, Md.: University Press of America.

Kant, Immanuel. 1990. *Foundations of the Metaphysics of Morals,* 2d ed., revised, trans. Lewis White Beck. Englewood Cliffs, N.J.: Prentice Hall.

Keller, Catherine. 1986. *From a Broken Web: Separation, Sexism, and Self.* Boston: Beacon Press.

Kuczewski, Mark G. 1996. Reconceiving the Family: The Process of Consent in Medical Decisionmaking. *Hasting Center Report* 26/2: 30–37.

Kushner, Eve. 1997. *Experiencing Abortion: A Weaving of Women's Words*. New York: Harrington Park Press.

LaFleur, William R. 1992. *Liquid Life: Abortion and Buddhism in Japan*. Princeton, N.J.: Princeton University Press.

Lauritzen, Paul. 1994. Listening to the Different Voices: Toward a More Poetic Bioethics, in *Theological Analyses of the Clinical Encounter*, ed. Gerald P. McKenny and Jonathan R. Sande, 151–70. Dordrecht, The Netherlands: Kluwer Academic Publishers.

————. 1998. The Knowing Heart: Moral Argument and the Appeal to Experience. *Soundings* 81/1–2: 213–34.

Lorde, Audre. 1984. Eye to Eye: Black Women, Hatred, and Anger. In *Sister Outsider*, 145–75. Trumansburg, N.Y: The Crossing Press.

McDonnell, Kathleen. 1984. *Not an Easy Choice: A Feminist Re-examines Abortion*. Boston: South End Press.

Midgley, Mary. 1986. *Wickedness: A Philosophical Essay*. London: Ark Paperbacks.

Milhaven, J. Giles. 1991. Ethics and Another Knowing of Good and Evil. *The Annual of the Society of Christian Ethics*, ed. Diane Yeager, 237–48. Washington, D.C.: Georgetown University Press.

————. 1993. *Hadewijch and Her Sisters: Other Ways of Loving and Knowing*. Albany: State University of New York Press.

Nelson, James Lindemann. 1992. Taking Families Seriously. *Hastings Center Report* 22/4: 6–12.

Outka, Gene. 1999. The Ethics of Love and the Problem of Abortion. The Second Annual James C. Spaulding Memorial Lecture, Iowa City, IA, School of Religion.

Reeder, John P., Jr. 2001. Are Care and Justice Distinct Virtues? *Medicine and the Ethics of Care*, ed. Diana Fritz Cates and Paul Lauritzen, 3–38. Washington, D.C.: Georgetown University Press.

Simonds, Wendy. 1991. At an Impasse: Inside an Abortion Clinic. In *Current Research on Occupations and Professions*, vol. 6, ed. Helena Z. Lopata and Judith Levy, 99–115. Greenwich, Conn.: JAI Press.

————. 1996. *Abortion at Work: Ideology and Practice in a Feminist Clinic*. New Brunswick, N.J.: Rutgers University Press.

Switankowsky, Irene S. 1998. *A New Paradigm for Informed Consent*. Lanham, Md.: University Press of America.

Taylor, Charles. 1985. *Human Agency and Language: Philosophical Papers* 1. Cambridge, U.K.: Cambridge University Press.

————. 1989. *Sources of the Self: The Making of the Modern Identity*. Cambridge, Mass.: Harvard University Press.

Taylor, Gabriele. 1985. *Pride, Shame, and Guilt: Emotions of Self-Assessment*. Oxford: Clarendon Press.

Thomson, Judith Jarvis. 1997. A Defense of Abortion. In *The Problem of Abortion*, 3rd ed., ed. Susan Dwyer and Joel Feinberg, 75–87. Belmont, Calif.: Wadsworth.

White, Becky Cox. 1994. *Competence to Consent*. Washington, D.C.: Georgetown University Press.

Winn, Denise. 1988. *Experiences of Abortion*. London: Macdonald Optima.

PART III

CARE AND NARRATIVE

7

God and an Ethic of Care: On Being Immanuel

Russell B. Connors, Jr. and Chris A. Franke

The waiting room of the pediatric oncology unit at the research center is far from warm and welcoming. Nevertheless, Brenda and James are glad to be there. The place is important because of what it represents for them: their continuing hope for their daughter Allison.

From the start Brenda and James could not believe what they were told by the doctors: the headaches and seizures their two-year-old daughter had been experiencing were the result of a tumor in her brain. Because of the tumor's location, surgery was not possible; the doctors recommended chemotherapy. Brenda and James prayed that their daughter would be rescued from this terrible disease. That was nearly two years ago. For many months the symptoms had disappeared, and the tumor was stabilized and reduced in size.

Four months ago, however, the situation changed: Allison's nausea, headaches, and seizures began to recur. The tumor had begun to spread again, and this time the physicians spoke of "comfort care." There was nothing more that they could do for Allison, they explained. Brenda and James refused to give up hope. They appealed to other doctors, who suggested the possibility of enrollment in a research protocol at the university hospital. Experimental chemotherapy, they suggested, might offer some hope.

Brenda and James are fighters; they say Allison is, too. The experimental technology was an answer to their prayers. "This is not over," they insist. "She just needs more time." They now believe more than ever that these new medicines are a gift from God, and are what their daughter needs to recover. Full steam ahead.

This story dramatizes many of the issues that we will explore in this chapter. It describes a common response to medical crisis: people expect that medicine will save their loved one. Brenda and James have put their faith in medical technology and hope that their daughter can be rescued by new medicines. When a disease is declared incurable, people often continue to hope that some miracle of medicine or some divine intervention will alter the course of the disease. We refer to this view of medicine and religion as "rescue medicine" and "rescue religion."

When Allison's doctors are unable to cure, they offer "comfort care," a sort of consolation prize awarded when medical technology fails or reaches its limits. Allison's parents reject this as inadequate. Care, in the minds of the doctors and the parents, is something to provide when "nothing more can be done."

This chapter expands the notion of what medicine and religion can and should be for those who suffer and those who provide medical care. The Bible presents an image of God that does not limit divine intervention to rescue, but envisions God also as "being there" with those who suffer, offering comfort through all stages of suffering, whatever the outcome. A biblically informed ethic of care thus provides a corrective to the notion that care and comfort are mere consolation prizes when medicine and God fail to cure. We propose that competent care givers are not only technically adequate, but are also able to be present to their patients throughout all the stages of treatment. We stress the importance of viewing healing as a response to the holistic needs of those who suffer.

In the pages that follow, we first explain and compare the notions of "rescue" and of "being there" as two different responses to suffering. We then describe what we mean by an ethic of care, after which we offer an in-depth examination of three biblical texts that illustrate our proposal about a different image of God. In that context we discuss the implications of these data for both patients and care providers.

On a personal note, as we were researching and writing this article, something occurred that dramatically altered and enhanced the process of our work. Chris discovered the evidence of an invasive cancer. Throughout the experience, from discovery to the surgery and its aftermath, as well as through the additional therapies, we had an opportunity to reflect together on what care giving could really be. Over the course of the treatment Chris shared with Russ her experiences with the surgeon, the surgery staff, and other care givers. We continued to think about and appreciate these experiences in terms of our expectations of what competent health care can and should be. This chapter relates some of these real life experiences.

IN THE PRESENCE OF SUFFERING: "RESCUE"

How do we deal with suffering? In particular, how do we respond when serious illness and the possibility of death face us, or (what may be worse) when such things face our loved ones, perhaps especially our children (Hauerwas 1990)? It seems to us—and to many others—that in the face of suffering, a variety of factors in our culture incline us to look for a way out, for rescue, indeed, for a miracle. Many of the threads in the fabric of both Judeo-Christian faith and contemporary Western medicine encourage us to look for a quick fix response to the problem of suffering (Connors and Smith 1996).

"Rescue religion" is a way of describing what has been the predominant mode of Judeo-Christian faith. In this view of things, God is the all-powerful master of the universe who sometimes intervenes directly in human affairs in order to right wrongs and ease suffering, particularly on behalf of those who live faithfully according to God's ways. Biblical evidence for this view is the spectacular intervention of God on behalf of the enslaved Israelites. God saves them from the perils of Pharaoh, leading them through the Red Sea and eventually into a land of plenty and a life of freedom. This God— the God of Brenda and James and many others—is a miracle-maker.

In the Christian dispensation, "rescue religion" is displayed by an especially strong emphasis on the divinity of Jesus of Nazareth. Jesus is the Eternal Son of God who has come down to earth to save humankind from sin and death. Many scriptural stories of the miracles of Jesus—particularly his healing of the sick and his restoration of the life of Lazarus—manifest his miraculous power. Those who believe in Jesus and follow his way believe they are able not only to share in his greatest miracle, resurrection from the dead, but also to be the recipients of Jesus' power over sickness and suffering. Jesus, the Son of God, is a miracle-maker.

In a different way, there is something about contemporary medicine that can foster similar hopes in the face of sickness and suffering. Many authors have called attention to this, often by noting that the predominant interest of medicine in our culture has been in curing, whereas attention to caring has been of lesser significance (Pellegrino and Thomasma 1997). In language that has affinities to religious faith, we speak of the miracles of modern medicine, and of drug therapies and genetic interventions that work wonders, eliminating illnesses and diseases once and for all. "Rescue medicine" is woven into the fabric of our death-denying culture. From Elizabeth Kubler-Ross to James Nuland, a host of authors have suggested that in the face of sickness and suffering we tend to look not for a way through, but for a way out (Kubler-Ross 1974; Nuland 1994). Not only for Brenda and James, but for many of us, if it is not "rescue religion" to which we have given our allegiance, it is "rescue medicine": medical marvels and miracles that we look to as our way of not simply coping with sickness and suffering, but escaping it.

IN THE PRESENCE OF SUFFERING: "BEING WITH"

Our proposal takes issue with the emphasis on "rescue religion" and "rescue medicine." Consistent with many of the elements of an ethic of care, we suggest that the ways we think about both religion and medicine be expanded, and that the expansion take the form of a shift from "rescue" to "being with."

To be sure, there are many biblical texts in which God is imaged as one who cures and saves people from dread illness, and even raises people from the dead. Elijah and Elisha in the Old Testament and Jesus in the New are depicted as curing people of terrible diseases (e.g., 2 Kings 5; John 5), and, through the power of God, even bringing people who have died back to life (e.g., 1 Kings 17: 17–24; John 11). The popular understanding of miracle seems to come from a reading of such biblical texts.

Miracle is most often understood to mean some spectacular and unexplainable (supernatural) act through which someone or some group is rescued from, taken out of, some dreadful situation. But in the Bible miracles are not limited to supernatural events. A miracle is any wonderful act that reveals something about God's purpose for people. The rainbow in the sky, for instance, is a miracle, a sign of God's covenant with humanity. A person finds water when thirsty—this is a miracle, a sign of God's loving care. Such phenomena are miraculous because they reveal God's presence.

The image of God as one who can perform spectacular, nature-suspending deeds has overshadowed another pervasive image in the biblical texts, which is that of a God who addresses the anguish of illness and death by being present with the ailing person, family, and friends. This feature of the divine image needs to be brought to the forefront because it can provide an important balance to the way that God is usually understood. God can be imagined not only as one who cures physical ailments, but also as one who heals (in a larger sense) whole persons by addressing other needs that go beyond physical illness. Physician Naomi Remens describes the reaction of hospital staff to an elderly woman who refused life-saving treatment

(Remens 1996, 201). They were outraged at her decision. No one understood her choice. Remens came to see that "the problem was that the doctors had known this woman's disease, but not the woman herself." Remens asks, "Can we know what is *best* for people, or . . . only what is best for the treatment of their diseases? Is it possible to improve someone's physical health and yet diminish their integrity?"

As we will see, the biblical name that best fits the image of the God who heals the whole person is Immanuel, God who is with us. We do not suggest that God is never a miracle-maker, that God does not cure. Rather, we propose that fundamentally God is Immanuel, and that the image of God as one who accompanies is most appropriate for an ethic of care. To explain why this is so, let us describe what we mean by an ethic of care.

AN ETHIC OF CARE

The idea that caring for one another is a good thing to do is not new. What is new, however, is the attention and analysis that caring has received as an alternative ethical pattern (Noddings 1984, 2). In his important book, *On Caring,* Milton Mayeroff describes what he calls "the basic pattern of caring":

> This, then, is the basic pattern of caring, understood as helping the other grow: I experience the other as an extension of myself and also as independent and with the need to grow; I experience the other's development as bound up with my own sense of well-being; and I feel needed by it for that growing. I respond affirmatively and with devotion to the other's need, guided by the direction of its growth. (Mayeroff 1971, 11–12)

At the beginning of *Caring: A Feminine Approach to Ethics and Moral Education*, Nel Noddings provides a similar and helpful description of the essential elements of caring. Characteristic of her emphasis on the mutuality of the caring relationship, her description is from the angle of the one-caring.

> Apprehending the other's reality, feeling what he feels as nearly as possible, is the essential part of caring from the view of the one-caring. For if I take on the other's reality as possibility and begin to feel its reality, I feel, also, that I must act accordingly; that is, I am impelled to act as though in my own behalf, but in behalf of the other. Now, of course, this feeling that I

must act may or may not be sustained. I must make a commitment to act. The commitment to act in behalf of the cared-for, a continual interest in his reality throughout the appropriate time span, and the continual renewal of commitment over this span of time are the essential elements of caring from the inner view. (Noddings 1984, 16)

Five things seem clear to us about these descriptions of caring. They capture the essentials of an ethic of care. First, caring presumes the phenomenon of being-with as a moral possibility. We take this to be very good news. Robert Bellah and colleagues may be right that a predominant characteristic of our culture's moral experience is individualism (Bellah et al. 1985), but the first presupposition of an ethic of care is that we are capable of recognizing and being with others. Our experiences are, indeed, marked by particularity, and experiences of suffering can have a devastatingly isolating effect. Even so, an ethic of care suggests that our experiences are marked by sufficient commonality that we are capable of recognizing others' experiences of need and "taking on their reality," responding in genuine human solidarity. The prayers and pleas, calls and cries of others can reach us.

A second feature of the pattern of caring is a paradox: to care is to commit oneself to the well-being of another and, in the same process, to commit oneself to one's own growth and well-being. Mayeroff does not ignore this dimension of caring, but Noddings places the paradox front and center in her analysis. Typical of a feminist approach to ethics, she stresses that there is a mutuality about the caring relationship. Although the caring relationship is not necessarily a relationship of equals, for it is commonly marked by asymmetry, it is nonetheless a relationship marked by reciprocity. The "cared-for" and the "one-caring" both stand to benefit from the experience of caring (Noddings 1984, 30–78, especially 48–49). On the road from Jerusalem to Jericho, more than one person gained from the Samaritan's caring deeds.

A third thing to note about the descriptions of the pattern of caring is the role of feeling. To care requires feeling what the other feels, as much as this is possible, and then being moved to respond. "The basic pattern" for both Mayeroff and Noddings presumes that caring involves the whole person, and that caring cannot get off the ground or be sustained without the significant involvement of our feelings. Our capacity to "apprehend the other's reality" requires that our hearts have not been hardened to the need and suffering of others. In other words, only those with a caring heart are likely even to recognize that there is someone to be cared for. Further, only those with courage are able to sustain genuinely caring activity (Mayeroff 1971, 34–35). Those making an appeal for an ethic of care are hardly the first to note the important role that the emotions need to play in the moral life, but the emphasis on the place of emotion is refreshing.

A fourth aspect of caring we see in "the pattern" is that caring is not passive or "wimpy." Mayeroff stresses that it involves "devotion" to the other; by that he means that to care, "I must commit myself to the other" (Mayeroff 1971, 10). Noddings stresses that caring requires a commitment to act on behalf of the other. In our view as well, caring should not be understood merely as being with the other in a passive manner, meeting the other and his or her situation as something that must be accepted on its present terms. Mayeroff says it this way: "The meaning of caring is not to be confused with such meanings as wishing well, liking, comforting and maintaining, or simply having an interest in what happens to the other" (Mayeroff 1971, 1). Rather, to care is to act on behalf of the other in a sustained way that may well entail strong, decisive moves to lead the other to a new place. In recent years care ethicists have stressed that caring must often include a passion to try to do something about whatever it is that is causing the other to suffer (Tanner 1996). In this manner an ethic of care is being situated more directly (and wisely, we think) within the context of feminist and liberation theologies. Extending caring into the broader social arena involves committing ourselves to the liberation of others from anything that oppresses or hinders them from the pursuit of human flourishing.

A final aspect of an ethic of care that we wish to note is emphasized by Mayeroff and presumed in the writings of Noddings: caring is a life pattern. Mayeroff stresses that caring is not simply what one is called to do, and it is more than one among other important virtues. Caring serves as a comprehensive way of ordering one's life. In his words:

> In the context of a man's life, caring has a way of ordering his other values and activities around it. When this ordering is comprehensive, because of the inclusiveness of his carings, there is a basic stability in his life; he is "in place" in the world, instead of being out of place, or merely drifting or endlessly seeking his place. Through caring for certain others, by serving them through caring, a man lives the meaning of his own life. In the sense in which a man can ever be said to be at home in the world, he is at home

not through dominating, or explaining, or appreciating, but through caring
and being cared for. (Mayeroff 1971, 2–3)

We, too, see that caring is a comprehensive way of realizing who we are
called to be and what we are called to do in this world. It is a comprehensive
way of looking at ourselves. To connect this with the renewed emphasis
on virtue ethics in recent years, to say that someone or some group is caring
is not simply to name a particular virtue; it is to name a constellation of
virtues that are ordered around a life pattern of caring. What and who it
is that we care about, and how well we sustain a life of caring is a measure
of our moral quality as persons.

A VIEW FROM THE BIBLE

In the pages that follow, we examine two biblical texts from the Hebrew
Scriptures and one from the New Testament. We focus on these three
passages because they are classic texts that relate to the question of how we
understand and image God in the face of suffering and death. People often
call upon these texts when they appeal to God as a rescuer. The book of
Job, as demonstrated by Harold Kushner, is often used when people wonder
how they should respond when faced with suffering and death (Kushner
1981). We suggest that there are other ways to understand these texts, other
ways to image God that are perhaps more fruitful and helpful to the healing
process. Following our exposition of the texts themselves, we attempt to
draw out some implications for contemporary theology within the context
of modern-day medicine. What emerges is an understanding of God that
is most compatible with an ethic of care—one that has challenging, but
also enriching implications for health care providers.

Psalm 23: Breaking Open the Text

For good reason Psalm 23 is one of the most frequently quoted texts in
the Bible. It is familiar to people of many different religions, as well as
those who have no religious persuasion. The text itself is brief, and it is
worth seeing it in its entirety.[1]

1. The Lord is my shepherd, I shall not want;
2. He makes me lie down in green pastures;
    He leads me beside still waters;

3. He restores my soul.
   He leads me in right paths for his name's sake.
4. Even though I walk in the darkest valley, I fear no evil;
   For you are with me;
   Your rod and your staff—they comfort me.
5. You prepare a table before me in the presence of my enemies;
   You anoint my head with oil; my cup overflows.
6. Surely goodness and mercy shall follow me all the days of my life,
   And I shall dwell in the house of the Lord my whole life long.

In movies, TV shows, books, and other dramatic presentations, people who are threatened by some deadly force recite the beginning words of this psalm, and when they do, we usually understand without difficulty the desperate state of the one praying. For most of us, suffering is not an abstraction. Some of us have voiced the words of Psalm 23 in our darkest hours. Let us look more closely at the text.

The psalm has wide appeal because it can be applied to a variety of situations. Note first that it can be understood as a prayer to God as rescuer. In several points in the text, the one praying asks that God restore her life (v. 3) and lead her through the "darkest valley." She asks that she be served by God in the presence of enemies (v. 5), from whom she will be rescued so that she might live a long life praising God in the temple. To paraphrase, the prayer asks that God rescue her from the dark and difficult valley and take her to "green pastures," to a different place, a better place. "Rescue me from this terrible spot, O God, and bring me to a better place." Many of us have prayed such a prayer.

Another situation in which this psalm is used today is in the funeral ritual. In this setting, God is seen not as a rescuer, but as a comforter, one who cares. At funerals, we often hear another translation of verse 4; instead of the "darkest valley," some translations, such as the King James Version, translate the Hebrew word as "the valley of the shadow of death." The text also expresses the conviction that God is the one who is present. In the face of death, the person nonetheless is aware of God's caring presence, and has need of nothing save that presence. Even in the presence of death the person fears no evil, *because you are with me*. God's shepherding presence is depicted in the symbols of the rod and staff, which function not as signs of rescue but of comfort. God's presence is meant to comfort both the person who has died and the bereft mourners. The deceased and the surviving community believe that they "will dwell in the house of the Lord" for a long time. Whether we understand this as an earthly temple or a dwelling place of God in the heavens, the sense of God's abiding presence is strong, even in the face of great evil.

Implications   Several things stand out for us as important implications of this passage. The first concerns God and how people pray. Note that for one who prays this psalm, God is affirmed both as a God of rescue and at the same time a God of comfort. Note further the connection between the two. The psalmist begins on a note of hope—that God will take the person out of this place to a new and better place. There is an unembarrassed expression of hope that God will rescue. But there is also something more, something deeper. Even if there is to be no rescue, there is a deeper expression of trust that God will be there—that God will be present in the deepest of valleys—and that God's comforting presence will be enough. The psalmist hopes that God will rescue, but at a deeper level the psalmist trusts that God will be present.

This two-fold view of who God is—sometimes a God of rescue, always a God of presence—is important for how we pray. Taking Psalm 23 as a model, we do well to pray in a both/and fashion, and not in an either/or way. It is important to present our needs before God in the hope that God's rescuing power may be made manifest, perhaps even in a dramatic way, but at the same time (we think, at a deeper level) we do well to pray for God to be present. We pray for the ability to experience God as Immanuel even in the darkest of valleys, whatever the outcome.

A second implication of this view of Psalm 23 concerns how we see the categories of cure and care in health care. Whether it is intended or not, too often when the ethic of care is discussed in medicine it has something of the feel of a consolation prize about it. When all else fails, when cure is obviously not going to happen and there is nothing else that can be done, then we must care. That is not as it should be. It is not the way suggested by Psalm 23. The most profound thing that God is for us and can do for us is to be present, to be Immanuel. At times—but not all times—God's care may manifest itself in a dramatic way, as a rescue. But whether that happens or not, Psalm 23 invites us to trust that God is always Immanuel, the one who is with us. God's care does not kick in when rescue has failed to happen. God's care is with us always.

We suggest that this is the right way to understand the relationship between curing and caring. The predominant call is for health *care* providers to do just that, to manifest genuine care for their patients by their attentiveness and responsiveness, to attempt to be with their patients in and through the dark valley of their illness and suffering. Much of what we are calling for here is captured in a patient satisfaction questionnaire that Chris received after her cancer surgery. She was asked to rank the surgeon and office staff on the following items:

> Were you satisfied with this visit?
> Was the receptionist polite and attentive to your needs?
> Were you able to schedule appointments within a reasonable time?
> Was lobby waiting time acceptable?
> Was nursing staff polite and attentive to your needs?
> Did the doctor do the following?
> • make you feel important?
> • talk down to you?
> • take enough time for you?
> • ask if you understood what was being said?
> • pay attention to what you were saying?
> • sometimes interrupt you?
> • act as though inconvenienced by talking to you?
> • seem annoyed?
> • respect your feelings?
> • answer your questions about your problem?
> • clearly explain what your troubles were?
> • tell you exactly what he planned to do next?
> • explain side effects from medicines?
> • tell why certain tests would be done?
> • explain why you should do the things he asked you to do?
> Do you feel that you can do all the things this doctor asked you to do?
> Would you ask to see this physician again?
> Would you recommend this physician to a friend?

These are good questions. They stress the importance of attentiveness and responsiveness on the part of health care professionals.

This kind of health care is the deepest and most important manifestation of care that we can offer. If it is possible to provide a cure for the patient's illness, then indeed all reasonable efforts should be made to bring that about, to help the patient move to "greener pastures." As they do in relation to God, patients look to health care providers in the hope of a cure. At times that may happen. But at a deeper level patients often look to health care professionals for something more; they look for presence, for care. This care is not a consolation prize when a cure is not forthcoming. Rather, comforting care is the deepest and most important form of health care that providers can offer.

A third implication of this view of Psalm 23 concerns who we think we are for one another, and it makes explicit what was hinted at above. Who might health care providers be for their patients? They might indeed be instruments through which the rescuing power and the consoling presence of God are made manifest. We do not wish to limit the way that God is "entitled" to be present in this world. God's power and presence are larger than our categories. Nonetheless, for people of faith, human beings are regularly experienced as the primary vehicles through which the (sometimes rescuing) power and (always consoling) presence of God is made known in this world. It is no wonder, then, that people of faith may experience God's power and presence in and through the health care providers who minister to them. That is as it should be. We do not wish to feed the monster of single-focused rescue medicine; nor do we wish to fuel the fire of perfectionism and the resulting burn out of health care providers. This is why a different version of what God provides (at times rescue; always presence) is important. It is all the more important for this faith-inspired view of health care providers. Sometimes they may make rescue happen. Always they are called to be present.

The Story of Job: Breaking Open the Text

The story of Job and his great suffering is familiar to many people—witness the best seller by Rabbi Harold Kushner, *When Bad Things Happen to Good People,* which uses the book of Job to grapple with the problem at which the title hints. People know all too well about bad things happening to good people. What many people want to know is why bad things happen. The question is most pressing when the good person is yourself or someone you love.

After breaking her hip in a bicycling accident recently, Chris received a get well letter from a student. The student said, "Maybe this is your test from God like we have been reading about; I hope this will make you even more determined to recover quickly and start training again."

A test from God—this is one of the common explanations for why bad things happen to people. It is a common interpretation of the story of Job in the Bible. God was testing Job to see whether he would be faithful. We do not believe that the details of the story of Job lend themselves easily to this interpretation (nor do we believe that this cycling accident was a test from God, "like we had been reading about" in Job!).

The story of Job can be summarized briefly as follows: In the heavens, God bets Satan that Job will be faithful to God whether or not Job has a comfortable and happy life. To win the point, God allows Satan to do every manner of evil to Job, except kill him. On earth, Job is afflicted with terrible misfortunes: death in his family, loss of all his worldly goods, and terrible disease. Job does not know about the bet between God and Satan, and he seeks an explanation for his desperate plight.

Job explores the depths of his dilemma by appealing to his friends, by sharing with them his desire to die (or his wish to have died at birth). He challenges his friends to tell him where he has gone wrong. He repeatedly asserts his desire to have a hearing before God, to present his case to God: "Let me know why you contend against me," he says (10:2), even though he has come to believe that God is not listening to him (9:16). Job is willing to wait for God to make God's presence known; he wishes that God would call so that he, Job, could answer him (14:15).

Job's friends are not helpful. They blame Job for his dilemma, and tell him that he has sinned, that he has done something wrong. They assert that God never punishes good people, but only those who do evil. They insist that Job admit his guilt and repent of his evil deeds. They urge him to call upon God, saying that God will answer his pleas. Here is the very problem that disturbs Job to the core of his being. He has been calling upon God, asking for a response to his cries for help, but God has not answered. Throughout chapters 3–42, Job bewails the fact that he is suffering unjustly. Repeatedly he asserts his desire to hear from God as to why this is happening to him. He complains that God has not answered his plaintive and pitiful cries.

Job has the opposite complaint about his friends. Their answers are all too numerous! He calls them "worthless physicians" who "whitewash with lies" (13:4). Their words are used to shore up their comfortable religious formulas about the causes of good and evil. It is easier to blame Job for his misfortunes than to admit the frightening possibility of the inadequacy of their cherished beliefs. Job recognizes that his friends are afraid of what has happened to him: "You see my calamity and you are afraid" (6:21). Job's friends cannot accept Job's experience. They cannot go into the dark and frightening unknown with him, and be with him on the deepest level of presence.

Throughout the long dialogue between Job and his friends, what Job wants most is a response from God. He is not so much interested in a cure or a return to his prior state of comfortable existence as he is in hearing God defend or explain these terrible occurrences. He wants to know that God hears, that God is there.

The conclusion of the dialogues between Job and his friends comes in chapters 38:1–42:6. God speaks to Job out of the whirlwind. In God's first long speech, God demonstrates the divine power in a rapid-fire series of rhetorical questions, and asks if Job has such power. "Can you command the morning, and set the days in place?" "Who brings rain on the land?" "Can you send forth lightnings?" "Is it by your command that the eagle soars?" Throughout this, there is a sarcastic tone to God's response to Job. "Where is the way to the origins of light and darkness? Surely you know— you were born then!" (38: 19, 21). At the end of the speech (40:1), God challenges Job saying, "Anyone who argues with God must respond."

Job's answer comes in chapter 40:3-5:

> *See*, I am of small account; what shall I answer you?
> I lay my hand on my mouth.
> I have spoken once, and will not answer;
> Twice, but I will proceed no further.

Most people interpret this as Job's pious answer to God. He is of little value or strength in the face of God's overwhelming power, and will speak no more.

Our interpretation of the meaning of Job's words differs in light of two factors: (1) the lengthy dialogues between Job and his friends, and (2) our translation of the verses. First, Job had asked repeatedly for a response from God and a chance to plead his case. He does not now suddenly give up this longed for chance to speak with God. This is his opportunity to be heard, and he begins by challenging the way God treats him.

Second, our translation of the first line differs from the New Revised Standard Version. The Hebrew can also be read as follows: "*If* I am of small account, what shall I answer you?" We then see that Job is not giving a respectful, humble answer. In these verses Job is responding to God in kind. Just as God spoke sarcastically to Job, Job now retorts, "Well, if I am of such little value, what is the point of my answering you? How can I respond to this kind of answer? I might as well shut up!" Why should Job respond at all if the meaning of God's words is to tell him that he is small and of no real value? This is not a pious assertion of Job's smallness before the awesome deity. Job is not giving up his chance to plead his case, but challenging God, in a surprisingly defiant tone, to explain further.

Indeed, God does respond to Job's challenge, not with punishment for Job's defiance, but with further explanation. God recognizes that something was amiss or lacking in the first speech, so Job gets the response he so desperately wants. God has heard him; God cares enough for Job to give him a further explanation. God tries again in a second speech, and after this, Job is satisfied. He says,

> I know that you can do all things,
> And no purpose of yours can be thwarted
> I had heard of you by the hearing of the ear,
> But now my eye sees you,
> Therefore I *despise* myself,
> And repent in dust and ashes. (42:2, 5–6)

Most readers interpret Job's second response to be a pious, self-effacing, humble admission of his smallness before a powerful deity. However, the usual translation of this passage is filled with difficulties. These difficulties are underlined above. Our own translation follows the Hebrew text closely and does not try to make Job into a pious, downcast mourner. Job does not say, "I despise myself." Most translations add "myself" to make sense of a difficult phrase. The Hebrew text simply says, "I despise." The word that is translated "despise" can also be translated "reject." What is it that Job despises or rejects? The answer is found in the next line. The Hebrew text is often translated, "I repent in dust and ashes." Sitting in dust and ashes is a common mourning activity. We know that Job has been in mourning. If we stay with this translation, it seems that Job is saying that he will mourn anew, or continue to mourn after hearing from God. Another translation is, "I repent of dust and ashes." This changes our understanding of the sense of Job's words. Our translation of the text is, "I reject and repent of dust and ashes"; that is, I have had enough of mourning. Now that Job has been made aware of God's presence and has had a chance to speak with God, he no longer needs to mourn.

Nowhere does Job ask to be healed or to have his family or possessions restored. Job wants to hear from God, to know that God is there, that God cares enough to respond. The content of the "answer" Job gets from God is admittedly problematic—an assertion of God's power and the power of creation. But it is the *fact* of the answer, the reality of the divine presence, that makes all the difference to Job. God has heard Job's anger and despair, has accepted it, and has given it legitimacy by God's very presence. God shows care for Job, and this is what matters the most.

Implications Although the story of Job's encounter with God is important for many reasons, there are two implications of the story that seem particularly important for the ethics of care, especially within the arena of medicine. Let us look more closely at the relationship between Job and his friends, and then consider how God performs in this great story.

First, Job's friends. Let us not be too hard on them. They do not have an easy time of it. How many of us have been in situations in which a friend has suffered some sort of tragedy, and now he or she cannot stop talking about it, complaining about it over and over again? Sometimes suffering can consume a person, and those nearby can find themselves bearing a good deal of the brunt of it. Further, Job's complaint is often expressed in the form of questions: Why is this happening? What have I done to deserve this? Where is God in all of this? Job may intend these to be rhetorical questions, but the friends feel a need to answer, as many of us do. In their desire to help, they provide answers to Job's questions, and they do so using the only categories they know. Despite Job's protest to the contrary, they suggest that in some way the bad things that have happened must be deserved. After all, bad things do not happen to good people, they insist. In all of this, let us not miss that the friends do show up and, at least in the beginning, they try to listen. They do not listen well enough, to be sure. They cannot hear their friend's experience; they cannot be with him in that dark and scary place from which his anger and despair come. They give too many speeches and provide too many explanations. They cannot abandon the traditional and comfortable explanations that have worked so well for them. But at least they are there.

We hope the implications for health care providers are clear. Such people, by their role and profession, often find themselves in the presence of those who are suffering. We do not mean here simply those who are experiencing pain, but, to use Eric Cassell's definition, those who find themselves in a "state of severe distress associated with events that threaten the intactness of person" (Cassell 1991a, 33). Suffering can have a devastatingly holistic nature. It can occasion distress at the deepest of levels, threatening one's identity and view of the world. As Job's friends and all experienced health care providers know, it can be difficult to be in the presence of such suffering.

What do those who suffer need? Perhaps Nicholas Wolterstorff says it best in his magnificent little book *Lament for a Son,* written after the sudden and tragic death of his son in a skiing accident: "What I need from you is that you recognize how painful it is. I need to hear from you that you are with me in my desperation. To comfort me, you have to come close. Come sit beside me on my mourning bench" (Wolterstorff 1987, 34). Arthur Frank describes his book, *The Wounded Storyteller,* as a "survival kit, put together out of my need to make sense of my own survival" (Frank 1995, xiii). He relates his own experiences with cancer and heart attack and emphasizes the need for the voice of the ill person to be heard. The sufferer is made whole in "having her own story not just be listened to but heard as if it were the listener's own story" (Frank 1995, 183). In more philosophical terms, this is what Nel Noddings suggests by saying that in caring we must "apprehend the other's reality."

This is what Job and all those who suffer need at the deepest of levels. They need others to try to enter their space, to "sit with them on the mourning bench." Health care providers, when they care most deeply, are able to do this. It involves first listening and genuinely hearing the patient in his or her suffering. Ironically, silence is often most eloquent here. Caring silence can validate the experience of the sufferer and let them know that they are taken seriously in their suffering. Then, to the extent possible, this kind of "being with" involves attempting to respond by acting on behalf of the other in a committed and consistent way. Put differently, it means "journeying" with the other, knowing that in some manner we are in this together.

Is this possible? We think it is. Chris's recent experience suggests that although it does not happen easily or automatically, such caring presence by health care providers happens with regularity, and when it does, it can have a kind of miraculous power. Here is her story about that experience.

Last summer I had a biopsy and discovered that I had an invasive cancer. I learned the results of the biopsy while I was away from home, teaching in Los Angeles. I was very upset and agitated over the news. It was necessary for me to make arrangements back home in Minneapolis for a meeting with a surgeon, and for another biopsy. Making these arrangements by phone was complicated. I had to coordinate adjustments to my teaching schedule and change airline tickets as I scheduled appointments with the surgeon. The office manager, Betty, and the nurse, Janet, were very helpful and patient with me in my agitated state, and kept calling to make changes until all arrangements were set. They were very reassuring and sympathetic. At that time, I had no idea how important these people would become to me. All I was thinking about was that I did not want to die soon!

After the mastectomy, I made many visits to the office and came to know Janet and Betty. They helped me to realize how important being present is to the healing process. At one point during this process I had had a very bad week, and was really down. I called and talked to the doctor, and after he talked to me about what I might do, he also suggested I call Janet, the nurse, the next day to see how she might help me. When I called the next morning, still in a low mood, Carol, whom I did not know, answered the phone. I identified myself and asked for Janet. Janet was not in. It was her day off. Carol suggested I talk to Elaine, whom I did not know. All of my experiences had been with Janet. What I wanted was my familiar nurse, not some stranger! I just grumbled something, said maybe I would call later, and hung up.

Five minutes later the phone rang. It was Betty, the office manager whom I had come to know well. Carol had told her about my call, and she wanted to know how I was doing and what she could do for me. Would I not like to talk with Elaine? I still did not want to talk to a stranger, so I tried to put her off, saying I would wait until Janet got back. She kept urging me to talk to Elaine. She was quite persistent, though in an understated way. Finally she said she could have Elaine call me. "Oh, well, why not?" I thought. I still was not very open to this, but Elaine did call and made a lot of good suggestions to this unhappy person at the other end of the line. The next day, I returned home after a long day, and found on my deck a huge bouquet of dahlias with an unsigned note. I knew immediately that Betty (she was an expert gardener and always had a bouquet from her garden on display to brighten up the office) had taken the time on a Saturday afternoon to deliver these flowers to me.

The best thing about this experience was that I was bombarded by this atmosphere of competent, compassionate care. Carol did not simply drop the phone call as she could have. Elaine did not drop this crabby woman on the other end of the phone. She too was persistent in trying to help. What I appreciated most from all of these people was that they were there. They knew there was a need and they wanted to help. In this office, health care means care for the whole person, body, mind, and spirit. It is much easier to heal and be healed when one is surrounded by people with such an attitude.

Let us return to the performance of God in relation to Job. In our view, God moves a bit in the story. God does not stop being God—God does not refrain from letting Job know of God's power—but God does seem genuinely moved by Job's cries of complaint and his understandably angry questions. As we have noted, God's first response to Job has a sarcastic tone to it; at least, that is how Job hears what God had said to him: "Well, if I count for so little, then what is the point of talking with you! I'll just shut up." But God is not satisfied with that. God seems touched by Job's in-kind sarcastic remark, and seems to feel that God needs to say more. That is what is significant. God does not stop being God, but in the story God is also very willing to take Job seriously, to take time for Job, to be with him enough both to listen and to respond, more than once, if need be.

What do sufferers need from those around them? What do patients need from their care providers? They need many things, of course, including technical competence. Among the other things that sufferers need is to be listened to and taken seriously. Sadly, the common complaint among patients is that their doctors (and perhaps other care providers) do not listen to them. It is frustrating and maddening to feel that one's questions have not been heard, much less responded to. This is not an argument that somehow physicians must find leisure time to chat with their patients or that they will always have things to say that their patients want to hear. Rather, it is an appeal to recognize the significance of genuine attentiveness and responsiveness (Cassell 1991b). Physicians and other health care providers have the opportunity and, we believe, the call to be nothing short of God-like in their encounters with patients. What is most striking about God's performance with Job is that God recognized God's miscommunication with Job and cared enough to try again. Health care professionals need to do the same. When they do, their patients, some of whom suffer deeply, may feel like they have been listened to and responded to by God. That is the way it is with religious faith: when we are cared for by other human beings we often feel cared for by God.

The Curing and Caring of Jesus: Breaking Open the Text

The stories of Jesus curing people from illness and disease are familiar to Christian and non-Christian audiences, believers and nonbelievers alike. Some modern-day healers claim to model their activities on the healing ministry of Jesus. Some Christians claim to have come to belief after seeing or experiencing a miracle. Non-believing skeptics challenge or even scorn such ideas, denying the reality of such miracles. Irreverent filmmakers make fun of these stories about Jesus. In varying degrees, most of us are familiar with these stories, although we may interpret them in different ways. In these pages we seek to uncover what we believe is the deep significance of the miracles and cures that the New Testament describes.

The gospels in the New Testament are filled with stories of Jesus's miracles. Mark's gospel, for instance, narrates numerous miracles in quick succession—so many that one imagines Jesus's life moving at a furious pace to accomplish works of wonder. Jesus calms the tumultuous wind and sea that threaten to break up the boat of his followers and drown them (Mk. 4: 35–41); he has power over the forces of nature. He cures a woman of a hemorrhage that she had had for many years (5:25–34); he has power over illness and disease. He drives demonic spirits out of people who are possessed (5:1-20); he has power over evil and evil spirits. He brings a little girl who had died back to life (5:21–24, 35–40); Jesus has power over death itself.

Many of these deeds, especially those involving the cure of diseases, are accompanied by Jesus's announcement that the sins of the person cured have been forgiven. The enemies of Jesus are most offended by this claim to be able to forgive sins, and they accuse him of blasphemy, of claiming to be God (Mk. 2:7). In a telling discussion with a group of religious authorities, Jesus asks them if it is easier to forgive sins or to cure people. He then explains the real reason why he cures people—not to show his power over nature or disease, but to show that he, like God, has authority to forgive sins.

Although it is true that the gospels show the power of Jesus by relating a variety of stories—calming the seas, driving out demons, curing ailments, raising people from the dead—these stories are not meant to present Jesus as a magician, someone who can do better "tricks" than others. There is a deeper significance to it all. These deeds are signs of a more enduring and potent reality that underlies what is narrated in both the Old and New Testaments. The power of Jesus is identified with the power of God, and the power of God extends beyond people's earthly lives.

The Gospel of John also speaks of the awesome deeds of Jesus. Unlike the gospel of Mark, which piles miracle upon miracle in quick succession, John's gospel contains only a few of these acts, and describes in much greater detail the underlying meaning of Jesus's healing power. John wants his audiences to know not only what Jesus did, but also the deeper significance of his actions. Readers of the gospels—especially John's—are challenged to think about how and why these events of the distant past are important to them in their own time and place.

The first part of John's gospel (chapters 1–12) is often called the Book of Signs. The signs in John's gospel include changing water into wine in

Cana (2:1–11), the healing of several people (4:46-54, 5:1–9, 9:1–41), the multiplication of loaves (6:1–14), Jesus walking on the sea (6:16–21), and the final sign, the raising of Lazarus from the dead (11:1–43). In some cases the significance of the deed is explained. The multiplication of the loaves, more than satisfying a temporary hunger, is meant to point to Jesus giving himself as the bread of life that would last forever. Jesus gives sight to a blind man (chapter 9) not so much to perform an impressive trick, but to talk about the deeper reality of looking and seeing with the eyes of faith. In other cases, the signs are left unexplained, but they are meant to catch the attention of the readers who must explore the deeper meaning for themselves.

The sign in John's gospel that illustrates most dramatically how God's presence becomes real to people in the person of Jesus is the last, raising Lazarus from the dead (11:1–43). The story in brief is as follows. Lazarus, a good friend of Jesus, becomes ill, and his sisters, Martha and Mary, also beloved friends of Jesus, tell Jesus of their brother's plight. Jesus does not immediately come to the aid of his friend, but waits several days before making the trip to Bethany, where his friends reside. Mary and Martha are now mourning. Their brother has been dead for four days.

When Jesus meets Martha on the way, she chides him: "If you had been here my brother would not have died!" She tells Jesus she believes that her brother will rise from the dead on the last days, but Jesus changes the conversation to talk about himself. "I am the resurrection and the life. Those who believe in me, even if they died, will live, and everyone who lives and believes in me will never die."

On arriving in the village, Jesus sees Mary (who chides him as her sister did) and other friends of Lazarus, all weeping. At this, Jesus is "greatly disturbed in spirit and deeply moved." He too weeps for his friend Lazarus. He then commands that the stone be removed from the tomb. Martha reacts with a very practical concern: "There is already a stench because he has been dead for four days!" Jesus reminds her of her belief, and the stone is removed.

Jesus prays aloud to his heavenly father, thanking God for always hearing him. He wants people to know that his deeds come from God, so that people will believe that God sent him. Then Jesus calls to Lazarus, who walks out of the tomb. Many come to believe in Jesus as a result, but others fear that these signs will cause such an uproar that the Romans will destroy the temple and the nation itself.

What does John want his readers to understand about Jesus? The Lazarus story suggests a number of things. First, we see that Jesus has friends. They care about him, and he cares about them. They feel free to ask for his help, and they also feel free to chide him when he does not come to their aid. Secondly, the story displays that Jesus has deep feelings, and he is not reluctant to express them, as in his weeping at the death of his friend. Thirdly, the story dramatizes Jesus's own belief in God's presence. He believes that God listens to him, and he has a sense that God can and will do good deeds for him and, through him, for others.

The story has several mysterious features. Why is it, first of all, that Jesus does not come immediately to the aid of his friend, but waits for several days before arriving on the scene? Why not come and save his friend from death and save his family from suffering and grief? Then there are those paradoxical sayings of Jesus about life and death. What does John want us to understand by sayings like, "Those who believe in me, even if they die, will live"; or, "Everyone who lives and believes in me will never die"? How does John want his audience (us) to respond to such sayings and stories?

We will not attempt to answer these questions in a complete way, but one thing seems clear. The story presumes the conviction that death—the end of life as we know it on this earth—is not the worst thing that can happen to a person. Jesus does not seem compelled to prevent his good friend from dying. Lazarus is brought back to life through the power of God made manifest in Jesus, but the earthly life that is restored to him is a temporary one. Eventually Lazarus does die. What Jesus seems driven to do is to make clear that physical death is not the end. John wants his readers to believe that those who live a life like Jesus's—a life of love and care—share the same destiny as Jesus, namely, risen and eternal life. Physical death is not the worst thing that can happen to us, the story seems to say. Life disconnected from the care and power of God, life without meaning, life without hope—that is what is really to be feared.

Implications   What we have uncovered about the curing and caring of Jesus in the New Testament is important for how we understand God in relation to an ethic of care and also for how we understand what care providers might do and who they might be for their patients. First, our reflection on the story of Jesus and Lazarus causes us to conclude that we do not do well to image God only as a rescuer. If God is only a rescuer who delivers us from suffering (and death), then God is a failure. We all die. Lazarus died. Jesus himself died. God, according to the story from John's gospel, is not driven to prevent death, but to see people through it.

This is what the author of the fourth Gospel wants us to believe, and it is the core of the Christian faith: yes, we all die; no, death is not the end. Faith in Jesus, the incarnation of the care and power of God, leads believers through death to new, risen life. God, in and through Jesus, is Immanuel, God is with us. God's care sees us through even death.

This view of God suggests to us something important for care providers in the arena of medicine. Death is not the worst thing that can happen to us. Rather, life disconnected from the powerful caring of others—suffering and dying without the attentiveness and responsiveness of others—is what must really be feared. All this is not to say, obviously, that if medical intervention can cure or at least extend life in a reasonable and qualitative manner, then such "rescuing" interventions should proceed. But rescue is not always possible. It need not be considered failure when the cancer returns, when the surgery is not successful, or when there are no more drugs or interventions that one can offer. It need not be called failure when the patient dies. Real failure—at its most devastating depth—happens when a patient's suffering goes unrecognized, when genuine human care is absent. Like Brenda and James in our opening story, many of us have come to expect rescue, and others of us too often expect to provide it. But rescue is not always a realistic expectation. Being with those who suffer, however, though a challenging expectation, is a consistently appropriate one.

A second connection we propose between the biblical story of Jesus's care for Lazarus and the care that medical professionals provide their patients concerns the affections of Jesus. Jesus is both the son of God in whom God's rescuing power is sometimes evident and, at the same time, a human being who is vulnerable enough to weep for his friend. The two are not incompatible.

What this suggests for health care providers is that the culture of modern medicine needs to change so that the human vulnerability of care providers can find appropriate expression. This is not easy. The professionalization of health care has brought with it the tendency for care providers to bracket their own feelings in regard to their patients, particularly in regard to the suffering of their patients. Some of this is both understandable and necessary. But care providers can become too good at such bracketing. At times it is important for both patients and care providers to find appropriate ways to express their feelings of love and care for one another. These relationships are, after all, human relationships. Rita Charon speaks of the need of physicians to allow their personal experiences to increase the power of their patient care and strengthen their empathic bonds (cited in Frank 1995, xii).

Without proposing that all boundaries between patients and care providers be erased, we propose that no one is well served by a health care culture in which the expression of human emotion, an essential part of care, is disallowed.

The recent experience of Chris is relevant here.

When Russ and I began to talk about writing this piece, I had no idea what was to come, how directly I would be involved with health care in the coming months. Since beginning this chapter I have undergone surgery for breast cancer, 18 weeks of chemotherapy, seven weeks of radiation therapy, and then a bicycle accident in which I broke my hip in four places. I needed implant surgery, and am still hobbling about on crutches due to a delayed union of the femur. I now think about the ethics of care from a vantage point informed by these experiences.

One of the most important factors in the healing process was my encounter with the surgeon who did the mastectomy. At our first meeting I had a hint of what would prove to be an extraordinary relationship. He came in, introduced himself to my friend (who came along to help me process all the information) and me, and then sat down. He was interested in knowing what I knew about my condition, answered our many questions, and explained (and re-explained) what could be done, and how and why. His manner was one of complete attentiveness to the two people with whom he sat. I had no sense that he was in a hurry to be on to the next patient. He didn't glance at his watch, shift around in his chair, or move to the door to indicate he was on his way to someone else. He was there for me. He told me that he considered it a privilege to be able help people in the work that he did. This seemed almost too good to be true. It was a remarkable thing for him to say, and to mean. It was a remarkable way for me to begin my relationship with this doctor, and in the following months I saw how he lived out the reality of these words. I continued to have the feeling that this physician was there for me.

When I came for the biopsy to see how extensive the cancer was, I was frantic with worry. I imagined the worst. During the course of our conversation, the surgeon not only explained what he was going to do, he began to tell me a story. It was about an experience he had while waiting for a flight that had been cancelled. I was drawn into this story and curious about the events he described. I was taken out of my immediate worry for the moment. This person is a great storyteller; he has a soothing voice and a calm demeanor that put me at ease in spite of my worries. I also wondered to myself as he spoke: Where is he going with this? What is this all about? In the end he explained that some things, like cancelled flights and diseases, are beyond our control, and that it is useless to spend time worrying about them, that worry will change nothing. One should do what one can, and spend energy on what will be fruitful. Even though the results of the biopsy were not as positive as I had hoped, I was able to take these words to heart. This was not easy. I did not like the idea that something so important was beyond my control. But I went home and threw myself into my work. To some degree I was able to keep myself from wringing my hands over the upcoming surgery by recalling his story.

After the surgery I was concerned about whether I would have the energy to go back to work. The surgeon knew that I love what I do, and he encouraged me by telling me of other women who had had similar surgeries and went right back to their work. I was energized by this, and by his positive attitude and encouragement. My appointments with this surgeon functioned as a lifeline as I healed from the surgery and adjusted to the reality of having had cancer. His office was a sanctuary for me. Before the surgery, I had wondered how I would respond to the results of the mastectomy. How would I feel about my changed body? At one point, while watching him perform a procedure, I made a comment about this. The surgeon said, "This is you." His manner was one of respect for the body in whatever condition it was. At no time did I feel ashamed or uneasy about my body or the results of the surgery.

I once asked him how it was to see the results of his work written on another person's body. He answered that he did not think of it in that way, and said, "I work on people's minds." Indeed, his dealings with me and with others had the element of care that went far beyond curing the body. We talked about the importance of support by family and friends. We talked about our beliefs. He told me of his gratitude and belief that God's providence had protected him from a number of dangerous situations that could have threatened the work that he loved, helping people as a surgeon.

He once told me that having cancer was a gift. He was right. It was an experience that transformed my life. An essential part of that transformation was the gift of having met this person who helped me through it, who taught me by what he said and did how to work through and accept life's experiences. What I learned from him also helped me through the difficulties of a badly broken hip and the prospect of having to hobble about on crutches for five months. Even more, my relationship with this remarkable person helped give deeper meaning to my life, to transform how I looked at myself, my friends and family, and the world around me. His being present with me, sitting with me, and sharing experiences with me have given me the power to be more present to myself and to the people I love. His care has also given me a certain freedom from worries about the future. Needless to say, those are important gifts.

A story told by Tolstoy seems to be a good way to conclude. A king wanted to know three things: What is the most important time? Where is the most important place to be? And who is the most important person? He received the answer from a peasant: The most important time is the present. The most important place to be is the place where you are. And the most important person is the one who stands before you. This chapter has been about care. More precisely, it has been about being-with. In our view, the most important thing that we can say about God is that God is the one who is with us; God is Immanuel. When we become aware of God's caring presence in the midst of difficulty and suffering, the experience can be transformative. God's caring presence does not fall from above. Rather, it emerges from below. God's caring and transformative presence can be glimpsed in the caring presence of our fellow human beings, including our health care providers. When a nurse or physician makes it clear that the patient is not only the most important person, but in some way the only one that matters, something awesome can happen: the caring and healing presence of God can be revealed.

Endnote

1 Except where otherwise indicated, Bible passages are cited from the New Revised Standard Version.

References

Bellah, Robert N., et. al. 1985. *Habits of the Heart: Individualism and Commitment in American Life*. New York: Harper & Row Publishers.

Cassell, Eric. 1991a. *The Nature of Suffering and the Goals of Medicine*. New York: Oxford University Press.

———. 1991b. "Recognizing Suffering." *Hastings Center Report* 21/3 (May-June): 24–31.

Connors, Russell B., Jr., and Martin L. Smith. 1996. "Religious Insistence on Medical Treatment: Christian Theology and Re-Imagination." *Hastings Center Report* 26/4 (July-August): 23–30.

Frank, Arthur. 1995. *The Wounded Storyteller: Body, Illness, and Ethics*. Chicago: University of Chicago Press.

Hauerwas, Stanley. 1990. *Naming the Silences: God, Medicine, and the Problem of Suffering*. Grand Rapids, Mich.: Eerdmans Publishing Company.

The Holy Bible. The New Revised Standard Version. 1993. Nashville, Tenn.: The Catholic Bible Press.

Kubler-Ross, Elisabeth. 1974. *On Death and Dying*. New York: Macmillan Publishing Co.

Kushner, Harold S. 1981. *When Bad Things Happen To Good People*. New York: Avon Books.

Mayeroff, Milton. 1971. *On Caring*. New York: HarperCollins Publishers.

Noddings, Nel. 1984. *Caring: A Feminine Approach to Ethics and Moral Education*. Berkeley: University of California Press.

Nuland, Stephen B. 1994. *How We Die: Reflections on Life's Final Chapter*. New York: Alfred A. Knopf.

Pellegrino, Edmund D., and David C. Thomasma. 1997. *Helping and Healing: Religious Commitment in Health Care*. Washington, D.C.: Georgetown University Press.

Remens, Naomi. 1996. *Kitchen Table Wisdom: Stories that Heal*. New York: Riverhead Books.

Tanner, Kathryn. 1996. "The Care that Does Justice." *Journal of Religious Ethics* 24/1 (spring): 171–91.

Wolterstorff, Nicholas. 1987. *Lament for a Son*. Grand Rapids, Mich.: Eerdmans Publishing Company.

8

Communities of Care, of Trust, and of Healing

Paul F. Camenisch

News of a potentially serious threat to one's well-being, to one's life, even to one's self precipitates several more or less parallel series of events. Some of these events are quite predictable and their significance generally obvious. Others can be identified and understood only in retrospect, after the frenzied period of imminent threat has passed. When the threat is a health crisis, the central events are usually thought to be the physiological events occurring in the body of the threatened one, and the responses of health care professionals to those bodily events. But a health crisis also triggers psychological and emotional, familial, economic, institutional, communal, and sometimes legal and religious responses that ought not too quickly be discounted as peripheral to the "real" events.

Looking back at my experience with coronary artery bypass graft (CABG) surgery eight years ago, I now realize that a number of events that at the time seemed secondary and peripheral to the crucial issue of the health of my heart were important factors in the healing I sought. In reflecting on those events, I have become convinced that: (1) healing, understood as becoming or being made whole again, is a much larger and more complex thing than we usually assume when we think of such sharply delineated therapies as medication or surgery; (2) much of this often ignored complexity consists in the fact that many of the ways we foster healing, the ways we help make each other whole, are communal in nature; and (3) for the kinds of communities integral to my healing—what I will call personal communities and professional/functional communities—trust is crucial to the healing enterprise.

THE SELF UNDER SIEGE

When life runs along well-worn tracks, most of us think little about the variety and number of relationships that make up the fabric of our lives.

But when some obstacle in the road suddenly throws our wheels off onto unfamiliar territory and shatters our assumptions about this journey and our control over it, we suddenly realize that we will have to supplement the resources we have relied on in ordinary times. Only by relying on others can we survive.

It was just such an obstacle I encountered on a warm May afternoon, when my cab stopped at the hospital's emergency entrance, and I was helped into a wheelchair, rolled into the emergency room, and ensconced in a curtained alcove. As I watched my wife Bonnie carry away my clothes and valuables in a plastic bag, I felt more exposed, vulnerable, and alone than I had ever felt in my life. Being stripped of my clothes was a minor thing, but with them had gone much of who I was: driver's license, credit cards, and social security card had gone with my wallet. With my twenty-five-year service watch went the only other tangible evidence of my link to my university, my profession, my CV! Sitting there alone and worried in my anonymous, short, open-backed hospital gown, I also felt at least momentarily bereft of other less tangible, but more crucial elements of who I was—my relationships with people—family and friends and colleagues—and communities which to a large extent defined who I was. I knew that all those roles and relations that made up my life, made up me, had not yet been permanently lost, but if my heart stopped . . . ? Even a temporary separation seemed bad enough, especially in a situation that was already so disorienting. Furthermore, how would all those strangers in soft green, scurrying about checking my symptoms, assessing my current discomfort, starting IV's, and hooking me up for an EKG, know about all these things, know me in the absence of those indications of who I was? How could they care for me properly if they didn't know who I was?

Some will suspect that this last question reflects my concern that I receive the treatment properly accorded a well-educated, middle- to upper-middle-class white male living in a comfortable suburb. Tragically, a number of studies do show that who one is can affect the amount and quality of care one gets (Wolf 1996). But without claiming any particular virtue on my part, I must insist that my concern that the professionals know who I was was much more complex. The sense of foreboding, of the threat that had made itself known earlier that morning when my new HMO physician had told me of the results of my thallium stress test, had slowly grown during the day. When I later sat at my desk reassuring myself that the vague discomfort in my chest was only my imagination, my fear was palpable. My father had died from his first and only heart attack when he had been just five years older than I was, as had his younger brother just a year before that. That is why I had sought out the most obviously needed resources—the expert staff and well-equipped emergency room of a 500-bed teaching hospital affiliated with a highly ranked private medical school. But those resources could meet only some dimensions of my problem. The threat I felt was a diffuse, even comprehensive one, not confined to a single organ; it was a threat that made me vulnerable on a number of levels. As I look back, I realize that some of those levels had to do with my capacity to continue being who I was, and to relate to those professionals, those strangers, as the person I had been and still was, and not as some generic coronary problem. Richard Zaner captures something of my feeling about the possibility of losing my self at that time when he writes:

> With these telling glimpses of loss and death, illness confronts the person with what and who she is, was and hopes to be, with finality. Wanting to know and wanting to be cared for are thus special appeals through which the person seeks recognition, affirmation, and appreciation of this singular person she is or hopes to be. To want to be cared for, in this deeply personal sense, is to want fundamentally to be this self in the presence of those who take care of her precisely in her vulnerability and suffering. (Zaner 1994)

Somehow, during the following pre-surgery week of tests and of waiting, my feelings of being so exposed, vulnerable, and alone diminished significantly. I came to feel elaborately, even exquisitely, supported, affirmed, and cared for, and reassured that I still was and would continue to be who I had been when I entered the emergency room. I had, in other words, begun to heal. The nature of the chemistry, of the alchemy that effected that healing transformation and put me back on the road to wholeness, even before surgery, is the subject of this essay.

KEY CONCEPTS

The concepts most basic to this experiential or bottom-up analysis are healing, care, community, and trust. I here offer what I take to be generally commonsense understandings of these terms arising from the ordinary experience of people, even if my definitions are sometimes burdened with the stilted, self-conscious language of the academy. These definitions, however, are only starting points to be tested and elaborated in the following discussion.

Healing

Given the roots of the word, it should not be startling when I suggest that our understanding of "healing" or "being healed" should begin with the idea of becoming or being made whole. The very impressive, but usually very focused and limited triumphs of highly specialized, modern medicine in healing specific illnesses, have seduced many into surrendering the larger sense of healing and wholeness that should guide any humane medicine. From the knitting up of torn tissue or broken bones, and the treating of specific lesions, we need to reclaim something like the larger sense of wholeness that the law seeks to recover for the victim of a crime as it tries to determine what is required to return the wronged one to his or her prior, pre-injury state. In this, the law goes beyond correction of or compensation for the very specific loss or injury to include elements such as the emotional harm done and the disruption of other dimensions of one's life. In both law and medicine, the precise prior state cannot be recovered when something truly irreplaceable has been lost or destroyed, such as one's sight, a limb, or a life. In such cases the closest possible approximation is sought, to which the law will then often add additional compensation. In similar cases, medicine and health care have to rely on their educative/rehabilitative function to try to bridge the gap between what was but can no longer be, and what now is. Part of this function is moving the patient toward what a friend, speaking of his daughter, born with spina bifida and learning to live with her "normal" friends, called her new or different "normal." Even when a prior condition cannot be fully restored, we know that the healing we seek must involve the maximum possible degree of autonomy, of control over our life and life-shaping decisions, and the greatest possible ability to resume or sustain our prior roles and relationships, restricted as little as possible by bodily or mental dysfunction, disability, and discomfort.

This broader view of healing as regaining wholeness does not mean that the specific medical "problem" that brings us in search of healing ceases to be important, but only that it is now put in the larger context of the patient's wholeness, where other dimensions of the patient's situation come to our attention and prompt us to consider the fuller significance of the patient's particular problem.

Care

For most of us, the idea of "care," especially when included in the phrase "medical care" or "health care," has been similarly narrowed. This, too, we need to expand. "Care," as in "caring for someone," refers on the most basic level to being well-disposed toward the one-cared-for. Caring means wishing to meet the cared-for's needs and to protect and further his or her interests. Where the means are available for doing so, caring also means carrying out those activities of protecting and furthering.

"Being well disposed toward" the one we care for is the foundation on which the other elements of care rest, and is itself a complex reality. Although it grounds all the actions that give form and shape to our care, it is itself not an action, but a disposition of the self toward the other, a disposition that is sometimes best characterized as attitudinal, and sometimes as affective. Here I mean an emphatically positive attitude toward the other.

We also need to speak of affection, or an affective orientation toward the other. Attitude may seem a bit remote to some, a bit distant, whereas affection sounds warmer and more personal, and certainly these latter are important and desirable elements. I believe we should retain both terms, attitude and affection. In most usage, affections cannot be commanded either by the agent or by another party. They seem to have a life of their own. In contrast—and this seems to be particularly important in health care professional-patient relationships—we do seem to have some control over our attitudes. We can at least work on them, and are more likely to be held responsible for them than we are for our affections. Thus, where there is neither time nor grounds for my health care professional to come to feel any affection for me, I still expect him or her to nurture a caring attitude toward all who seek care.

Clearly, then, there is an attitudinal/affective dimension of care and an actional dimension. A third dimension might be called the modal dimension, referring to how one carries out the relevant activities: with due attention, precision and deliberation—that is, care-fully—or casually, indifferently, and perfunctorily—care-lessly. This last is an important matter in many kinds of care, but it is a minor issue in this essay. Many of the puzzles about care and caring involve, I believe, the relations among these three dimensions or forms of care, the attitudinal/affective, the actional, and the modal. Most obvious, perhaps, is the question of whether one who is deficient in attitude/affection is likely to give the best actional care, and to be sufficiently careful, in the modal sense, in doing so. The relevance of these matters to many health care issues beyond the ones discussed here, including training and educating health care professionals and understanding health care professional-client relations, is too obvious to need comment here.

COMMUNITY

By community I mean here an association of persons joined not only by functional interconnections, but also by their shared commitments to each other and to certain values or certain highly valued tasks/goals. Community-constituting commitments join persons together as persons in ways that involve not only their similar technical competencies and institutional functions, but the values that make community members who they are as personal, moral, and even spiritual beings (Camenisch 1986).

The primary agents and catalysts in transforming my situation as a sick, threatened, vulnerable, and potentially lonely and isolated individual into a comforted, supported, well cared for, and already healing person were the various parties who came to my aid and support who cared for me at my time of need. Each brought a very individual and personal form of care that grew out of the carer's own identity and style, and out of the relationship between us. Crucial to my focus here, however, is the fact that these persons were not random, unassociated individuals who just happened to walk into my room, dial my phone number, or send me cards. These were people who shared with me membership in one or another community. Without in any way detracting from the uniqueness and individuality of the care offered by each person, my major concern is with the communal dimensions of the care they brought—with how their care represented and reflected the values and commitments of particular communities, how these communities were supportive of the care given, and how the care tied me back into those communities.

Kinds of Community

Two major types of community were of primary significance in my healing. One kind, represented by family, church, and friends, I will call personal communities. The second kind, represented by the health care institutions and professionals, I will call professional/functional communities. Although there are other kinds of communities, these are the kinds of most interest here. I acknowledge that the lines separating various kinds of community are not sharp and clear. For example, my own professional/functional community, the university and my academic department, has, over my thirty years in it, also become a very personal community.

One major difference between my relations to these two types of community is that I was fully a member of the personal communities prior to and independently of the health care needs that prompted me to seek out the professional/functional health care communities to which I came largely as a stranger. Whatever connections I had with them by the time I left their care, I still did not hold membership in those communities in the same full sense that I enjoyed in the personal communities. This difference was reflected partly in the fact that my relationship to the health care communities was economic to an extent not true of my relationships with the other communities.

Communities and Their Characteristic Values   Although the above differences between communities are important, they are less significant for our purposes than are the differences between the values that ground, unite, and animate the different communities, and the different kinds of care that consequently characterize each community. For many the idea of family initially refers to a shared physical basis of community—expressed in the past as kinship or blood, but increasingly thought of in terms of genetics. But considered more carefully, and certainly in relation to the issues addressed here, families are held together most fundamentally by their commitment to each other as persons. Intertwined with that commitment and supporting it is usually a complex set of other values and commitments that has some continuity across most instances of family, but which also varies from instance to instance. Major elements usually include a shared heritage, history, and tradition that helps members understand who they are and why. Also important are time spent together and shared experiences, through which current members help shape each other into the persons they are, and by which they add to the heritage and tradition they share and pass on to succeeding generations. The specific tradition or heritage members of a given family share can itself involve particular values, such as national origin, religious or political affiliation, and specific values or traits that have characterized key members of the family, such as commitment to the public good, patriotism, loyalty, and generosity. Taken together, these values and commitments are generally thought to mean that family members are committed to, value, and care for one another as total persons, in a kind of inclusive, and, as some now prefer to say, unconditional way, not predicated on or limited to specific qualities or traits possessed by a given member. Whether "family" is appropriately and helpfully applied to groups that encompass these latter elements but which lack the physical basis of family and even the formal or informal adoption procedures that in many ways can stand in the place of that basis is a complex and important question, but one which need not delay us here.

Compared to the community of family, the community of friends is more voluntary, its members being freer to cultivate or to dissolve the relationships and the commitments that bind them together. Although this may make the relations and the caring among them seem less broad and inclusive and less firmly grounded than we ideally find in most families, in genuine friendship the relations and care among the parties often approximate or even surpass those found in the family. This does not mean that friendships do not often begin with some specific and limited factor—a shared love of fishing, golf, or classical music, or even simply living next door to each other—but if that starting point does not lead to a broader, more complex relationship between the two people, then we properly speak of fishing buddies, fellow classical music fans, or next door neighbors, rather than of friends.

Ultimately, whatever values or other factors members of a family might cite as underlying their commitments to each other, and whatever shared interests initially brought friends together, if family members and friends are not finally committed to each other simply as the persons they are, then the relationship of both family and friendship have stopped short of their richest possibilities. This being linked and committed to the person of the other is part of our reason for calling these communities personal communities.

Religious communities are even more complex in their grounding and in their members' commitments to each other. In voluntary religious associations such as those that dominate in the West, most members choose to affiliate with a given religious community or to remain affiliated with one into which they were born because of its theological, ethical, or ritual tradition, rather than because of commitments to its other members. Yet given the way the tenets of most major religions claim some relevance to, if not sovereignty over, the entire person and life of the believer, members sharing a commitment to those tenets or practices and attempting to be faithful to them often find themselves involved with other members of the religious institution in ways that approximate the relations found in families and among friends. This, no doubt, is one important reason family imagery is often one of the major rubrics by which religious communities understand themselves.

Ideally, then, all three of the personal communities mentioned aspire to cultivate in their members a sort of general and inclusive care for each other. A professional/functional community, by contrast, begins with a much more focused, even narrow base. Ideally and traditionally, that base point is the professional's desire to become an agent through which a particular good is made available to the professional's clients and society at large. A real legal community, for example, is not just a group of individuals who happen to practice law and pay membership dues to a professional association, but a group that practices law in the hope of making justice more accessible to their clients and to society. Similarly, community among health care professionals arises from their shared concern about the quality of and access to health care and the benefits it can deliver, the professoriate from a similar commitment to knowledge and understanding, and the clergy from concern about spiritual well-being. Thus the ties among members of a professional community as such are related to the good that defines that profession and the skills and knowledge needed to cultivate that good. Similarly, the professional communities' initial links to laypeople who come seeking expert assistance begin with the focal or defining and thus limited good in which that profession specializes (Camenisch 1983a, 1983b). This does not mean that the relationships or the community that develops among professional colleagues, or between professionals and their clients, cannot extend beyond that focused starting point and come to encompass the entire persons of the parties involved. But at that point, I believe we need to speak also of a community of friends among the colleagues or between the professional and his or her clients.

It should be clear that, as I am using "community" here, not every person with blood relatives will be a member of a familial community, nor will every person with the requisite skills, knowledge, and license be a part of a professional community. Being a member of a community is not like being a member of a species, or simply having certain interests and skills; community membership is added to or built on these various foundations, but it is always something additional to them, something defined primarily in terms of certain kinds of values and commitments.

On most ideal understandings of family, friends, and, at least as some view them, religious communities, the care most fundamental to their self-understanding and practice is what I have called attitudinal/affective care, which is often extended to persons outside as well as inside the community. By contrast, professional/functional health care communities specialize in and are sought out because of their members' expertise in a particular form of actional care. Most of us hope that professional care will be delivered in an atmosphere of attitudinal care, but our central concern is usually the adequacy of the actions taken to care for us. To make this distinction is not to imply that personal communities care for us only attitudinally/

affectively, but it does suggest that we need to make a distinction within actional care.

Members of the professional health care community responded to me initially and primarily with the kinds of caring actions around which those communities are organized, the sort of care they are trained to deliver, and the sort I came to them to receive. This was the care that directly addressed and, we hoped, would correct what was happening in and to my body. I will call this technical care. As my stay in the hospital lengthened and my health care professionals and I became better acquainted, I believe the care among at least some of us also became attitudinal/affective. It is clear, however, that it was the technical care and their capacity to deliver it that remained at the center of our relationships, even as those relationships became supported and enriched by other forms of care.

Members of personal communities also acted out their care for me, but in ways that from the beginning addressed a wider variety of needs. Most obvious among these ways of caring were visits, phone calls, cards and flowers, offers of various kinds of assistance to my wife Bonnie and me, and, more important than it might sometimes seem, simple reminders that they were thinking about, praying for, and available to us. Although it desperately needs a better name to assure it the standing it deserves, I will call this care general personal care. It is general in several senses: it takes many different forms; all of us stand in need of some forms of this care repeatedly throughout our lives; and most of us are capable, without special training, of rendering several forms of this care. It is personal because its various forms address the many dimensions of who we are and do not focus primarily on a single, easily circumscribed dimension of us, such as the physiological. It is personal also in that it comes from and reflects the full person of the care giver, rather than reflecting primarily a single, specific, and sharply focused commitment, as is often the case in professional care.

Trust and Community

The connections among the three concepts or realities already listed—healing, care, and community—and the last one, trust, are complex and elusive. The general connection between trust and personal community can initially be rendered plausible by asking ourselves if we would speak of community among a group of people who did not trust each other. It might be possible for a small number of untrustworthy people to be included in a community, but if there were little or no trust among the members at large, it would be hard to know what "community" meant in that instance.

From the positive side, where trust, especially in important and potentially costly matters, has begun to emerge among parties, there it seems are at least the beginnings of community.

Assuming that "community" in part means shared commitments to certain values and tasks, and assuming that there is a general consensus among the members of the community about the meaning and importance of those tasks and values, and further that the commitment of most community members to those values and tasks is sincere, it would seem reasonable for members to trust one another to pursue those tasks or defend those values even at some cost, and to let those shared values guide their conduct toward and caring for each other.

I here assume a general and what I consider to be a commonsense definition of trust. However, there are many levels of trust that vary in terms of the extent or depth of one's trust, the complexity of what we mean by trust, and just what we are willing to entrust to the other. On the simplest level we may mean by trust the expectation that the one I trust will act in a situation the same way he or she has acted in similar situations in the past, so that trustworthiness may mean little more than consistency in one's patterns of action. On a somewhat deeper level, trust is my expectation that the trusted one will act according to those values that have guided him or her in the past—values which, in most of the cases that concern us here, represent the shared values of a community to which the trusting and the trusted one belong. Trust at this level introduces more flexibility or freedom of action, more *spielraum*, for the trusted one, because most such values are not articulated in precise rules. Thus I do not know exactly how a trusted one will apply a given value to a particular situation, or even to which of the several values we share he or she will give priority. An even deeper level of trust goes beyond consistency and predictability, and even beyond expectations that the trusted one will apply values we share, to trusting that person as such. At some point in our acquaintanceship—and this sort of trust surely must, in most cases, rely on extended acquaintance so that I truly know who the person I trust is—I come to trust the person to do or to have done the right/appropriate/proper thing partly by selecting which values should guide that action and determining how specific values apply to particular situations. At that point I trust the person, I trust that person's judgment or character. This leaves maximal freedom for the trusted agent to decide and act autonomously while still retaining my trust. The person may, of course, exceed the limits of that freedom and forfeit my trust. The person may do something that I can see only as a departure from or even a contradiction to the values I thought he or she held and the person I thought he or she was, and, unless that person can show me the continuity, the trust is probably gone.

Some complex medical situations would seem to require at least trust at the second level and perhaps at the third. Unfortunately, "textbook" cases are seldom met in living patients, so the surgeon who takes informed consent seriously, having encountered in an anesthetized patient something other than or in addition to the expected condition, would have to either perform a needed but unanticipated procedure, or to close up the patient, secure the patient's consent, and then subject the patient to the trauma of a second surgery, unless such a situation had been provided for. The advance provisions for such eventualities that have become routine in most hospitals clearly rest on a foundation of trust, not only trust in the surgeon to do what is needed, but more problematically, trust in the surgeon to decide what is needed, or even what this patient would most likely see as being needed. Can there be any other option for the patient than to trust the neurosurgeon who attempts to excise an acoustic neuroma that has engaged the facial nerve? The surgeon must be trusted to weigh the likelihood that the tumor will recur because of a remnant left in place against the likelihood of facial paralysis from trying too hard to remove all of the tumor. Without at least the second level of trust, the positions of both the patient and the surgeon become untenable.

None of the above implies that members of my family, my church, or my other communities are guaranteed to be trustworthy and caring in their dealings with me simply by virtue of our membership in the same community. Nevertheless, because the values and commitments that tie each of us to the community would seem at the same time to tie us to each other as members of the community, I believe that we rightly base a *prima facie* assumption of the other's trustworthiness and positive disposition toward us on our common membership. Similarly, these same facts would seem to be *prima facie* grounds for my own readiness to trust and to care for the community's other members. So fundamental is some level of trust to personal community that I would have great difficulty separating the two to see what such community would look like in the absence of trust.

Trust and Care

There is a fairly obvious link between trust and care in the attitudinal/affective sense, but it does not prevail in every instance. Nor is the relationship symmetrical, because truly caring for someone implies trust and trustworthiness between the two parties more clearly than trusting someone implies that I care for them. I may trust the police officer or fire fighter who answers my call for help without in any way implying that I am attitudinally or affectively tied to him or her. I may simply trust the institutional mechanisms that create, qualify, and oversee such professional public servants although knowing too little about this particular public servant to trust him or her as an individual.

By contrast, consider the incongruity, if not the sheer contradiction of the following statements: "I really care for you, but you cannot and should not trust me"; or "I know she cares for me but I cannot trust her." Obviously we can imagine instances where such statements might make sense and where the inability to trust or to be trusted did not totally defeat the claim to care. Think, for instance, of the caring one caught in the grip of some substance addiction or other compulsive behavior, or of the caring one who, by such a statement, is acknowledging his or her weakness of will, or lack of moral fiber. Still, such cases do not defeat the general assumption that attitudinal and affective care and trust normally do and should go together; people who truly care about each other normally trust each other and strive to be trustworthy. A parallel case can be made for a tie between these two elements and modal care. If A truly cares (attitudinally and affectively) for B, and there is mutual trust between them, we expect that A will deal carefully with B and B's interests. Again, exceptions abound for all sorts of reasons, but they remain exceptions to what we ordinarily and rightly expect.

Here I note only the most relevant dimensions of the possible ties between trust and actional care. With regard to many kinds of care, some level of trust must precede and ground our willingness to permit others to take care of us. We quite properly speak of entrusting ourselves to another's care. As the stakes in such care increase, as they clearly do in many forms of medical care, even more trust will be required. If the connections suggested above between trust and community hold, such trust will come more easily if the relationship between the care provider and the one-cared-for is encompassed or undergirded by some sort of community tie. In the absence of such a tie the question of why I should have entrusted my well-being and health, even my life, to that group of professionals I met for the first time during my hospital confinement becomes very serious. Where the rules of consent are followed, care givers, except in emergency situations, will get no chance to care for me unless I have some degree of trust in them. Although such questions of personal trust between care giver and recipient are becoming increasingly complicated not only in emergency situations but in much of our current highly specialized style of medicine, I believe many of them can be illuminated and even largely resolved by the following analysis of professional communities.

One final link between trust and actional care should be noted here, even though I will not treat it at any length: there is good evidence, both anecdotal and otherwise, that trust between care giver and care-receiver enhances the efficacy of the care given.

Trust and Healing

It is reasonable to assume that health care givers who are sensitive to the broader human and personal dimensions of their calling wish to be trusted by their patients, and that all patients would like to be able to trust their care givers. Although the suggestion that trust facilitates healing would be very difficult to document, it remains persuasive both conceptually and practically. Conceptually speaking, and recalling the connection made above between healing and wholeness, it would seem that a patient in a threatening situation who can truly trust his or her care givers has already achieved a kind of wholeness, including a realistic acknowledgment of the situation, an assessment of his or her resources and options, and a kind of cohesiveness of the self in spite of the forces threatening to disrupt and fragment the self, which permits the patient to place himself or herself trustingly in the hands of another. Thus the one who can trust seems already to have achieved one important form or level of wholeness, of focus, of centeredness. On the other hand, one riven with doubts and uncertainties, haunted by an inability to trust or by active distrust, pulled in various directions simultaneously by competing hopes and fears, obviously suffers from a lack of wholeness at some level.

Practically speaking, parties to a trusting medical/therapeutic relationship would seem to have a better chance than those in a nontrusting relationship of setting aside peripheral and distracting matters between them and focus-ing on the main concern that brought them together, namely, the patient's need for competent and effective health care. Furthermore, all the attitudinal elements often cited as enhancing the chances of a good outcome—a positive mental attitude, a will to live, keeping hope alive, being a "fighter," and so on—would seem either already to contain an element of trust or to be susceptible to having their positive impact further enhanced by such trust.

The continuing, even increasing insistence on securing informed consent to health care seems to reflect a growing recognition on the part of health care professionals and legislators, patients and patients' families, and ethicists as well, that a patient's informed, and I would add trusting, consent to a proposed therapy is important legally, morally, and therapeutically. Some relatively simple and straightforward medical problems may be easily and adequately managed with minimal concern for the issue of trust, but with more complex problems in which the stakes are higher and which involve greater uncertainty, an absence of trust on the part of the patient makes it difficult, if not impossible, for the patient to give himself and all of his physical, mental, emotional, and psychic resources over to the healing process.

THE COMMUNAL DIMENSIONS OF HEALING: PERSONAL COMMUNITIES

Much of the above will be obvious to any of us fortunate enough to be part of communities that rally around their members in times of serious crisis. But what was not obvious to me at the time of my hospital admission, and what I believe many people have forgotten, is that general or personal care and support such as I received are not important simply because they help the patient and the patient's family deal with the threat posed by the patient's condition and with modern medicine's often traumatic way of dealing with that threat. Communal presence and support are not confined to the minor supporting role of making more bearable the medical professionals' technical interventions. In my case, that presence and support in all their forms were important parts of the healing itself—if not of the organ, the heart (although I would not automatically discount that)—then certainly of the patient, Paul. As the threat loomed ever larger, as various findings confirmed my condition, I felt my ties to these various communities stretch and then hold firm against the weight of my situation, which had seemed about to hurl me into an abyss—an abyss from which I was not so sure those flimsy wires and tubes running to and from my body could protect me. Somehow, through their interventions, my personal communities armed me well to face my situation and the challenges it presented.

One might begin to understand the healing power of these personal communities by referring to the distinction between illness and disease invoked by Arthur Kleinman (1960) and others, and applied by John Dominic Crossan to some of the New Testament accounts of Jesus' healings (1994). In general terms, this distinction suggests that "disease" be used to refer to the pathology, whether physiological or psychological, experienced by the patient—in my case hypercholesterolemia and arteriosclerosis—which, in our time, we believe to be best addressed by the technical care of health care professionals. "Illness," by contrast, should be used to refer to the often diffuse social, cultural, communal, and perhaps psychological repercussions of the disease, and of the ways the patient and the patient's various communities perceive and respond to those dimensions of the patient's situation.

I welcomed these various communities' activities as comfort and support for me and my family, but I was slow to realize that they also contributed to my healing, a failure I strongly suspect is not unusual in the United States today. Contemporary high-tech, invasive medicine and its practitioners have, in relation to many ills, become so impressively successful and therefore so influential in choosing and delivering the care we presumably need that the rest of us feel like untutored and largely helpless laypeople, like amateurs in the pejorative sense, playing our little peripheral games while the real action occurs in the surgical suite or other highly specialized, even exotic settings. We can get some idea of the price this loss imposes by consulting any of the numerous accounts of traditional healings in which the community's involvement in a patient's problems and its support of the patient's struggle were crucial to the patient's returning to the community whole (e.g., Covington 1995; Knab 1995; Murphy 1993; Powers 1982). Instructively, this resort to the assistance and support—including the rituals and medications—of traditional, non-technical communities often continues even after the patient and the patient's communities have begun to avail themselves of the advantages of modern "scientific" medicine.

Although the distinction between "illness" and "disease" accounts for some of what I wish to affirm here, standing alone it is inadequate. It makes some dimensions of healing ceremonies and other practices of traditional communities, both religious and otherwise, comprehensible, even palatable, to many scientifically oriented moderns. However, it may also serve to discount such phenomena, because this explanation often seems to rely on and may perpetuate a dualism between the body on the one hand, and various other dimensions of who we are on the other. Although such a dualism has been variously and vigorously challenged, it still dogs far too much of our thinking.

The Healing

There are at least three crucial questions to ask about the healing I experienced from these communities: Did healing occur? What did those communities do to effect healing? And how did their actions result in healing?

I feel fully qualified to assert that healing did occur. I am less confident in saying exactly what I mean by such healing, and in proving that it occurred. I can say only that my perception of and my response to my situation was radically transformed between the time I entered the emergency room and the time, one week later, I entered surgery. I do not believe that a second angiogram would have shown that the plaque in my arteries had been reduced by such healing and that surgery was no longer necessary. I do believe that I—the total "I," including body, as well as mind, psyche, spirit, or however one wishes to parse this complex thing we call the self— was better prepared for the surgery and other healing processes. I had, in fact, already begun to heal, to be made or to become whole.

Looking back, something of the extent and the effects of that transformation first came home to me when, as surgery drew near, one of my children commented that I seemed awfully brave. "I am going to go to sleep and expect to wake up in better shape than I am now, but if it doesn't turn out that way, then things are in other hands, including yours," I responded. At the time I thought I was simply being realistic, although I may also have been ducking the issue by focusing on possible factual outcomes, which on the surface of things can be described without reference to such intangibles as courage or fear. I may have been in denial, somehow believing that the information about CABGs I had received from doctors, nurses, and instructional videos applied to other people, but not to me. Whatever the role of courage and denial in my response, the fundamental reality was that I felt a calm confidence that surgery was the best route for me to follow, that we—including all the communities involved—had done all we could to prepare for it, and that life would continue, whatever the outcome of my surgery. Not only would my loved ones survive the outcome of my surgery, but their lives would retain much of their current richness and fullness, in part because the communities that had surrounded and supported us together would continue to do so for them. Furthermore, in ways that words capture poorly, I had become convinced that I would somehow participate in the continuing lives of my loved ones and their communities.

Most of the actions of the communities that brought about this healing were predictable and unexceptionable, although that does not mean they were any less welcome, appropriate, or effective. Included here were the acts of paying visits, making phone calls, sending cards and flowers, offering various kinds of assistance to Bonnie and me, and simply reminding us that they were thinking about and available to us, which I have already mentioned. Other responses of these communities and their members were supportive, reassuring, and healing partly because of their unexpectedness.

Within a half hour of arriving in the emergency room, a familiar face—
that of a nurse and fellow Cub Scout den leader from fifteen years earlier—
appeared through my curtain wall to express her concern and to assure me
that I was in good hands. When nothing conclusive showed up on the
monitors or tests, I was wheeled to the CCU, where more nitroglycerin
brought me to the verge of unconsciousness until the nurse tilted the bed,
sending the blood rushing back to my brain. When I awoke from a brief,
phantom-ridden sleep, one of my pastors sat quietly across the room, his
presence driving home the possibility that this could be serious, but also
eloquently testifying to the fact that I was not in it alone. Later in the week,
while I awaited a verdict on surgery, one of the Vincentian priests with
whom I had worked in several capacities visited me, reflecting the Vincentian
personalism that continues to inform De Paul University's life, and enlarging
the foundation that was supporting me.

When surgery began to look like a certainty, a university colleague in
computer science called to express his concern, and upon learning which
surgical team I was with, assured me, as did many others, of their excellent
record. Although my colleague's medical credentials were not impressive,
he could vouch for the computerization of some of their procedures that
he had helped design. Another university colleague—it may be worth noting
a male chair of a department other than my own—called to extend his
greetings, concluding our conversation with the very un-academic and,
some might suggest, very un-male, "We love you, man." My own department
responded—not only, I told myself, because I was chair at the time—in
some predictable ways, but also in others that were especially sensitive to
my particular situation, and creative in terms of our shared interests. I
received from one departmental member, recently returned from Japan, a
small wooden plaque portraying a Japanese *kami* or god whose powers I
gladly added to my armamentarium. Another colleague, our visit interrupted
by a dietitian, patiently stayed for what seemed an interminable lecture,
having realized part way through, as I had, that she had been mistaken
for my wife and that walking out would have caused considerable embarrassment to me and to the dietitian whose uncertain grasp of the English
language and of American customs were already making her role awkward.
Another department sent me a small collection of wind-up toys to amuse
me during recuperation from surgery. These were small things, and yet
they made the setting in which I found myself less alien, and tied it and
me back into the familiar and reliable world that I thought I had left—or
had left me—at the hospital entrance. Whatever was happening to who I

was in the hospital, there was no doubt that outside the hospital, I very much remained who I had been.

Of course the family rallied round. Bonnie and our three children, two in from out of town, were present, loving, and supportive in more ways than I can name, some of which were significant beyond the acts themselves. As soon as the surgeon had left the room after we had agreed to surgery, Bonnie said she would call the church. I was puzzled. Both pastors had already visited, and other church members had called and sent cards. "The blood," she explained, "for transfusions." I had been content to leave such matters in the hands of the professionals. She had immediately seen good reason to enlist additional support from a community that had already extended itself in other ways. Seeking donors from among our presumably clean-living fellow Presbyterians may not have been the most ecumenically inspired thought of the week, but looking back, I see that it was important to us far beyond simply securing a presumably safer-than-average blood supply. Bonnie's suggestion and follow through on the blood prompted me to ask another friend, a surgeon in another major hospital, to mix personal and professional duties and to inquire of his colleagues whether surgery seemed to them the best course in my situation. These were the first truly active steps we took to shape the course of the entire experience. They reminded us that we were not restricted simply to responding to the options presented by others, waiting passively for the professionals to do their thing. By reclaiming some of the initiative and setting limits to just how disabling we would permit this crisis to be, we took back into our own hands part of the future that had seemed to be slipping away from us. The healing had begun. The fact that we could also intentionally marshal some of the resources of our communities to aid us in this effort was even more important at a time when we badly needed to exercise some of the diminished powers left to us.

The response of church members was also therapeutic in unexpected ways. Among the church members who responded was a former student of mine—in biomedical ethics, as it happened—who came with sister in tow to give blood. Early one morning a woman from the hospital's blood bank called my room to ask if I needed blood. I explained the situation and then asked how she had known to call if they had had no information on me. "Well," she explained, "there's this elderly gentleman down here who refuses to leave until we take his blood for you." Later, when I learned the identity of the donor—a truly gentle soul several years my senior—I knew his uncharacteristic assertiveness was a barometer of just how determined he was to help. These and several other church members—including one who, in his effort to donate blood for me, learned of his own previously undiagnosed hypertension, and so in caring for me was better equipped to care for himself—enabled us to put aside any concerns we had had about the blood supply. Giving blood is not offering up one's life for another. In fact, until my surgery, giving blood was for me, as it is for many, a minor inconvenience usually undertaken with little thought about its real significance. But in my situation and state of mind that simple gesture was transformed into an act of healing.

My peril was further domesticated and put in the context of my family when we considered my situation in light of my forebears' health history. My paternal grandmother had died from heart troubles at the age of 75, her keeping by her bed a small bowl of coarse barn salt that she was convinced helped her through the "bad spells" apparently not having solved her problem. My father, not so lucky, succumbed to his first and only heart attack at 57, following his younger brother's fatal attack by only thirteen months. My older brother had had a nearly fatal attack at age 42. All this was attributed by the family to the in-laws, my paternal grandmother's family, the Seewers. The local paper reported the death of my grandmother's father at age 63 as having come "as thunder from a clear sky to his family and friends." "That old Seewer heart!" the Camenisches had exclaimed upon each such calamity. That, of course, is not an entirely happy and reassuring context, and yet it undercut the isolation I felt, and challenged the whimsy with which I initially felt I had been selected to be so afflicted. It also made me feel fortunate, by comparison, and grateful to have access to kinds of care not even dreamt of by prior generations.

Family members near and far offered to make that family context physically present by coming to be with us, and staying with Bonnie and the children during surgery. Although we declined those offers, it was not because the family links and context were unimportant. In fact, my spirits were significantly buoyed when the initial frenzy of my admission had receded enough for a nurse to take my family history. Even though I knew the carefully focused reasons for taking such a history, I also felt that the process of reconstructing the me who had been reduced to a set of symptoms had begun. Some connections with the real, more complex me were being made. Strangers who encountered my history would now not only be better equipped to help me, but they would also be brought to the edge of what could become a relationship between them and me, a communal tie. I could now be seen as part of the most primal of communities—a family—which was a status that they and I shared.

As a life-long, active Presbyterian Christian in more or less good standing, I should acknowledge that thus far I have treated the church simply as another human community, and certainly it does function on that level. At the same time, some of the values and commitments around which that community is organized involve beliefs about a divine being who is generally well-disposed toward humankind and therefore is seen by many as a resource, not only for helping one get through difficult situations, but also for changing their outcomes. Although there may have been somewhere in my many-layered response to this crisis some element of reliance on God's will and on God's benevolent disposition toward me in life, in surgery and even in death, it was not, to my knowledge, significant in the healing I am trying to understand and describe. As one of the fortunate to whom this life and world have been very good, I do live with a poorly articulated conviction that the ultimate powers behind the universe are well- rather than ill-disposed toward us. I have great difficulty, however, with any theology that envisions a God who would take care of me because I asked, because others asked, or even because I had a reasonably good service record, but would do less for equally needy people for whom no one had thought to seek such intervention. At the same time, of course, from a Christian perspective, the human presence and actions of my several caring communities can be seen as channels of grace, of God's intervention, through which my situation and perhaps even my understanding of myself and of life were significantly transformed. Such a religious or theological interpretation of the care I received from my various communities seems to me to confirm and to enrich what they did, without in any way undercutting or challenging what the nonreligious observer sees in such community actions.

How and Why Healing Occurred

Although the care and support of these personal communities sometimes came in unexpected forms, the fact that they extended to me came as no surprise, as others similarly blessed will easily understand. Members of these communities simply continued doing what they had always done for their members, giving that care new shape and energy according to my changed circumstances. What did come as a surprise, although I realized it only later, was the extent to which that care and support were therapeutic and healing in deep and complex ways. I am convinced that their actions were healing, and that they helped return me to wholeness, but I still struggle to understand and articulate just how those actions effected such healing. Sometimes the best we can do is to resort to images and figures that may do little more than restate in other words what has already been said. Some of those images may, however, prove to be wedges with which we can pry open the mystery ever so slightly.

There are several potentially helpful themes or images that can perhaps be separated conceptually, even though they are so complexly interwoven and even interdependent that any analysis separating them makes them seem like artificial constructs. I have already said that my personal communities of care pulled me back from the abyss and armed me to face the challenge ahead. This may suggest to some that we have already abandoned reason and analysis for poetry, poor poetry though it be. Perhaps we can have— perhaps we need to have—both. I believe the healing I experienced arose in large part from my being reassured that the various communities of which I had been a part still held me, the person I had been and continued to be, as a member, and expected to continue to do so, whatever the outcome of the current crisis. They assured me, in other words, that they were prepared to assist me back to health and wholeness, perhaps not the precise wholeness I had known before, but to whatever wholeness would remain possible and appropriate for me. This may strike some as disingenuous; how can I call someone's state one of health and wholeness if it turns out to be only part of what one enjoyed previously? But health and wholeness for an eighty-year-old person is never what it was for that same person at eighteen, so why should we feel dishonest when we speak of health and wholeness after an illness, even if it varies from the patient's state before the illness? By assuring me that I did remain a part of the community, even if my old familiar role was changed by the current crisis, and by helping me to prepare for any revisions in that role, the community demonstrated to me that my value to them was not limited to the roles I played, that underneath those roles was a self they continued to value, to nurture, and to make a place for.

On one important level, the language of wholeness should be taken quite literally here. The human self we wish to heal and to be healed is not just a body. That is the crucial underlying physical platform from which a human life is lived. But it is the multiple, complex relations to others, both as individuals and as members of a community, that make one a distinctive and irreplaceable self. Relationships or connections to others are not add-ons or options; they are our very essence, the core of who we are.

Thus the communities in which most of those relations occur and are lived out have a kind of custody over crucial parts of our selves. When, through their caring actions, members of my own communities assured me that these relations, these parts of my self, remained intact, they were helping me to heal, to become whole again after the initial, fragmenting onslaught of potential disaster.

In remembering me with cards, calls, visits, and prayers, the members of these communities were not just calling me to mind again; they were literally re-membering me in two important senses. They were making certain that I knew that I was still fully a member of the community that they represented, that I was still a part of them, that that part of who I was was not at stake in this crisis. In doing this, they also re-membered, or re-constructed me by assuring me that those crucial parts of who I was were still alive and well, that I could and should go on being precisely who I had been.

They did not, in other words, come to comfort the individual, Paul, floating in regal and devastating isolation in some otherwise uninhabited universe of his own. They came as persons, to me as a person, one to whom they were already connected, with the message that we were still connected to each other and simultaneously to numerous others, and that the life we all enjoyed was not a fragmented life parceled out separately to each incidentally connected but ultimately individual entity, but a life that flowed between, among, and around us, so that the loss of any one of us was a loss for all. They were themselves living lifelines to me, and I to them, so that if any one of us was removed from that network, all our lives would be diminished. I was not, they were saying, one of those most isolated and isolating of entities known to and too often cherished by the Western mind, an individual pared down to the simplest possible entity, cut off from all else that it is related to, but not part of. In that case, were I to die, they, in their sovereign individuality, would have gone on essentially untouched, because we had never really been part of each other.

Another message, embedded in the others, was that any loss I suffered would be a shared loss. These caring persons could not remove the possibility of loss, nor could they take my place in the distribution of that loss should it occur. At the same time, I did not face it alone. Were I to die in surgery, these communities would also feel the loss. This also meant that the loss could not be total, because in feeling a loss, in remembering me, those communities would continue to affirm, and therefore in some sense preserve, what I had been, what I still was to them. The threat I faced was, to be sure, still serious enough, but it could not wipe out the entire me.

These communities, then, by caring for me in these and other ways, helped cut the threat that hung over me back to its true dimensions, and helped me see that serious though it remained, it was a more limited and focused danger that could not obliterate all that I had been, was, and hoped to be. With those assurances, and my restored sense of wholeness, with my having been re-membered and returned in most respects to my pre-emergency state—possibly even to an enhanced state because of my refreshed awareness of all these truths that, on some level, I had surely already known, but had not fully appreciated—I could turn with confidence and trust to seek the other sort of healing and wholeness I needed.[1]

THE COMMUNAL DIMENSIONS OF HEALING— THE PROFESSIONAL/FUNCTIONAL COMMUNITY

I was slow to realize just how much those personal communities were doing for me, how much they were contributing to my healing. Like the twentieth-century American I am, my major focus was on the health care professionals who were delivering the technical care, which I assumed was the primary thing I needed. This would suggest that I saw the personal communities and their caring and healing activities as secondary or auxiliary to the "real" healing done by the professionals. Yet with the benefit of some distance from those experiences, I now wonder if, on some less than fully conscious level, I had not inverted that relation between the two kinds of communities, giving pride of place to the personal communities, and establishing their healing activities as the paradigm to which I wished the professional/functional community to conform. To be more precise, I wonder if I was hoping to see in the professional community some of the same elements of care, community, trust, and healing that were serving me so well in my personal communities.

Two years after my surgery, participation in a seminar on Religion and Morality in the Professions in America gave me the chance to investigate this question. I explored the events of those two weeks in interviews averaging two hours per person, with my seven major professional health care companions on that journey: cardiologist, cardio-pulmonary rehabilitation nurse, cardiothoracic surgeon, diagnostic (or invasive) cardiologist, internist, nurse/patient coordinator for the cardiac surgery team, and pre-op primary care nurse.[2] Initially the interviews had only the broad concerns of the seminar title to guide them, but gradually they came to focus on the issue of trust and professional community. The issue of trust did not arise because anyone I met during those two weeks in the hospital seemed untrustworthy, nor because any of the interviews gave me reason to be distrustful, but because when matters as momentous as suffering, disability, and even life and death may hang in the balance, the mere fact that I have no reason to distrust you does not justify my entrusting you with such weighty matters. One wants positive evidence of trustworthiness. In addition to distrust, there is a kind of passive trust, a readiness to take others' words and actions at face value when we have no reason not to trust and there is little at stake. There is also an active trust, in which I entrust to you something of great value to me because I want you to help me to protect it. This puts you in a position from which you may, out of incompetence, indifference, negligence, or even malice, harm what I have entrusted to you.[3] Active trust calls for positive evidence of trustworthiness. In the course of the interviews, I came to realize that an anxious desire for this evidence had hovered just below the surface as I moved ever closer to surgery.

This was the case in part because I was dealing overwhelmingly with complete strangers. I knew only two of my major health care givers prior to admission: my internist, whom I had first consulted a few weeks earlier when I began to suspect some heart problems; and the rehabilitation nurse, a fellow member of a local congregation. The possibility of grounding trust on long-term relationships with health care providers has been greatly reduced for many of us by our own mobility, by the transience of staff in many medical organizations, and by the increasing specialization of medicine, which means that in complex cases we often meet those presumably best qualified to help us only at the time of acute need.

In earlier reflection on many of these issues I suggested that patients had the option of trusting either their individual health care deliverers or the institutions in which we meet them—the hospitals, HMOs, and the professions themselves, as well as licensure and specialty boards. Because contemporary patterns of health care do not give many of us the opportunity to build long-term relations of trust with individual deliverers, we may now be left with what many will see as a second best option, of putting our primary trust in institutions (Camenisch 1998). It now seems to me that there is a third possible locus of patient trust, what I am here calling the health care deliverers' professional/functional community, which in several respects appears to fall between trusting the person of the individual professional and trusting the institutions within which we meet those persons.

I now realize that during that first week before surgery I was busy trying to identify a locus of trust, to discover if those who were to deliver the technical care I needed also constituted a community on which I could rely, and in which I was somehow included. Given the standing of the institutions I was dealing with, I assumed that the professionals were technically and educationally qualified, an assumption well supported by the subsequent interviews. Thus, matters of competence did not concern me to any significant degree. But what about commitment? Did these people also constitute a community, tied together by their commitment to certain values, including their dedication to caring for their patients as well as they knew how? Could the recipients of their care plausibly see relations with their care deliverers as more than an economic relation with highly trained professionals? That is, could patients trust that they were putting themselves into hands that were not only competent, but also morally committed to their patients' interests, hands that would therefore be guided by care and toward care in its fullest sense?

Reassuringly, even before I had begun to sort out and discuss with my health care providers these issues of community, care, and trust, some providers were already acting in light of those concerns, and others, as I later learned, had been puzzling over them for some time. Two professionals—neither, as it happens, directly involved in my case—reached out to me on the basis of rudimentary communal connections that we already shared. The first was the emergency room nurse/den mother who went out of her way to offer me reassurance in my new and potentially alarming situation. Later in the week, a member of the surgical team who had served with me on the board of an emergency shelter/transitional living facility dropped by one pre-surgery evening to extend his good wishes.

In retrospect, I realize that I was not content just to search for community and all it entailed among my health care givers, but that I even tried to create community by attempting to pull some of the professionals out beyond their usual roles. When I learned that the young cardiology resident, my most frequent visitor other than the nurses and their various assistants, was from Norman, Oklahoma, I asked if he knew very close friends of ours who had lived there at the same time. As it turned out, his younger sister and our friends' daughter had been best friends. That did not and should not have entitled me to any better care, but the knowledge of even that remote a connection was another strand tying that strange hospital world to my more familiar world. My relations with my health care givers did not have to be entirely remote from those I had with the personal communities that were serving me so well.

The patient coordinator for the surgical team reported even more direct ways in which patients and their families invite care givers to enter into more personal forms of community with them. She is in repeated contact with the patient and the patient's family as they move through the complex procedures of major surgery. Thus it is natural for a feeling of connectedness and community to develop. She notes that sometimes patients or their families ask her to pray for the patient. She wonders why they think she will be receptive to that request, but clearly they have read her well. In fact, when she has little other hope to offer a family, she sometimes suggests that they pray for the patient, reflecting her belief that they are all tied together in ways that go beyond the purely professional and financial, that they are all part of a caring community.

BUILDING COMMUNITY AND TRUST WITH PATIENTS

These examples of professionals carrying pre-existing personal relations and shared community into their professional setting and even entering into some limited forms of personal community with their patients are noteworthy for a number of reasons. But my major concern here is with the community and trust that is possible among professional health care givers as professionals. My concern is also with the community and trust that is possible between them and the patients who are at the heart of their professional activity.

In addition to being the dedicated professionals I already knew them to be, all of my health care deliverers showed themselves in the interviews to be sensitive and reflective people who think deeply about what they do as professionals. Thus the issues on my mind, including the matters of trust and community, were not new to them. Even as I searched during my hospital days for community among the professionals and for grounds for putting my trust in them, several of them were reflecting on these matters. Early in our interview, the surgeon commented:

> I am continually amazed that I can walk into somebody's room . . . and say, "Well . . . your angiogram shows that you have three vessels that are diseased, and we need to do heart surgery on you tomorrow, and there is a 4 percent chance that you may not survive the operation," and to have them say,

"Well, you do what you have to do, doc—I trust you. ... I really don't think there is anything I can do in the amount of time that I see the patient to be worthy of their trust or respect. I think I am worthy of it, but I don't think they [can] know it."

Whatever his intellectual position on the issue of building trust, the surgeon underestimates what he already does, perhaps through simple instinct, to build trust with his patients. After introducing himself to Bonnie and me as the newest member of the surgical team and as my surgeon, he commented: "The good news is that at your age and in your general condition you should stand the surgery very well. The bad news is that at your age you'll probably be back here in ten years or so. But perhaps we'll have something better for you by then." Whether intentionally crafted to do so or not, those comments already began to build trust, even community between us. Few people intent on selling a good or service, or simply on commending themselves and their skills to another, are likely to begin the first conversation with a stranger in this balanced and objective way. With his direct and honest comments he treated us as mature and intelligent adults, conveying the comforting feeling that we were all in this thing together, and that the patient's interests—my interests—would have priority.

If patients are to feel included as members of the team or the community, health care providers must not only take positive actions to invite and even usher patients in, but they must also avoid actions and language that make patients feel like outsiders. In the middle of the night before surgery, obeying an order to report any chest discomfort, I rang the nurse and mentioned a slight but unusual sensation. I dozed off for a moment and awoke to see six very serious people surrounding my bed with the young man obviously in charge asking me that perennial question of the cardiac care unit, "On a scale of one to ten how bad is the pain?" Not satisfied with my "one and a half to two," he responded, "Give me three deep inspirations." Confused by the late hour and the strange situation, I came up with only two— Martin Luther King, Jr. and Mahatma Gandhi—and momentarily feared I might die if I didn't get a third. Then I realized that he was speaking in the language of his professional community; he wanted three deep inhalations. Neither my slight discomfort nor my sleepiness kept me from feeling annoyed by that exclusion, inadvertent though it was.

It was the surgeon who most explicitly invited me into a kind of temporary membership in the community that had taken on my care. He dropped by at an unusually late hour the night before my surgery: "We've got a problem. I wonder if you can help." Puzzled, I nodded for him to continue. "We did an angiogram on a patient today and he's got 90 to 95 percent blockage in several arteries. We have to do him tomorrow morning."

Several things rushed through my mind: gratitude for being included in the conversation; a suspicion, later confirmed, that the patient was my roommate, a gentle and charming retired southern minister with whom I shared a couple of professional acquaintances; and the question of the wisdom of delaying my surgery. "You're in no danger," he assured me. "If you're willing to skip breakfast, then we'll do you in the afternoon if another OR opens up. Otherwise we can do you Saturday morning. The nurses don't much care for that, but I like it. You've got the place all to yourself." I permitted myself a small, only half-joking inquiry. "Just how much don't the nurses like it?"

A question, raising the issue of what my standing in that community of decision making was, occurred to me: What if I had said "no"? Confronted with this question later, the surgeon's answer was twofold: "I have never had a patient say no once I've explained the situation. Deep down I just think we're all good people, willing to do what we can to help others. . . . But I would never let another patient stand in the way of surgery for someone who urgently needed it. I would offer the reluctant patient another surgeon, or a later time the same day if possible. But I would not endanger the patient with the more pressing problems."

Thus the surgeon maintains the belief, or perhaps the hope, that we are all tied together in a caring community in which all agree that the most needy must be served first. That, no doubt, is part of why he approached me with a question and not a declaration. Conveying this sense of community to all patients early on could be a real boon to worried, hurting people suddenly thrown among strangers on whom they must rely.

Feeling included in this community, being treated like more than a paying customer, I felt free to reciprocate and to treat its other members as equals. As I lay almost immobile and sore in bed following surgery, a TV station promised to list that evening the 10 area hospitals with the best and worst morbidity and mortality rates for bypass surgery. On his afternoon rounds, I asked the surgeon, half facetiously, if I should watch. "Sure. We ought to do fine. If we don't, it's our own fault. We get lots of practice on patients who've had very good medical care and good lifestyles, so they are usually in generally good health and any problems are caught early."

I watched that night. The hospital and I did okay; we made the top five. As I fell asleep, I was buoyed as much by the surgeon's candid and undefensive response, his treating me as an equal and thereby giving me further evidence that I was in trustworthy hands, as I was by the TV's revelations. By the end of my hospital stay, I was so much a member of the team that one day on afternoon rounds, while the resident reported on my uneventful recovery, some of the younger members of the team played on the floor with the wind-up toys sent me by my political science colleagues.

COMMUNITY AND TRUST AMONG PROFESSIONALS THEMSELVES

Much of the above can be read as occurring between individual professionals and an educated, white, male patient to whom they could easily relate. I must wonder if these demographics don't also account in large part for what was perhaps the strongest indication of the professionals' openness to more than a purely functional/professional relation—their later granting, without exception, my request for interviews. But my question here is whether the above events reflect something like a community of values, commitment, and trust among the professionals, a community of purpose or function focused on serving an ever changing roster of temporary or associate members—the patients. The existence of such a reality would indeed be good grounds for patients to enter trustingly into community with those professionals.

The clearest testimony for the existence of such a community among the professionals at that particular hospital came from the surgical team's patient-coordinator nurse. Among her major resources in guiding the patient and the patient's family through the complex process of cardiac surgery was the cooperation and support of the team of which she was a part. This, of course, meant relying on each member of the team to do his or her own part, but also supplementing the task done by other members if a patient's needs had not been met, which sometimes led to a temporary re-casting of the team's immediate goals. When it became clear that an elderly patient was very fearful of undergoing the procedure in which her husband had died, the entire team, from patient-coordinator to head surgeon, shifted to a broader form of care, supporting and encouraging the woman until, a few days later, she felt ready to undergo the procedure.

Through the interviews I discovered not only a task-oriented team committed to cooperation, but a community of purpose requiring trust among its members. When I asked about her role in the decision to recommend surgery, my internist indicated that although she was informed about the results of the angiogram, she saw her role in such matters not as second guessing the specialists, but as being sure that she works only with specialists she trusts. Otherwise, she says, it would be "unethical for me to encourage my patients to trust them."

In the course of the interviews, it was perhaps among the nurses that the reality of a professional community of care became clearest, the result in large part, I believe, of the distinctive organization and nature of their work, especially its character as a collaborative undertaking among people who are, to a considerable degree, professional equals.

I also found among the nurses a shared concern that the most important dimensions of the relation between patients and their care givers, including a shared sense of purpose and community, not be obscured or distorted by economic considerations. The rehab nurse, for example, visits patients in the hospital after their surgery to make certain they understand the importance of rehabilitation. She knows the job involves recruiting as well as patient education, and she faces an issue mentioned by virtually all the professionals I interviewed—institutions' and funders' growing concern about the cost of care. The rehab unit must see that their client count stays above the break-even point, so, as an economic fact of life, her recruitment serves the unit. But she wonders about the long-range impact of such cost concerns: "If I have to look at you coming in the door as a dollar sign rather than as a person, that changes my relationship with you. And if you have to come into the hospital and look at me as a hired hand, then that changes your relationship with me. And I don't know where it's all going." She rightly senses that given the nature of what her unit tries to do for patients, their success rate will almost certainly suffer if the nurses do not relate to the patients in ways that go beyond the economic and technical. They must elicit from their patients—often seniors long set in their ways and frequently fatalistic about their future following various heart incidents—a long-term commitment to exercise, to an appropriate diet, and to a healthy lifestyle in general. This can be done only by cultivating in patients a sense of hope, bolstering their confidence in their ability to change their lifestyles, and, sometimes, by getting dispirited patients to share the professional's concern about and hope for the patient's future health. The need for a sense of community is especially urgent in the rehab unit because it is so closely linked to the nature of the care given.

Others among my care givers were sensitive to these concerns about the costs of care, which seem to threaten the kind of relations they seek with their patients, and thus possibly to undermine community and even trust. The diagnostic cardiologist struggles against pressures to use an older, cheaper dye in angiograms, which tends to increase uncomfortable side effects, or to routinely catheterize only the left side of the heart even though the right side yields more subtle but still important information. Although many of my professional care givers fear what these trends may mean in the future, none feel that either the care they currently deliver or their relations with their patients has yet been compromised.

CONCLUSION

My experience of by-pass surgery not only improved the condition of my heart, it also expanded my understanding of the meanings of care, of healing and wholeness, and of the roles community and trust play in our returning to and maintaining wholeness. In the care I received from the personal communities of which I was a part—care I now see as not only comforting and supporting, but as actually healing—I began to intuit a model of care that I tried inchoately at the time to apply to the rather different care I sought from health care professionals. Two major elements in that model of care were that it grew out of community and that it was significantly enhanced by, if not dependent on, trust.

In the section on personal communities I have sketched and then elaborated on that model of care and how I experienced it, drawing primarily on the numerous actions, large and small, of friends and family that mediated that care to me. Bolstered by that care and the sense of a self renewed and regenerated by it after my diagnosis and all of its foreboding possibilities, I turned, without fully knowing what I was doing, to the health care professionals, hoping to find in them a similar kind of care. I knew their care would differ in important ways from that offered me by my personal communities, but I nevertheless hoped it would conform in certain ways to the care that had already brought me so far.

Reflecting further on my experience and drawing on interviews with my health care professionals, I have also recounted my search for and offered evidence of the existence of community among these professionals that parallels in some significant ways the community I knew among my family and friends, and which therefore offered me good grounds to trust the strangers who cared for me. I also believe that that sense of community and the trust it engendered enhanced the therapeutic effect of what they did for me, but that is a more complex thesis that I cannot defend here.

The community I now believe I encountered among my professional health care givers conformed to some elements of the definition of community offered earlier better than others. For example, "shared commitment

to . . . certain highly valued tasks/goals" understandably seems more prominent in professional communities than are members' direct commitments to
each other as persons. Nevertheless, given the way their shared commitments
permeate their common enterprise and help define who they are as persons,
I am quite comfortable referring to my health care professionals as constituting a community, specifically a community of healing.

It may be harder for some to see the patient as a member of that
community, even as the associate or transient member I have suggested.
This raises the question of the boundaries of community, the criteria for
inclusion, and the indicators of one's standing in it. The variety and complexity of communities prevent any serious attempt to answer these questions
here. However, it was striking to me that no physician ever spoke of a
patient's making the wrong decision with regard to therapy. All acknowledged that the decision the patient makes is the right decision for that
patient, even when it goes against the professional's own best judgment.
The professional's task, assuming that the decision is well informed, is not
to persuade the patient to choose differently, but to make certain the patient
understands the risks of the option elected as well as of the one refused,
and to assure that the patient will still get the best possible medical care
consistent with the choice made.

This fact does not irrefutably prove patient membership in the medical
community. Explicitly asserting patients' full membership in the medical
community still feels forced and unnatural to me. Yet the observed fact
does suggest a deep respect for the patient and the patient's judgment, a
respect apparently not dimmed by the professionals' possible disagreement
with the decision, nor by some potentially condescending sense that they
really know better than the patient but unfortunately are helpless to administer the "right" therapy. Finally, little, if anything, in my position actually
depends on patients being fully included in the professional healing community, even as associate or transient members. It is enough for my argument
to see the community of health care deliverers as receiving the patient as
a guest, or even a respected and valued stranger to whom they, according
to the shared commitments that make them a community, have certain
clear duties and obligations. Put another way, it is enough to say that the
members of the various communities who meet in the patient-professional
health care deliverer encounter must realize that whatever specific communities each party belongs to, they as individuals and their communities are
encompassed by a larger, more comprehensive community that now informs
the ways they are to relate to each other and the ways the values that define

their various communities come together to guide them as they pursue their shared goal of securing the best care possible for the one in need.

Would antibiotics, radiation, and surgery "work" in the absence of the personal and professional-functional communities I have held up here, and the trust I suggest arises largely within and in relation to such communities? I am empiricist enough to think that if we could indeed construct a case where there were no remnants of these communities, we would not find either the physical properties or the immediate outcomes of those therapies significantly altered. However, I end with a question and an observation. Would the "working" of these therapies under such circumstances usually constitute what we mean by healing, by returning the patient to wholeness, or what we mean when we say the patient was well cared for or received good care? Finally, the fact that such communities may be neither necessary nor sufficient for some kinds of care and healing does not mean that they have not played an important, even a crucial role in the healing of those of us who have been blessed by their presence and their care. It should surprise no one if we who have been so blessed wonder how others can return to wholeness or feel truly cared for without healing communities to sustain and to care for them.

Endnotes

1 A number of these themes and dynamics find parallels in Mayeroff 1971, although our key terms differ: "In the sense in which a man can ever be said to be at home in the world, he is at home not through dominating, or explaining, or appreciating, but through caring and being cared for" (2); "The experience of *belonging* that stems from being needed by my appropriate others helps ground me; it is an ingredient of basic certainty. I belong because my appropriate others need me, because I have been entrusted, as it were, with the being of these others. . . . I have a need to be needed, and the need of others for me goes hand in hand with my need for them. Belonging, in this sense, goes with my own actualization" (49–50).

2 I am grateful to the Lilly Endowment for funding the seminar, Religion, Morality and the Professions in America, at the Poynter Center at Indiana University, which was the starting point for much of the work presented here and for which the interviews drawn on here were conducted. In spite of the barrier of anonymity, I express my sincere appreciation to the seven professionals I interviewed for the competence, commitment, and sensitivity with which they cared for me, for their willingness to participate in this study, and for their openness and thoughtfulness in the interviews. I am also grateful to the DePaul University Research Council for the Paid Leave grant that enabled me to bring this article to its final form.

3 This statement of some of the dynamics of trust draws on Baier (1994, 99 ff). There are different kinds of trust. Jay Katz catches the core of the kind I have in

mind when he defines the trust he hopes for in physician-patient relations as "trust based . . . on the confident and trusting expectation that physicians will assist patients to make their own decisions—-decisions that in the light of their medical needs and personal history *they* deem to be in their best interests" (Katz 1986, 101–2). He contrasts this trust with the formerly (and currently?) dominant "trust based . . . on Aesculapian authority and following 'doctor's orders' " (101). Katz, himself a physician, comments on the demands placed on physicians by the kind of trust he hopes for: "It is a trust that requires physicians to trust themselves in order to trust their patients, for to trust patients, physicians first must learn to trust themselves to face up to and acknowledge the tragic limitations of their own professional knowledge; their inability to impart all their insights to all patients; and their own personal incapacities—at times more pronounced than at others—to devote themselves fully to their patients' needs. They must also learn not to be unduly embarrassed by their personal and professional ignorance and to trust their patients to react appropriately to such acknowledgments" (102–3). All the professionals involved in my study seemed to me to have dealt well with these issues, with the possible exception of the last. Incapacity "to devote themselves fully to their patients' needs," obviously a very complex and sensitive issue, did not arise either in my care or in the interviews.

References

Baier, Annette. 1994. *Moral Prejudices: Essays on Ethics*. Cambridge, Mass.: Harvard University Press.

Camenisch, Paul F. 1983a. *Grounding Professional Ethics in a Pluralistic Society*. New York: Haven Publications.

———. 1983b. On Being a Professional, Morally Speaking. In *Moral Responsibility and the Professions*, ed. Bernard Baumrin and Benjamin Freedman, 42–61. New York: Haven Publications.

———. 1986. Confidentiality, Persons and Community. In *The Common Bond: the University of Texas System Cancer Center Code of Ethics*, ed. Jan van Eyes and James M. Bowen, 105–17. Springfield, Ill.: Charles C. Thomas.

———. 1998. Patient Trust in an Age of Institutional Health Care. In *Religion, Morality and the Professions in America*, ed. David H. Smith and Richard B. Miller, 10–28. Bloomington, Ind.: The Poynter Center.

Covington, Dennis. 1995. *Salvation on Sand Mountain: Snake Handling and Redemption in Southern Appalachia*. New York: Penguin.

Crossan, John Dominic. 1994. *Jesus: A Revolutionary Biography*. San Francisco: Harper.

Katz, Jay. 1986. *The Silent World of Doctor and Patient*. New York: The Free Press.

Kleinman, Arthur. 1960. *Patients and Healers in the Context of Culture: An Exploration of the Borderland between Anthropology, Medicine, and Psychiatry*. Berkeley: University of California Press.

Knab, Timothy J. 1995. *A War of Witches: A Journey into the Underworld of the Contemporary Aztecs*. Boulder, Colo.: Westview Press.

Mayeroff, Milton. 1971. *On Caring*. New York: Harper & Row.

Murphy, Joseph M. 1993. *Santería: African Spirits in America*. Boston: Beacon Press.

Powers, William K. 1982. *Yuwipi: Vision and Experience in Oglala Ritual*. Lincoln: University of Nebraska Press.

Wolf, Susan M., ed. 1996. *Feminism and Bioethics: Beyond Reproduction*. New York: Oxford University Press.

Zaner, Richard M. 1994. Experience and Moral Life: A Phenomenological Approach to Bioethics." In *A Matter of Principles: Ferment in U.S. Bioethics*, ed. Edwin R. DuBose, Ronald P. Hamel, and Laurence J. O'Connell, 211–39. Valley Forge, Penn.: Trinity Press International.

9

Doubled in the Darkest Mirror: Practice and the Retold Narrative of the Jewish Burial Society

Laurie Zoloth

Medicine is about the gesture of healing, and bioethics is about the moral witness, the embodied narrative, and the complex reasoning that surround this gesture. As ethicists and storytellers of medicine, we ordinarily structure the story around some optimistic possibility, and we end the story, the witness, and the reflection when the person who is the patient at the center of the narrative dies. Medicine tends to turn away from the body at this moment, and gives the lost body over to the invisibility of orderlies, the morgue, the silence of the autopsy. The body, once the site of so much frantic and calculated attention, is left waiting on the gurney, and all of the things that matter so urgently in medicine—the measures, the numbers, the pain, the chart—cease at that moment to be important.

This essay is about that moment, the time shortly after death, and the ritual practice of one faith tradition, Judaism, which makes a particular meaning emerge from the ritual act of preparing a body for burial. It is about what does matter in the time after medicine and before remembrance. It is about the story of the ones who are *shorim* (guardians for the dead body), and about those who care for the body, thereby shifting the genre of the story from medicine to community. It is a different sort of reflection on death, one that suggests that there is a need in bioethics for situating reflections on dying and death within particular contexts of meaning, not only for the sake of the patients whose lives we hope to affect, but for the sake of their care givers, who will each, one by one, inevitably follow them into death.[1]

This volume is an effort to consider how narratives of care, of remembrance, and of personal practice effect our thinking and discerning in bioethics. When the editors asked me about the use of narrative in bioethics,

I sent them this (odd) piece, an essay that began as a series of letters to friends about how my involvement in a traditional Orthodox Jewish community was changing my thinking as a feminist philosopher. It was odd because it was not about caring for patients in a clinical context, but about meaning after the clinical story.

A call to reflect on care and medicine is often a call to recreate moments of the triumph of the body. This essay explores another sort of triumph of healing and recovery, which takes place in the performance of a traditional Jewish ritual. Looking at the specific acts surrounding the *taharah* (purification), which is the preparation of the dead for burial, is a way to begin a larger conversation about morality and mortality, and to situate a feminist praxis for Judaism and for bioethics. Through careful attention to this act, we can comment fruitfully on the discourse that has emerged about death and dying, and the ethical obligations and choices that a community faces in its confrontation with death. Because *taharah* is based on the essential commandment to practice *gemulut hasidim* (acts of loving kindness) without regard for reward, it allows us thoughtfully to consider how the gesture of care differs from the gesture of power in medicine, how the gesture of altruism differs from acquisition or control, and how the constancy of the ones who care for the body creates a narrative frame for this care. This essay is also, and perhaps most centrally, about how the moral deeds of the narrator are carried along in every subsequent deed, and how the stories of a complex practice of a community shape the practitioners and shape the scholar as the teller of the tale.

Of all the ritual acts that are a part of the community life of a commanded faith tradition, none is as covert as the work of the *chevra kadisha*, or the Jewish ritual burial society (literally: the "blessed comrades"). Operating in most Jewish communities, the *chevra* is a group of women and men selected to prepare the bodies of the dead according to rabbinic tradition, with a liturgy based in the *Song of Songs* and a practice that forces the abstract discourse of embodiment into intimate, tangible detail.

The laws of ritual burial are straightforward: Every Jewish person completes his or her life in the same way: washed clean, with a specified amount of running water poured from the hands of his or her *chevra*, gently patted dry, dressed in simple unbleached linen shrouds that have been sewn by hand. The same is done for all—the rich and the poor, the powerful and the powerless. Each is wrapped in linen with small handfuls of dirt from Jerusalem placed at their heart, eyes, and womb or genitalia, lifted into a pine box made without nails, the lid closed and a candle lit on the top, and watched until carried to the grave. Women prepare women for burial, men prepare men.[2] The term *chevra ḳadisha* is an Ashkenazi one. Sephardic Jews refer to the group as the *lavadores*, those who wash. Having a separate group that is assigned to this work is one of the oldest traditions in Jewish life, and it is referred to in the Talmud.[3]

Like many rituals in Jewish life, this practice must be performed within modernity. For American Jews, it is removed by years, exile, and continents from the cultural origins of the practice. When a postmodern Jewish feminist joins the *chevra*, how is this act both preserved and revisioned? This essay presents not only an analysis of the development of the ritual through a participant description that rethinks the ritual itself, but also a methodological claim that participation in this ritual is at its heart a deeply feminist, caring act. Reflecting on the ritual affords us a chance to think about the nature of mandated, obligatory nurturance. Like the act of mothering or of nursing, it allows a tangible and sober manifestation of the theoretical commitments that feminism has claimed as its own unique insights.

THE *TAHARAH* AS A FEMINIST PRAXIS

How can I make such a claim? How can one of the most ancient and traditional practices in Jewish life also be considered a feminist practice?

First, such a practice calls upon participants to build a small community whose work is based in the recognition of obligation. The selection of the members of the *chevra* is traditionally an honor reserved for the most mature and pious within a community. Once asked, it is considered improper to refuse. When a call from the *chevra* leader comes to prepare a body, in the midst of other tasks, other moral appeals, and other relationships, it is considered imperative to respond affirmatively. In other work, I have spoken of the theological meaning of the act of interruption. To be interrupted is to reawaken to the contingent and frangible nature of human existence. The interruption of one little master narrative—what each of us thinks of as the terribly important story of our daily lives—reminds us of the absurdity of the narrative, its narrowness, and its negation of possibilities. To be a member of the *chevra* is to be willing to allow the dislocation of death to stop the business of ordinary life; with a consideration of sacred time and the insistence of the Other, the needs of the Other become paramount.

Second, the practice impels a recognition that whatever we are theologically, as persons, we inhabit the frail and limited human body. At the time of our birth and our death we are fundamentally in need of others. Just as each child is born from the body of a woman into the waiting arms of others, the ritual of the *chevra kadisha* affirms that each will die surrounded by the waiting arms of others, who will quite literally lift and carry him or her from the ritual bath into the coffin—bearing the weight of the body's last ride, the last time the body will be held to the body of another. In the tradition of the Jewish community, this will not be a matter of luck or chance; it will be the result of a conscious choice on the part of certain members of the community to respond to a divine command and to fulfill a promise. If the language of health care decision making is self, autonomy, and control, then the language of the *chevra* is other, dependency, and powerlessness. The practice reminds us that there is really not a possible turning from the face of death, or from the dead one in our midst. Because death will come to us all, this practice reminds us that, ultimately, we all need each other. In the face of death all we have is the love of neighbors and the simple gestures of a ritual washing—gestures made moral by their responsiveness to human need.

Third, the practice holds the notions of finality and fragility in tension with a lifelong attention to the external embodied self. Because women prepare only the bodies of women, and men only the bodies of men, cleaning and dressing the body provides a mirror for our own fears and projections about our bodies, our beauties, and our deaths.

Finally, seeking to reenvision this particular ritual requires raising broad questions about the nature of the *brit* (covenant) in a Jew's life. To what acts of the flesh are we bounded and promised? What is the relationship between the inescapably obligatory and the chosen? Inescapability is underscored in this practice by the nonvoluntary tradition within which the voluntary act of service takes place. What is the moral meaning of a call (from the dead) that cannot be left unanswered (because the dead, paradoxically, cannot wait)? To answer that question we must examine the nature of urgent commandedness within Jewish life and its parallels to the boundedness of normative secular communal life, especially the lives of women in families.

The *chevra kadisha* means the "blessed" or the "holy" fellowship. But how, exactly, is the fellowship a holy one? How is this holiness enacted amid the pragmatics of the ordinary world, especially the world of modernity, virtual reality, and electronic distance? What is the moral meaning of such a fellowship? How can the responsibility for the specific tangible details of cleaning a body translate into religious and theological reflection on the usually gender-bound roles of cleaning and re-ordering the world after death?

This essay is intended to challenge the distance between the scholar and the religious life. I ask you to begin your engagement with this piece by imagining yourself into the story that I am about to tell you. I ask you to imagine that you must turn to your neighbor, and take his or her hand. I would give you a small wooden stick, a toothpick, that intimate tool, and ask you to clean the other's fingernails with complete care and utter dedication. Your life depends on this task, in a way that is both complex and ordinary.

A NARRATIVE ACCOUNT

I wrote the following letter to a friend after my first *taharah*:

There is a door to the back room of the mortuary you must open. The door is to teach you about death.

The hallway, and the quiet, you will not speak once you pass this door. I have a secret to tell you, your mother would say, and after that, the world changes, and your body will take you there, whole. This is that moment again: now the door opens, the ordinary mortuary sign says, "Keep Out." You know this room, you know it waits. The small Jewish women in the scarves and the skirts, they will come at night and you will know them, and you will join them.

During the *taharah* we read: "And the angel of God raised his voice and spoke to those who were standing before him saying, 'Remove the soiled garments from them,' and he said to him, 'Behold, I have removed your inequity from you and will clothe you in fine garments.'"

We start with the fingernails, the blue hands, the blue toenails. Cleaning under each nail, we note the blood on the toothpick, note the strength of the last grip, the curve of the fingers, her last little gesture. Every fleck of body, off, into the small, muslin bags, this woman's last dirt scraped in the bag. It feels like cleaning marble, that cold, that heavy, the chips that small, the sweat of her last desire, gone into my bag. Does this seem strange, the attention to detail? We are accepting the way of the world, now the nails are perfectly clean.

Now the face: ah mother, ah sister, ah self. You are so beautiful and so dead. The blue edges of your ears, your blood all fled to your blue back, the earth beginning to pull you in already, blue blood first, and your hair is dark, soaking seeping blood, *let me go*. We save every bit of blood. We cut the old stains and the new stains from the sheets, save the blood on our gloved fingers. We wash you over and over.

Then we read verses from the *Song of Songs*:

"Oh, your hair is like the most fine gold, black and curling, oh heaps of
dark curls are as black as a raven.

Eyes like doves beside the waterbrook, bathing in milk and fitly set.

Cheeks like a bed of spices, towers of sweet herbs

Lips are roses dripping flowing myrrh.

Arms are golden cylinders set with beryl

Body as polished ivory overlaid with sapphires

Legs are pillars of marble, set upon foundations of fine gold.

You are like Lebanon, as rare as her cedars

Your mouth is most sweet, and you are altogether precious

This is my beloved, and this is my friend, daughters of Jerusalem."

We take off the sheet, and it is at precisely this moment, when we can
see the face, the body—the moment when we would turn away in the
secular word—that we are told to remember that each person is made in
the image of God. We recite verses of love and praise of the beautiful,
sensual body: hair, eyes, breasts, thighs. We say verses from *Shir haShirim*
[*Song of Songs*]. A stunning moment: the poetry of love and desire at the
moment of distance.

We continue, we know her body, we are her body.

You are so beautiful, my sister.

The distance between us and the dark night of East Oakland. We work
until midnight, washing and pouring, lifting the buckets over our heads as
high as we can reach. The water must be poured like a continuous river;
each of us has a bucket. Specific details call us back and back from our
thoughts to the work at hand. Turn her gently to dry her back, her belly,
her legs, the childbirth marks, her soft breasts, her vagina, her scarred knee.
We dress her in the simple clothes, twist the cloth into bows and knots that
look like the letters of God's name *shin*; four turns of the knot, *dalet*. And
you, dear dead one, you will be the *yod*. And we lift you through the air
in our arms, your sacred flight, your sacred fellowship, your blue hands in
the plain white muslin. We find the bag of earth from Jerusalem, and
we place some on your eyes, your heart, your womb. Now we are your
sacred fellows.

THE *TAHARAH* AS ETHICAL PRAXIS

As I wrote this letter I told the story of how it became clear that the *taharah*
was both a spiritually deepening and enriching act and something that I

was obligated to do. I wondered in the letter about how we create norms and obligations both within secular culture and within the culture of Jewish faith and practice. What are the sources of ethical norms if they are not based on desire? And what happens if we as a society or a particular community need something done that no one particularly desires to do?[4]

The *chevra kadisha* is said to be a "hard *mitzvah*" (commandment) that is "not for everyone." In framing the performance as chosen, ritualized, and mandatory, a social contract is created in which role-specific duties emerge. The fulfillment of these duties is an ethical gesture and not merely an act of faithfulness. The moral agents who perform the ritual must not be related to the dead person, nor can they be students of the deceased. They must be as strangers, yet they must enact the most primal of interactions: the primate bonding that marks the beginning of the first human relationships at birth. This bonding takes the form of skin-to-skin touch (or, since the AIDS epidemic, skin-to-glove), grooming, and the face-to-face gaze.[5] These behaviors are initiated at birth by all primates, and it is these acts that are re-created by strangers toward the *metah* (the dead one) at the moment of transition from death to burial, light to darkness, being to unbeing.

I described my initiation in another letter to my friend:

The first time members of my Orthodox synagogue spoke to me about it, I was at a Purim *suedah* [festive meal during which Jews masquerade, at the end of the Jewish holiday that celebrates the legend of Queen Esther]. I was dressed in a rather silly costume, gunning for *homentashen* [sweet, date-filled pastries made especially for this holiday]. It stopped me cold.

"You want me for what?"

"We want you to be in the *chevra kadisha*, the burial society. You were a nurse, right? You dealt with bodies, right?"

"I don't know if I am your guy," I say. "I don't know enough."

"We'll teach you what you need to know."

"Am I ...?" I do not finish. Am I good enough? Strong enough? Intentful enough?

"We'll teach you," they say. And they say it is a mitzvah.

Later, I tell my cousin. She sighs.

"You are not supposed to tell me. See, already you aren't right. It is supposed to be secret, supposed to be for very pious women. Hah."

"I told you they only got me because I was a nurse," I mutter.

Reflecting on this work more than a decade later, and thinking about how my telling of this work in a series of letters was integral to my understanding of Jewish bioethics, I came to see that both the content of the story and the background of the ritual were important. Inherent in the practice is the notion that Judaism is concerned with the "beloved stranger." Jews are obligated, as part of their duty to promote social justice, to care for the stranger in need.

In the textual account of Jewish life, one can see the display of the preferential option for the poor, the marginalized, and the powerless. In the largest arenas of public policy, one is obliged to seek justice, and in the arena of social welfare one is responsible to act as God would act. In the care of the poor, the sick, and the bodies of the dead, the ritual enacts a textual doubling, in which the acts are performed and the justification is reflected in the mirror of the *midrash* (exegetical story) that has God doing the *taharah* for Moses. The *midrash* provides a textual justificative template for the community's praxis.

The following *midrash* on the verse "and he buried him in the valley" is a narrative commentary on the preparations for death. The text imagines God paying tender attention to the body of Moses.

All creatures go down to the grave with their eyes dimmed, but as for you [Moses] your eye is not dimmed. All mortals are disposed of in vestments made by man, namely coffin, bier, and shrouds, but you are disposed of in shrouds made in heaven, a coffin made in heaven. Another explanation: When all mortals die, their relatives and their neighbors attend to their burial, but as for you, Moses, I and my Court will attend to your burial. Whence this. For it is said, And he buried him in the valley [Dt. 34: 6]. (*Rabbah* 19)

In another talmudic discussion, two rabbis discuss the meaning of a verse describing the creation of Eve from Adam. Here they are asking what God did with the opened body. The discussion shifts to the nature of God's care of his creature's body:

And he closed up the place with flesh instead of thereof [*tahtennah*]. R. Hanina b. Isaac said: He provided him with a fitting outlet for his nether functions, that his modesty might not be outraged, like an animal. Rabbi said: Jannai and R. Jannai differed thereon. One says: He provided him

with a lock and a saddle cloth pressed over it, so that he should not suffer
pain when he sits. The other said: He provided him with cushions. R. Ila
and R. Ammi disagreed. One said: He instituted burial for him; while the
other said: He made shrouds for him. (*Rabbah* 19)

What is occurring in these odd texts about burial is that the rabbis are
using stories to tell their hearers something about the details of ethical
practice. They are conversing and disagreeing about the relationship between
the corporeal and the spiritual, and they are linking this discussion to the
problem of the care of the dead. In the first narrative, God is described as
providing the *taharah* for Moses, a *taharah* in which Moses is washed in
rainwater and shrouded in white clouds. God attends to every detail.

In the second narrative, the rabbis describe the duty of the care of the
dead and the burial of bodies as a key component of what separates us
from animals. How is it that we are not regarded "like an animal"? This
is a central question of the Genesis narrative. It is by the act of burial, the
ritual and care that such an act involves. It is not, of course, only the ritual
itself, but the radical recognition that such a ritual allows us. By retelling
the narrative, the rabbis double the potency of the loving ritual act, not
only re-membering it (by providing an imaginative account), but also man-
dating its repetition with the authority of *halachah* (law) and justice itself.

The call to do specific acts of embodied love toward the ill, the dying,
and the dead is a privileged call that is linked textually and socially to
larger public acts of justice. Responding to the call is required as opposed
to optional, both in a social and in an ontological sense. Without a community
that acknowledges this obligation, this marker of humanity is not possible.
Being human involves not only the foreknowledge of one's death, but the
construction of a community that is prepared to handle the specific, difficult,
embodied details of death.

In this second narrative, the act of the creation of the other, of Eve from
the side of Adam, is linked not only to death, but also to the necessity for
taharah. Creation and birth are linked to death and the care of the dead.
Flesh of flesh, bone of bone, birth, bodies, and ethical choice are all linked
to the act of covering the body of the dead one in her shrouds. Before the
human world is even finished—before naming, or call, or response—this
relationship between the care of the body and the task of the human
is established.

The rabbinic texts that refer to the caring actions that surround death
are not limited to these *midrashic* passages. In a longer talmudic discussion

about the duty to restore lost articles to their owner (focused around the temptation to keep that which is valuable), the rabbinic talk turns to the problem of what one does if one finds an article that seems to be of no worth, or is repulsive. Does one have an obligation to return it, or does the handling of such a thing transfer its worthlessness to the moral agent? Can one avoid the whole matter if this is the case? Does the worthless nature of the article eliminate the finder's responsibility? In the following text, we can see how the moral language of one problem (returning articles) is applied to another problem (providing for the burial of the dead).

> Yet was not R. Ishmael son of R. Jose an elder for whom it was undignified [to help one to take up a heavy load]—He acted beyond the requirements of the law. For R. Joseph learnt: *And thou shalt show them*—this refers to their house of life (work); *the way*—this means the practice of loving deeds; *they must walk*—to visiting the sick; *therein*—to burial; and *the work*—to strict law; that *they shall* do—meaning actions beyond the requirements of the law. (*Metzia* 19)

The explanation is important for it is from this verse that the need to provide for the burial of the destitute is rationalized as a duty beyond the call of duty. Directly out of this teaching, the *chevra kadisha* achieve their centrality. To hold up the duty to do the difficult act, to go beyond the letter of the law, raises the standard for community norms. In the discussion that follows this passage, the rabbis explore the relationship between this compassionate stance and the commitment to social justice, laying the blame for the destruction of Jerusalem on the inability of the justice system to go beyond the requirements of the law. In this textual modality, then, the acts of supererogatory compassion that are part of the *taharah* are not only linked to justice and to proper judgment, but also to the literal redemption of the community. Our life, in this textual account, depends on whether we will tend to the sick and to the burial of the dead. Our life in a just world depends on the world's attention even in death.

THE *TAHARAH* AS AN ACT OF THEOLOGICAL RENEWAL

This claim lies at the heart of normative Jewish practice and of theology as well. The creation of the *chevra kadisha* represents a critical shift in people's thinking about how a community relates to the divine. Unlike parallel practices within Egyptian religions, the mediation of the death process within Judaism was and is both simple and unadorned. Jewish law insures that all members of the community receive a ritual burial. The act of burial is thus linked to the larger notion of a just human order. Like many practices in early rabbinic Judaism, the *taharah* encourages the community not to spend time decorating the dead, or obscuring the reality of death (Astren 1999).[6] Burial is put into the hands of the laity; priests (*cohenim*) are forbidden to touch the dead, which insures the democratization of the practice. The members of the *chevra kadisha* are secret, known only to one another. Yet in at least some periods, the society consisted of a rotational membership that afforded each member of the community with the opportunity to confront death.

Let me return to another of my letters. In this account, I am struck by the very starkness of the practice. Like the rabbinic discourse noted above, I retell the story of the care as a way of encountering the spiritual and intellectual issues of death. It is later in the year, after I have been a member of the *chevra kadisha* for a while. I have begun to lead the ritual myself:

It is the buckets and the wood, the 2 × 4s that start the grief in my heart, and it is because they are so clumsy, and they are the stuff of the poor laborer, steel buckets for water, wood for under the body, like lumber for a fragile poor woman's shelter. I think that they are the same tools that my Litvak great grandmother took into her hands as she went out into the Lithuanian night to wash the dead of her shetl. Around her, the black earth smells of cow dung, the path to the room for the dead was ankle deep in mud. And I do not know one thing about her, she, her family, the muddy shetl long burned in the Shoah, but I can know this central thing about her life, that she went out in the night to wash the bodies of her dead *chevra*, because, as I do, she knew that she must. It is raining and raining as she walks, and the buckets bump at her legs a little, the edges cut. And it is raining here in California tonight, and the buckets fill a little with rainwater as we carry them into the car.

So here is the moment that we all like to pretend doesn't exist, and here is the truth that for all our fussing will happen with certainty: each of us, and one by one all of us, will die. The people we love will die, and the people we hate will die, and people unknown to us will die; each of the strangers will be us as well. And each of them, because we are so fundamentally tied to them, will be forever lost to us. We cannot breathe, if we think of it, for the loss of it. So that is a very good reason, that stopping of the breath, to live out our lives as if it were not there, the door that leads to the room of death.

Traditional practices of death need a community of respondents. Someone must clean the body, someone must dress it, someone must watch the body until it can be buried, someone must dig a grave, and someone must fill it. In traditional communities, all of this work is done by members and mourners, not by invisible workers. As a scholar, I became curious about the historical evolution of the practice that I was engaged in. Such activity stops the ordinary work of the world. In antiquity, it was clearly mandated to be the work of all, but as communities grew larger, the need arose for a group that was specifically obligated.

All who pass by one who is buried must accompany the funeral [but] on occasion, Rabbi Hanuna came to a certain place and heard the sound of the funeral bugle. When he saw that members of the community continued on with their work, he said, "let them be placed under a ban." They informed him, however, that there was a *havurah* which occupied itself with this duty and he permitted the others to continue work.

In this passage, it is clear that the general practice of the rabbinic period underwent a change at a certain point, which became codified in the text. The *Shulhan Aruch* describes the formalizing of the practices:

At the beginning the departure of the dead [the burial] was more difficult for the relatives than his death because they used to take him out for many departures until they laid him in his grave and fled from him. Until Rambam Gamiel the elder came and behaved in lenient manner in the *halachah* and they took him out in a linen garment, and after him everyone did the same thing. (*Aruch* 19)

The details of the practice evolved over time. The essential idea is the same in many death rituals: to wash and re-dress the body. But how, and with what accompanying liturgy, is a matter that developed; hence this passage in the *midrash*:

When R. Johanan was departing from the world, he said to those who were to attend to his burial: Bury me in dun colored shrouds, neither white nor

black, so that if I stand among the righteous I may not be ashamed, and if
I stand among the wicked I may not be confounded. When R. Josiah was
taking leave of the world, he asked those who were standing around him
to summon his disciples, and he said to them: Bury me in white shrouds
because I am not ashamed through my deeds to meet my Maker. (*Rabbah* 19)

These passages mark the decision of a community to rotate the duties
involved in the *taharah*, allowing various groups to play a role, and the
decision to formalize the rituals of *tachrinin* (the making of the shrouds of
linen) and the use of the Jerusalem earth. From the first to the seventeenth
century, the *chevra* remained essentially a closed society, with members
caring for the burial of other members. But in the seventeenth century,
Jews began to urbanize, and formal *takkanot* (regulations) were drawn up
on the subject to establish regularized *chevra kadisha* with services that were
available to all, without attention to membership or dues.

Because I was a participant in the practice, I developed a further interest
in the role of words and narrative in the careful ritual. What is striking is
the silence of the ritual and the way that the silence allows for the most
intense inner reflections. This makes the spare and beautiful verses from
the *Song of Songs* even more potent. The practice evolved in large part out
of community custom. I explored this tradition because women in my
community were curious about how fixed the custom was, and whether it
could be changed from what was printed in the mortuary books that we
copied and passed around to read as we worked. Could we be permitted
to change the verses, using different parts of the *Song of Songs* (for example,
using parts that referred to women's bodies in particular)? Or was the
switching between differently gendered texts a carefully considered part of
the controlling legal texts that determined so much of the practice? Was
there a linguistic re-framing that we wanted to pursue as feminists, as had
been done in other rituals?

Research indicated that there is very little in the classical rabbinic literature about the liturgy recited at a *taharah*.[7] It is traditional to recite certain
psalms, verses from the prophets, and selections from the *Song of Songs*.
However, this is not codified in the traditional literature. The *Kitzur
Shulchan Aruch* (an authoritative book of legal summaries) does not mention
it (suggesting that when he is asked, the modern *psak* or rabbinic decisor
in traditional communities leaves it to the discretion of *minhag,* which are
local community customs and practices, and personal choice). The liturgy
is not mentioned in other classic commentaries such as *Sefer Chochmat*

HaAdam (a commentary on *Yoreh Deah*), and nothing is found regarding it in the *Shulchan Aruch*, *Turh*, or *Gemara*. In such cases, on other issues, communities were allowed a degree of innovation. There was no ironclad *halachic* standard specifying the sections of the *Song of Songs* that were to be read or whether the traditional readings could be replaced with different ones.[8] American communities tended to share and exchange common *taharah* handbooks, or have their own customs.

As I wrote of my experience in the *chevra* it became clear that it was not a widely known practice in American communities, where much of the ritual was performed by Jewish employees at funeral homes, or was abandoned altogether. It is not unusual for small Jewish communities not even to have a *chevra*. Even in Chicago, with a large Jewish population, the *chevra* was not established until 1950. In Berkeley, the *chevra* began with the death of a child in a newly established Orthodox community in the 1960s. A child died, and the family simply could not bear to turn her over to the mortuary. They asked if there was another way, if friends could perform the *taharah*. One woman I spoke to reported about that first night:

> She looked like a very tiny angel. Perfect. We sat and looked at her. One woman knew what to do, and she showed us how to begin. From then on, we began to be called more, at first only people we knew, then strangers. They had died in all kinds of ways, murders, the unfair deaths, babies. And when we were finished, I think, they are all very beautiful, all the pain, the grasping, all the trouble, gone from their faces.

From this first *taharah,* the *chevra* grew slowly. When I joined, it had been in existence for 10 years.

In a later letter, I referred to the way that the details of preparation both interrupt the secular flow of time and create a new temporal space that allows for the reflection on death.

> When the phone call comes, I am stopped, I know I should say yes. The premise here is simple: as in the talmudic dictum, a death in the community ought to stop us all, in the middle of the work of production, the bugle of death.
>
> We work out a time. The person must be attended to and buried quickly, ideally before sunset, surely within 48 hours. The Shiva period, and the grieving rituals associated with it, do not begin until after burial. We work out a place to meet. We need at least 3 women, 5 is the best. We drive out

to the mortuary, and we talk. Nobody is happy, we complain about our interrupted lives, our children left behind, the work we have left. In some communities, we reason, this work must have been done only by older women. We know that the *tachrechim*, the burial shrouds, must be sewn by post-menopausal women. But in our community we are mostly young, and pregnancy pulls women out for a time. The tradition here is not to have a pregnant women do this: the work is hard, physical, but that is only a part of it—it is the visual contradiction that is impossible to bear.

The mortuary is always odd, flashy, and falsely adorned, fake wood, fake opulence. It looks like a lobby of a cheap hotel. But they show us to the back room and it is always grim, a lab, with its metal tables, and big sinks; there are drawers full of theatrical make-up, and false hair, and curlers and spray. We walk in, buckets clanging, heads covered. We usually are in the middle of East Oakland. The man who runs the place is a sweet man, 6'3", helpful. He has read about us. He is good to us.

People at other places are more curious, they want to talk to us, we are the first Jews that they have seen, and clearly we are out of the mortuary class, right out of the picture in the book. We begin by ripping the satin lining out of the coffin and politely handing it over. We gown and glove now, we are aware of AIDS, herpes, the scars that mean she had surgery and maybe a blood transfusion, the marks of the chaotic world, it is the Bay Area.

Then all that is needed to work is assembled. We all wait outside. Once we enter and begin, after we ask permission to begin from the *metah*, we will not speak at all until we are finished. We wash without a blessing. It is the silence that is the most difficult part of the ritual. The theological construct is clear; the *metah* cannot speak, so to speak of her would exclude her. There are other reasons. Death is a world we cannot enter. We obscure the reality of this with talk, we turn desperately from silence to speech, and in the clinical world, to jokes. If it were not prohibited, I would chatter the whole time. We would argue about the method, guess about the narrative that the *metah* bears on her body. The silence forces presence, concentration. Now we are all without words, beyond a rational structure of response.

"Now may she tread with righteousness into the Garden of Eden," we say.

After, we thought about this.

"I find myself thinking about the clothes I have sewn. I find myself thinking about my body as my clothes," says one of us.

Another woman says, "In a way, we are all dressed in a kind of new clothing, the *chevra* wearing the skirt that one begins to set aside for this work, the head cloth, and now the gowns and gloves; the *metah* wearing her special garb as well."

I tell them that because there are no words, I make a story inside as I work.

A woman's hair must not be braided, clipped, tied or pinned; it is uncombed, rinsed. I unbraid the thick black hair, it is nearly waist long, only a little gray, very full. I unbraid her hair and unbraid her into her death, uncoiling her thick, beautiful hair. I work in silence, and my *chevra* watches in silence. I imagine the voices that surround her hair in her life. I think of her Hebrew name, the name that she has used only in childhood and in death: "Enya, sit still, I never get this hair done." "Enya, my sweet, look how your hair shines this morning." "Enya, get the hair from your face." I finish and I look up, and I see the *chevra* smiling. It is a corollary to this work that most of my friends think it ghoulish, and are afraid to talk about it. Historically this was not the case: Moses Montifiore was a *lavadoro*. But for many whom I have asked to join, it is too much to imagine, and unless they are bound by the sense of a committed life, they say no quickly. It is true; it is hard work. It means dealing with blood, lifting the body, twice: once onto a board, and once into a coffin. How can we go on, I sometimes think, in the middle. But this is a task that we must complete, and when we have done it, she is pure, transformed.

After we close the lid, we take our gloves off, and we ask forgiveness, in silence, from her. We are sorry, our human selves, we are tired, we are clumsy, we drop things, we are sorry beloved stranger, please forgive us.

And we step out, whole and living, into the black rain of Oakland. It is cold and it is lonely. We realize we miss the intense presence of the one in our midst who does not leave with us. We huddle closely around the tap outside the building. We wash our hands hard for a last time. Finally we talk. They tell me that they smiled at how beautiful her hair was. We think that Enya was proud of her hair, and it makes us smile to think of this. It has been three hours.

We drive home, shaken each time. Each time you are changed. We drive back, go home to the usual world. That night is taken up where we left it. But the next day I find myself thinking about this one that I have met, known, touched. We often call one another to talk about it.

CONSTRUCTING THE SOCIAL BODY

The act of the *taharah* is taking the body of the dead and returning it ritually to a human and particular self. Looking back on this later, after formal academic training as an ethicist, allows me to see what a powerful answer this deliberate care and reenactment of the ancient ritual is to death. Let us reflect on what precedes this in the clinical context, which is the usual site of medicine and bioethics' reflection on medicine. In many cases, death in modernity is a battle lost. Death is seen as the problem, the structural enemy that is engaged by the moral gesture of medicine itself. But medicine is both a moral gesture and an act in the marketplace economy. Hence, when the body is no longer a patient, with all that status entails, it is ordinarily discarded by a certain prestigious sector whose attention can no longer be repaid—certainly not financially. The body then is treated as though it has returned to an animal state. It is wrapped, refrigerated, and handled by the clinical world in this way, like a piece of refrigerated meat, cared for by the lowest status person, not even gowned in any garb, only wrapped in a sheet.

But the first gesture of the *taharah* is the creation of a different tangible relationship, a ritual and temporal space in which the body is named, with the name of the child self, given in infancy,[9] and invited to the act of care by the community. The dead's utter inability to respond means that the act will have no direct benefit to the participants. There will be no compensation. Caring for the dead is given as an example of working beyond the line of the law. It is important to see how this act—a religious act, and a moral one—thus differs in tone from the act of medicine. We, the participants, regard and so construct a "social body" over and against the body of our ordinary practices of caring and medicine.

Catherine Bell, a sociologist, comments in her work on the practice and theory of ritual (Bell 1998), and she pays special attention to the ritual body. Her reflections create a useful frame. Bell reminds us of the way that all bodies are "social bodies." The body is the social location that encapsulates the principles that organize society. The body serves not only as a metaphor, but also as a carrier of the postmodern idea of the necessity for articulating tangibility, location, and context.

The body of the dead one (the *metah*) is a body that is, as much as is possible, a pure, irreducible "body." Because we know only the Hebrew name of the *metah*, and because she is a total stranger to us, naked, without title, clothes, or history, we receive her without the trappings or illusions of power or linkages to politics. She cannot speak, and we cannot (in large part) speak. Our interactions with her are entirely embodied, tangible ones. Yet she will be re-constituted by the ritual. She will be washed of all the last indignities of dying, and she will be re-dressed in the stylized garments unchanged in shape or construction since the first century, a tunic and a shirt, a bonnet for her hair. Because this act is done in silence, and its perimeters are not subject to negotiation, it is an example of what Boudieu describes as "a dialectic of objectification and embodiment" that makes it the locus for the coordination of all levels of bodily, social, and cosmological experience (Bell 1998). She may have died as a body, ravaged by the travails at the nexus of modernity, medicine, and illness, but she will be buried as a Jew, in exactly the ritualized body of the Jew of two thousand years previous to her particular story, thus relinking her and the ones who prepare her with other, replicated selves.

But the body of the *metah* is not the only "ritualized body"—the bodies of the *chevra* also become ritualized by the process of the *taharah*. The ritual is a series of physical movements. Ritual practices spatially and temporally construct an environment organized according to schemes of privileged opposition. The construction of this environment and the activities within it simultaneously work to impress these schemes upon the bodies of the participants. For example, there is tension between pollution and purity, death and love, blood and water, nakedness and clothing, the poetry of the liturgy and the starkness of the directions (place the feet toward the door), all of which potentiates the essential contradiction: the *chevra*, alive, and the *metah*, dead.

The logic of ritual acts that are embodied in complex physical movements returns the participant to a logic of the body, a logic that is "thereby lodged beyond the grasp of consciousness and articulation" (Bell 1998). Hence the acts of silent care taking, the act of cleansing with water and lifting the person, once onto boards, naked, and then again into the coffin, clean and re-dressed (and the injustice of death, also redressed) imprints on the *chevra* the intimacy and the compassion of friendship. In the face of the stark horror of death, and in the midst of the great mess that it is to die, one acts *as if* the world of chaos and contingency are not all-powerful, to recreate a space of order, cleanliness, and reciprocity. As Bell reminds us, ritual is an act of production—the production of a ritualized agent who is able to wield a scheme of subordination or insubordination (Bell 1998). It is a strategic act, meaning that it is an act directed at a goal: It is meant both to accomplish something for the *metah*, her purification, and to offer a complex strategy to the members of the *chevra* for returning to the world after the starkness of the confrontation with death. By doing this act, we produce ourselves as moral actors. We are the ones who can do the act of stopping for the other, and we can return, internally shaken but heroicized, a rare moment for women. It is here that the simple power of that which is traditionally the work of women is most fully realized: washing and cleaning the body is a metaphor for that which must be done to remake the world morally after the loss and unfairness of mortality.

But the reality of our situation is a sort of binary opposition: we can leave, you must stay. This can lead to resolution through the reestablishment of hierarchical needs, or it can lead to a deeper appreciation, through the ritual, of the play of differences among related elements and persons who are in different positions in the ritual. Here, we turn to Derrida's insight that ritual acts can produce a "grammatology" or notice of signification, which rests on an open-ended social contradiction. One is drawn into a series of unanswered questions that lie just below the surface of the act. We are, after all, preparing a dead body for burial. But for most of the participants, the work of the *taharah* is accomplished by the difficult physical gestures, actions that actively create a safe, controlled, and faithful place within a difficult physical environment, within the most difficult of human narratives. That the actions themselves are in large part that which would be done to one's own body, or to the body that one loves, marks them as both intimate and mundane, and hence sacred and profane.

The strategies of even the most traditional of rituals are often resistant to larger cultural themes. In the act of the *taharah*, one can clearly locate this resistance in texts and actions used in the service of the theoretical metaphorical acceptance of death. For example there is the use of the *Song of Songs'* erotic love poetry as text, and the act of ritualized control over the earth on the body—earth taken from Jerusalem has always been required in such a gesture, defying both time and venue. For many participants, the act of the *taharah* is both socially redemptive and personally redemptive, in precisely the way that Bell notes. By this act, we acknowledge both the finality of death and the power of God, yet we are arranging the earth in patterns, and we are saying words to remake the ill and injured body as beautiful.

In her work on the ritual life of elderly Jewish women, Barbara Myerhoff notes similar themes. The work of the *taharah* is done by both men and women, but it is quintessentially women's work, is done in private and in secret. "Women," she writes, "are kept humble by the nature of their everyday activities. They are immersed in unglamorous stuff—the mess of life itself, bodily excretions and necessities, transit and trivial details that vanish and reappear every moment. ... I would claim that there is a set of understandings, regularly stated and shared among women, concerning the meaning and value of their conventional functions" (Myerhoff 1978).

Much is in fact "understood" in this way. Even though the *taharah* is associated with traditional women's work, it is also, in my view, a feminist gesture—a gesture of care without mutuality. Both men and women alike can cultivate such care; indeed, by requiring that men and women alike pay careful attention in the *taharah* to the most needy, messy, and voiceless, Jewish practice has compelled compassion from each to each (Boyarin 1998). Much more research will have to be done along these lines. However, Daniel Boyarin has argued that many of the required practices of rabbinic and medieval Jewish culture resisted gender-based determinations of roles. Boyarin argues that the ideal Jewish man in the Talmud is not the Roman warrior, and that this difference in gender position is one of the distinctions between Jews and early Christians.

The understanding that Myerhoff refers to also marks the first-person accounts that are beginning to be published in the literature about the *chevra kadisha* as a new generation of Jews begins to join, and to speak and write of the transformative possibilities of the ritual. In account after account, participants speak of the beauty and peacefulness of the *metah* after the ritual is completed, and of the shift in the self that the act demands, the ability of both women and men to enliven faith in the act of honoring the daily and mundane. Here again much more research is needed to understand how newly imagined Jewish life, just now undergoing a renewal of attention and of traditional practice, will regard this "hard *mitzvah*." Not all of the *chevras* that exist are Orthodox. In Berkeley, for example, there are now two: a Conservative and an Orthodox one. Because the practice is largely shaped by community practice, the work of the participants will continually recreate the practice itself, within the essential constraints. This process of tradition-constituting renewal, as Boyarin and others remind us, has been a continual part of Jewish life over the last three centuries. It is important to note that this renewal takes place against the textual grounds referred to earlier.

Where do considerations of the ritual event of the *taharah* and of the *chevra kadisha* lead us as scholars (and as participants)? This directs us toward several possible next steps, useful and fruitful directions toward new theoretical developments and new practices that are rich with ethical implications.

First, as communities of modern Jews reflect on the way that traditional *mitzvot* are reconfigured and expressed, the attention to the embodied experience of the *taharah* allows Jews to pay attention to death and the confrontation that it requires. Rather than a simplistic and cheery attention to joyfulness, celebration, and festival, this *mitzvah* insists on the silence and mundane necessity that death requires. Communities that take on the requirement of participation in the *taharah* are asserting their willingness to provide the necessities of adult life. It is the ultimate expression of intergenerational responsibility.

Second, in asking the question about whose obligation it is to care for the bodies of the dead, we begin to understand why the act of caring for the dead one transforms us. Rather than reifying the horror of death, we work ritually to prepare ourselves to face death nobly—one of the key tasks of a human life. It is one of the tragedies of modernity that in our eagerness for the triumphs of medical science, we rarely witness birth and death first hand. We live as if the great mess and tumult of the ending and beginning of life is best handled in a separate, clinical arena. But the concept of the *chevra*, as one in which each is obligated to participate, deconstructs such a distance. The starkness and the nakedness of the *metah* impose a great lesson of death—that possessions are in the deepest sense pointless. We see instantly that what is left to you is literally the company of community, and the last hand that will touch you will be empty of all but the moral gesture of *chesed* (compassion).

Third, it is at the *taharah* that the sense of the utter otherness of the stranger is most strongly felt. The gaze toward the beloved stranger cannot be returned. Silence surrounds his or her narrative, and it is at that moment, in the fictive, imagined, and internalized conversation that one is unable to remain entirely discreet. The power of the work of the *taharah* is that the participants must touch the person and make him or her the center of intense and highly detailed activity. The act is not over when one is bored, or tired, or no longer entertained as in so much of modernity.[10] It is over only when all details are perfectly complete. And this intense focus on the utterly other reveals in the encounter a moment of radical recognition that this one will be you. Otherness is both total and vanquished, because although I may never literally be the other that I meet—I may never really be this powerful one or that vulnerable one except in my moral imagination—I will in fact be exactly as dead as this other at some point. I may not ever fully understand the situation of the other, I might never share her life circumstance. But there is one way in which we are exactly, and inescapably alike. I will be a dead Jew, just like this.

The dead one, who is other-than-self, is not faceless or abstract. One by one, the dead will be carefully dressed, and the encounter will underscore the uniqueness and the difference of each. The other is irreducibly herself and irretrievably gone, but is incontestably you, as well, because you, too, will be as dead as she is dead. What the act of the *chevra ḳadisha* offers is the inescapable recognition that this is the road for all of us, no matter who else we were, or what else we wear.

Fourth, the act of the *taharah* offers an extreme and final comment on the oddity of the American culture of the body. One is directed to say a passionate liturgy of love as they clean a dead, often aged, broken body, and to come to see it as beautiful and pure by virtue of their account and attention. This loving attention in death repudiates the culture's hatred of the old—especially women's old bodies. For each participant, it reveals the emptiness of the yearning toward the perfection of modernity; the costume and the made-up self are washed away. At some point, the beautiful body will be this body. We are the last ones to see the vulnerability of the breasts, the genitalia, the belly-house of the children. The task of the *chevra* is to remake this body one last time, to create human order over the chaos of death without obscuring death. This is what love does: it allows for the essential core self to be intimately and nakedly gazed upon, seen in all of its vulnerability, and found utterly and completely beautiful. We see, when we see the *metah*, a double visage, ourselves in the darkest mirror of our own death.

BIOETHICS AND THE STORY OF COMPASSIONATE ACTION

Finally, the discourse surrounding the *chevra ḳadisha* has implications for our approach to the subject of death and our attempts to order and control it. As a bioethicist who studies the social construction of policies and practices of death, I think it is critical that we allow the insights gained in the particularized experiences of the *chevra* to shape the social debate, to remember the textual link between justice and redemption, between the care of the least of us and the fabric of the whole. Death cannot be controlled, it can only be witnessed, and in that witness, we must love the other enough to stand through and past the leave-taking.

The ritual act of care and the retelling of the act create a literary paradox akin to the problem in bioethics of the framing of a story based on some event. The problem of the tension between text, context, and moral meaning occurs whenever the narrative is about death. In her reflection on the *Aḳedah* (the Biblical account of the near-sacrifice of Isaac), Aviva Zornberg asks the question of why the Jewish *midrashic* narrative tradition insists that Sarah dies because of the *Aḳedah*. It is a paradox, a final joke on death—

Isaac is not dead, so why does the *midrash* recount an imagined story of him coming home to her, and of her death when he tells her of his rescue? The idea is of a self that can be torn from the world. Abraham tears himself from the world, and this is an act of faith. Seeing the dead self, who is still utterly and inescapably that particular self, reminds us of the core at the center of the world of the constructed self. What is then startling is how death replicates this tearing from the community to an unknown distance. (It is notable that one of the key Jewish mourning rituals is that some article of the mourners' clothes is torn at the funeral and worn all that week to make this "tear" visible to all who see the mourner.) It is this sense of contingency that creates for Sarah a sense of vertigo, as described in Ricouer, the insight that one lives by the breath of chance, and that nothing can protect one from this. Modernity represents the idea that all can be chosen. "If you can be born again, you can be unborn," notes Peter Berger; even religion is so much costume to be taken on and off (Berger 1998).

But you cannot be unborn from death. It is the unchosen nature of the event, the torn-ness that is repaired by faith and by solidarity alone, stitched together by hand, like the shrouds of our burial *tachrehim*, that makes human life possible again. We can leave the stranger and go back into the night and our lives because she is accompanied by our mundane, com-manded, moral gesture, a small good act. She is lit by the smallest flame, by the lifting of the body into the air, the tying of her bonnet just so, the buckets and the wood.

As a bioethicist, I write an essay that tells you, the reader, of how the act of compassion toward the dead transforms my gaze toward the dead, toward the living, and finally toward myself. This is the nature of story, the moral of story. It is why narrative ethics is in part about how to pass on the truthful, and in part about how telling what is truthful is itself a transformative act. We are made whole again after caring the *metah* back into a wholly clean state. She is clean, "sanitized," and we are sanctified—the same root word.

I place story against story against story, word against word against word, to alert you to the possibility of disarmament of the powerful master narrative of medicine. This idea of narratives of care serving as cultural forces and foundational stories operates in ways that are completely unparochial as well. My narrative in this essay, presented through letters and then reflections on the letters, about the peculiar death practices of my Orthodox community, seems particularistic in the extreme, so much so that I wonder how well it can serve as a shared cultural metaphor in bioethics. However, the resonances are unexpected, even serendipitous. Across years and cultures, I later come across a scene in the novel *Blindness* by Nobel laureate Jose Saramago that fully elicits this response (Saramago 1997). It describes the aftermath of a mass epidemic of blindness; it reflects on disease and clinical treatment, on death and redemption, and on moral relationships between neighbors when speech and action are all that matter. The idea that words told in the correct way can be disarming is his insight. At the core of the novel are the daily details of caring for the utterly vulnerable and for the dead. Ritual/real bathing is used twice in the novel, and both times the cleansing is a purification and a real cleaning both, exactly as in the *taharah*.

In one passage, Saramago describes the response of women, held in a hospital during a medical quarantine, to a brutal gang rape. During the rape, one of them has died, and one—a woman who has not been blinded by the epidemic—must care for all of the others. In his account, one can see nearly every detail—the buckets, the cleaning, and the transformation that takes place when one attends to the cleaning of the dead. It is an indirect parallel, a mirror of my account. As Saramago tells the story, we as readers of the events in his fictive universe are given what we need to be moral actors in our own world, the alchemy of ethics and narrative transforming deed into word (in the case of this essay) and word into the possibility of deed again (as in the novel), transforming the world on behalf of the other's needs.

> She knew what she wanted, she did not know if she would find it. She needed a bucket or something that would serve the purpose, she wanted to fill it with water, even if fetid, even if polluted, she wanted to wash the corpse of the woman ... to wipe away her own blood and the sperm of others, to deliver her purified to the earth, if it still makes sense to speak of the purity of the body in this asylum where we are living, for purity of the soul, as we know, is beyond everyone's reach. ... When the doctor and the old man with the black eyepatch entered the ward ... they did not see, could not see, seven naked women and the corpse of the woman ... stretched out on her bed, cleaner than she had ever been in all her life, while another woman was washing her companions, one by one, and then herself. (Saramago 1997)

Near the end of the novel, there is another "*taharah*," another ritual/ actual total purification. Saramago writes a scene which comments on and redeems the desperate and isolated *taharah* in the first part of the novel.

Here, these same women, covered in the filth of weeks of incarceration, have escaped the hospital that has become literally a prison, and they burn it to the ground. Afterwards, they slowly create a small, just, and loving social world amidst the despair that has engulfed their city. They find a new way to transform through moral activity and compassion the epidemic blindness that has overtaken them ("we are still blind—blind but seeing"). They return to the home of the woman who is the protagonist, and the one who has cared for and hence saved each of the others from death, and they stand on a balcony. There is a sudden, drenching and steady rainstorm, and they strip off their filthy rags and stand naked in the downpour, "buckets and buckets" of rain covering and cleaning them. It is as if God is doing the *taharah*, and the cleaning is utterly redemptive. It is "the most beautiful thing in the history of the city" that somewhere in the darkened night, women see each other's beauty in the moral commitments that have been made. The other women are thanking the first woman by seeing her as her moral activity has constructed her. They see only her social body or rather her "ethical" body, and it is beautiful. Instead of mirrors, what is seen of the body is only the acts of loving-kindness, which in the Jewish tradition are all that we have after death, all that we can say of heaven, the word Jews use to disarm death's power. The life of the person continues on in the presence of the deeds of care.

In a scene in which care, feminist commitment, and narrative language are all visible, the narrator begins as witness:

Perhaps we have judged them wrongly, or perhaps we are unable to see this the most beautiful and glorious thing that has happened in the history of the city, a sheet of foam flows from the balcony, if only I could with it, falling interminably, clean, purified, naked. Only God sees us, said the wife of the first blind man, who despite disappointments and setbacks, clings to the belief that God is not blind, to which the doctor's wife replies, Not even he, the sky is clouded over, Only I can see you. Am I ugly, asked the girl with the dark glasses, You are skinny and dirty, you will never be ugly, And I, asked the wife of the first blind man, You are dirty and skinny like her, not as pretty, but more than I, You are beautiful, said the girl with dark glasses . . . but at my age . . . that's what happens to us we were more beautiful once, You were never more beautiful, said the wife of the first blind man. Words are like that, they deceive, they pile up, it seems they do not know where to go, and, suddenly because of two or three or four that suddenly come out, simple in themselves, a personal pronoun, an adverb,

verb, an adjective we have the excitement of seeing them coming irresistibly to the surface through the skin and the eyes and upsetting the composure of our feelings, sometimes the nerves that cannot bear it any longer, they put up with a great deal, they put up with everything, it was as if they were wearing armour, we might say. (Saramago 1997)

We might say this about medicine as well, and certainly about the alchemy of his ethics, to turn deed back into word, act into story, and care into narrative. It is the intent of this essay, this "word pile," to create a method for finding such a moment—surfacing the excitement and the seeing that rise in us at our best, which is to say, at our most human and defining moments.

Endnotes

1 This language about the need to tell the narrative on behalf of the temporary survivors was suggested to me by the editors of this volume.

2 Earlier historical periods allowed women to prepare men for burial.

3 The *Talmud* is a compilation of law, commentary, and narratives surrounding the commentary that was collected and recorded from older oral traditions in the period between 200 B.C.E. and 500 C.E.

4 By this I mean to include the many things that medicine requires as well, like caring for the poor, the infectious, or the difficult, as well as for the dead.

5 All that is missing here is feeding. This list of primate bonding behaviors emerges from the work of Harlow, Klaus, and others. Primate infants deprived of these behaviors at birth become nonfunctional, exhibiting behaviors that are like those seen in autistic children. My point is that the body is re-humanized using the same behaviors that are normally performed at birth to initiate contact into the human family.

6 Astren notes that Jewish practice discouraged spending time at the graveside, as well as other behaviors that resembled pagan death rituals.

7 This research was done by Haggai Resnikoff, a Yeshiva student who was my research assistant in the summer of 1998. I wish to thank Mr. Resnikoff for his carefully conducted research into the Aramaic and Hebrew sources.

8 This is an important point, especially when we reflect on the fact that the liturgy that is recited is based on the section of the *Song of Songs* that describes a man's body. My research suggests that this focus could be altered through the use of other selections from *Shir*, keeping the traditional text in tact but adding other, more feministic verses to it. No *halachic* damage would be done thereby. This needs further research, but this is my conclusion at this point.

9 Jews are named at birth. Many American Jews are not addressed by their birth names again until they die.

10 Even in religious practice, some constantly try to make it "more enjoyable," as if it were a game or an event meant to amuse children.

References

Astren, Fred. 1999. Depaganizing Death: Jewish and Muslim Burial Practices. *Humanities* (spring).

Baba Metzia, 30b Soncino Talmud. 1973. London: Soncino Press.

Bell, Catherine. 1998. *Ritual Theory, Ritual Practice*. New York: Oxford University Press.

Berger, Peter. 1998. *A Far Glory*. New York: Oxford University Press.

Boyarin, Daniel. 1998. *Judaism and the Rise of Heterosexuality*. Stanford, Calif: Stanford University Press.

Goodison, Lusy. 1989. Death, Women and the Sun. *Institute of Classical Studies Bulletin Supplement 53*. University of London.

Hoch-Smith, Judith, and Anita Spring, eds. 1978. *Women in Ritual and Symbolic Roles*. New York: Plenum Press.

Midrash Rabbath, Soncino Talmud, Midrash Deuteronomy. 1961. London: Soncino Press.

Midrash Rabbah, Soncino Talmud, Midrash Bereshit. 1961. London: Soncino Press.

Myerhoff, Barbara. 1978. Bobbes and Zaydes: Old and New Roles for Elderly Jews. In *Women in Ritual and Symbolic Roles,* ed. Judith Hoch-Smith and Anita Spring. New York: Plenum Press.

Saramago, Jose. 1997. *Blindness*, trans. Jose Sanger. New York: Harcourt Brace.

Shulhan Aruch. 1984. London: Soncino Press.

Weiss, Abner. 1991. *Death and Bereavement: A Halakhic Guide*. Hoboken, N.J.: Ktav Publishing House.

10
AIDS in East Tennessee: Medicine and Morals as Local Activities

Ruth L. Smith

SITUATING MEDICAL ETHICS

Small local hospitals in the mountain counties of the Southern Appalachian highlands depend on doctors and interns who are willing to moonlight from the nearest regional medical center. In taking on extra work while an intern at the Johnson City Medical Center in northeastern Tennessee, Abraham Verghese gets to know Essie Vines, a highly committed lab technician at the Blackwood Virginia hospital. Several years later, Essie hears that Verghese has returned to a faculty position at the medical school just as her brother Gordon has returned home to Virginia in bad shape with HIV/AIDS. After a call to Verghese, Essie drives Gordon down that evening to meet the doctor at the emergency room (Verghese 1994, 73). Gordon is probably the third person diagnosed with HIV/AIDS in the Johnson City Medical Center and the first of what within five years would become a group of eighty patients for Verghese, whose interest in infectious diseases had already brought him some experience with HIV/AIDS patients in Boston hospitals. In the mid-eighties, drug therapies for the HIV virus were undeveloped, and sexual intolerance compounded the contemporary inclination to interpret those suffering from any feared disease through punitive metaphors (Sontag 1990). No hospital would be the same place for Gordon that it would be for patients whose illnesses could be better charted and who were not so vulnerable to hostility, though patients such as Gordon also signify the uncertain course of much illness and the power of any prejudice to jeopardize receiving even minimal medical responses. As it turns out, people with HIV/AIDS who enter the Johnson City Medical Center will be both shunned and extremely well cared for.

In *My Own Country*, Verghese's account of AIDS in East Tennessee, the official rhetorical practices of medicine and ethics flounder in the face of weak research and strong homophobia. I use this hiatus to raise and explore the question of how medical ethics happens, or more to my point, takes place as a rhetorical-spatial transaction. Because Verghese makes explicit his sensibilities to locations, I rewrite his practice as an opportunity to consider place relations as part of medical ethics, here in my study of three loci: bodies as sites of touch, Vickie and Clyde McCray's front porch, and The Connection, the local gay bar in Johnson City. The disciplinary production of medical ethics has been so routinely situated in the modern hospital that we forget that it is situated at all. As a consequence, context and practice indicate a-theoretical spaces, termed "background" or "application," to which theory may have reference, but which are not themselves spaces of theoretical knowledge. Deemed unphilosophical, context and practice cannot engage theory on its own terms, but can only fulfill or fail the theory overlaid on or applied to them. This problem is evident in the undeveloped character of notions that indicate the context of a situation, ethos in ethics and pathos in rhetoric, which are suppressed at least in part because they destabilize the kinds of claims about autonomy that mark much of modern moral and social theory. Modern claims to autonomy are at once secure in their authority to override any situation and insecure in their perpetual struggle with the monolithic determinism regularly assigned to context. Either way, context is presented in a dualistic relation with autonomy and as description that does not enter into the proper boundaries of moral consideration itself.

As feminists and African-American womanists have argued, however, accounts of contexts are accounts of relations and so are active, not passive. They do not simply describe but recommend; that is, they attempt to persuade regarding what merits acknowledgment and what does not. Any notion that context is prior to morality suppresses moral arguments and perspectives available only through considerations of context. What in modern views constitutes ethics proper is itself an argument that certain relations prevail over others. One way in which some feminists have developed contextual ethics is with notions of care that emphasize the primacy of relations in contrast to autonomy, which deprecates or silences them. Feminist arguments, however, often articulate care through a generalized context without attention to differential power relations in the rhetorical spaces of care. Traditionally, arguments for an ethic of care also identify ethics by a single term from which all else follows. I argue, instead, for a messier, more complicated view of ethics that is not summarized by a master relationship, virtue, principle, or rule. Ethics is elaborated, invented, and interrupted in activities and gestures (saying—being—doing) that indicate the uncertain character of moral territories and discourses and the place-rhetorical character of how morality is produced.

One may argue that any moral discussion of context presumes virtues, principles, and rules of conduct, and so we are back to customary terms anyway. I would say that these terms only sometimes signify, and always in and as a rhetorical-spatial context. My approach intensifies the stakes of virtues, principles, and rules by considering how they work when one takes place relations into account in the activity of ethics. My approach calls into question traditional moral codes as an adequate way of describing moral activity in situations in which so much is unknown (and these situations tell us about others we consider known). Accordingly, I work with Verghese's account not to establish the backdrop for moral action, but to explore and analyze how players transact situations of medical ethics at the junctures of HIV/AIDS. Here morality includes activities that expand a familiar modern moral lexicon of respect and compassion with older terms of consolation, assistance, and courage, and newer terms of resistance and solidarity. At the same time, the moral activities at the junctures of HIV/AIDS also exceed, contradict, and subvert all of these terms, pushing us not only to contest their moral discourse, but also to rework our notions of how morality occurs when it does occur. In the nexus of Gordon's being infected at all, Essie Vine's call to Verghese, and Verghese's response, vectors and strata cross and shift in exhibited movements that make their senses, moral and otherwise, in the rhetorical spaces these people inhabit. In the directions of their driving, walking, speaking, and gesturing, with and without an official moral lexicon, medical ethics occurs through situational exigencies, conventions and unconventions of language, and locations and times in linguistic and nonlinguistic features.

How medical ethics gets re-imagined when situated is currently under discussion in arguments that give priority to context and practice. In "Keeping Moral Space Open," Margaret Urban Walker elaborates a notion of context through narrative with the argument that ethicists who work in health care environments are better understood as architects of moral space than as masters of normative law and code (Walker 1993, 40). As a participant in a narrative, the ethicist helps design a way for things to happen through negotiation and mediation in the conversational space where different parties meet or need to meet. Looking out for moral interaction takes place not apart from but amidst the design process. Carl Elliot, also arguing against a medical ethic limited to principles and procedures, elaborates a notion of context that emphasizes the ways morals are located in ways of life, not as closed, symmetrical, whole entities, but as diffuse and overlapping in their social significations (Elliot 1992, 31). Though we may make decisions for how we negotiate morals as part of a form of life, the articulation of morals entails much more than a decision-making process. Elliot hints at the larger field with his argument that, among other loci, the baseball game and American church-small town relations participate in the moral shaping of "the right to die" debate in this country (34).

My approach has affinities with those of Walker and Elliot, but emphasizes geographies specifically as the spaces we articulate as and with bodies, words, institutions, dwellings, and migrations. This perspective runs counter to two related philosophical inclinations, each of which assumes hermetic autonomy and homogenous space. One is the inclination to denote space as a determining category outside human activity that posits and controls fundamental conditions of existence and meaning, as with Plato's theory of forms and some notions of Christian transcendence. An opposite and complementary inclination is to consider place as a determining category of the inert inside, in which no motion or only predetermined motion is possible, as is the case with notions that, like narrow empiricist understandings of reality as strictly predictable and fixed, ascribe mechanistic qualities to location. Attention to place relations in medical ethics indicates, however, that spaces entail aspects of life and death not well captured by either of these philosophical inclinations that leave ethics divided between formal and instrumental views of place, each with their notions of control. So, to bring Verghese's description and analysis of a situation into my considerations about ethics is not to deploy it as an alternative model that constitutes unproblematic moral perfection, or that constitutes a series of discrete, monolithic variables of imperfection, but to deploy it to think critically and inventively about the making of ethics *in situ*. If place relations participate in what ethicists conventionally call agency, then the boundaries of person and context are themselves a question. At the same time, the view I am exploring is not that of a closed, fused, symmetrical system in which moral or existential deliberation has no place, but one in which whatever is going on morally only makes sense as a context that makes a demand, what rhetoricians call the rhetorical situation. After spontaneously calling Essie Vines to check on Gordon late one night, Verghese comments: "I was developing a patient-physician relationship unlike anything I had known" (Verghese 1994, 137). Verghese's relations with his patients have little to do with a crisis decision made amidst the hypertechnologies of the modern hospital, and much to do with events and exchanges that are more transparently connected to the social experiences of illness, more variegated in their linguistic and nonlinguistic exchange, and more diffuse in their locations of place and time, aspects current theories of place help articulate.

SPACE AND PLACE AS PARTICIPATORY

At this point, readers may be wondering what such an approach asks them to commit themselves to, because I am not only asking readers to consider an argument, but to consider a kind of approach that I cannot fully demonstrate by measures conventional to ethics, and so must rely on other kinds of persuasion. Most notably, I must try to convey the performative character of medical ethics. In some sense, thinkers always ask this of each other, to go a distance further than the means of persuasion can adequately cover, but I am also proposing different sources of persuasion than are common to ethics. Verghese poses these issues in certain respects, asking his readers to have confidence in his version of things as reliable, even as there are other versions, and to have confidence in his medical practice, even as it includes a range of conventional and unconventional performances. Part of Verghese's figuration of self is his attentiveness to bodies, both his and those of his patients, as loci, and to the built and natural environments in which they move and which move in them. This does not mean he always knows where he is, but that he is aware of these facets and their shifting rhetorical registers. Their shifting is one I am particularly drawn into as a reader and writer, because I grew up in Johnson City and so see things with different and mutual recognition, sharing with Verghese the fragilities and deceptions of memory about place. Readers are accustomed to such orientations and disorientations in autobiographical-biographical writing, but we are less accustomed to this experience in reading and writing ethics. What we are used to is geometric space.

Gaston Bachelard takes issue with the inherited philosophical dualism of geometric and inhabited space with his argument in *The Poetics of Space* that sensory awareness and memory are kinds of knowing that can only be grasped through attention to the spaces in which we experience them (Bachelard 1994). Spaces are not the background or the occasion for memory and sensation but participate in their very existence, that is, in having them at all, and in the contingencies of their existence. The vulnerability of image, like the vulnerability of value, attests to its life (59), jogging verbs into action, as with any one event of "to emerge from" (109–10). Bachelard makes uncritical use of archetypes and northern European images; nonetheless, he opens up place not as an unproductive force, but as a plethora of images that make their way willy nilly into all knowing, although the knowing of philosophy is constructed to keep them at bay in fear that its narrow rationality will be undone (see Smith 1997–1998).

To extend Bachelard's focus on intimate sites, E.V. Walter advocates a philosophy of "topistics," in which the life of inhabited places emphasizes the wholeness and integrity, intact or broken, of all aspects of natural and built life in any given dwelling, be it the Aborigines' desert, contemporary urban street corners, or migrations of germs in fourteenth-century Europe (Walter 1988, 6, 204). Like Bachelard, who speaks of the well-being, recapturable in reverie, that precedes being cast into the world (7), Walter is after a frame of mind they both associate with earlier human consciousness in which the sensory communication between being and habitation constitutes a recognized, felt, fluid unity of experience and knowledge (18). Walter identifies this frame of mind with the older notion "theoria," for which place relations of sensed knowing are paramount. Although the notion of theoria tends to emphasize the more distanced senses of seeing and hearing, Walter argues that in Plato it constitutes a strand submerged by the other strand of Plato, the rationality that inhabits only geometric space (3–4).

Verghese's own spatial orientation is more tactile and participatory than either strand in Plato, and extends the aspects in Walter that indicate a more externalized, less finished view of people and their environments in the making. Yet Verghese's search for home indicates some notion of an integral experience of self with place and activity. The assumption of an earlier ontological or historical experience of an integral self and sense evident in Bachelard's and Walter's theories is important to arguments that emphasize the lost interactions of humans and places habitual to polytheistic or animistic cultures. David Abram associates this loss with the invention of alphabetic writing systems whose letters have no reference to sensate, physical life and whose primary figure is the individual who gains self-reflexivity but loses connection with the animal life of the human species and with other organic life (Abram 1996, 112, 121). Ecologically oriented feminists associate the loss of sensed place participation with the emergence of patriarchal institutions that instate violent notions of the sacred located outside and over the earth in opposition to its own polytheistic spirits (Lippard 1983; Spretnak 1991). However remote, the participatory character of place for these thinkers remains as a vestigial, potentially retrievable aspect in sensory and intuitive knowledge. Nonetheless, these proposals share some of the problems of care ethics. They are embedded in notions of an unfissured unity considered synonymous with an inherent ontological good that is without reference to power, memory, or plurality in place-sense experience, features that are always part of human experience and knowing. Self-described "art thinker" Lucy Lippard breaks through the controlling assumption of unity by considering place relations as a matter of changing and exchanging human and geological narratives. For Lippard, any one "here" is comprised of "the particular intersection of land, history, and—at once rotary and crossroad—culture" (Lippard 1997, 5), as are the "heres" of Verghese's places of Ethiopia, India, Boston, and the Appalachian highlands.

As an experience of the senses, place tells us where we are equivocally and unequivocally as we make our ways around. But it is not just sense reaching out for place; place reaches out for the senses in redolent, tactile, auditory, and visual significations that extend in further experiences of association, memory, and image with their familiarity, novelty, and shock, aspects that may or may not assume the shape of narrative with a beginning, middle, and end. These aspects feed inhabitants and their geographies what Walter calls a "topistic diet" (Walter 1988, 150). The tangibility of place, composed of its energy, its "intangible provisions" (150), may be located or constructed, as in sacred sites—the mountain as a locus of divine communication or mystical communion, the geomantic positioning of stone on a cave wall, the tree of life, or the building of a cathedral (Schama 1995). Sacred spaces are among the most direct ways to consider the performative character of place in the full range of the sensory, including the intellect and the "sixth sense" of spirit. Attention to behavior in a sacred space may be for many people their most self-conscious experience of the participatory character of place; it also highlights the performative character of place relations more generally as we reproduce, challenge, and elaborate them in ways that shift and change what we too simply distinguish as space and actor.

Regardless of how one answers questions of what constitutes barriers and conduits of place-knowing, the responses expand perception to include the imagination, intuition, and sensation that places evoke from us (and we from them) in the mingling of human with other life forms that have been largely banished from what is considered perception. Contrary to the modern view, the kitchen table where Verghese sits with Essie and her daughters putting together Gordon's medical history is alive in some sense, as is the site of Gordon's grave, further into the mountain, looking out on an extraordinary vista. In considering what has been banished, Lorraine Code observes that perception is the foundation claimed for modern rationality, with its Cartesian views of what constitutes authoritative evidence (Code 1995, 165). To qualify as a fact, any claim about the senses must meet criteria that evaluate the claim's capacity to satisfy an agreed-upon set of conditions for rationality; these conditions include the rhetoric of "sense-data," those abstracted pieces that constitute information. There is also an agreement here to withhold the evidence of the uncodifiable aspects of sense, marking off what is nonrational or irrational and unreliable, and therefore nonfactual. Verghese's medical knowledge is broadened and complicated by his more porous spatial orientation and at the same time looks less like what is professionally considered factual or procedural medical knowledge. In the modern framework, what is withheld is nonevident in rhetorical power, reinforcing among other things the separation of moral agency from the relations of places, including the relations of bodies, and also underwriting cross-referenced dualisms of geometric and inhabited space, idea and material, mind and body. As universal and incontrovertible, this notion of perception is not subject to evaluation; perception's epistemology is separated from ethics because its facticity is considered so unstable (Code 1995, 49–50). Still, ethics and epistemology have shared the rhetorical-spatial figuration of the normative male as the perceiver, the thinker, and the moral agent. Code looks to space and location as ways to reconsider the broader realms of perception and the connections between how we know and how we value and evaluate, enabling her to consider who it is who knows and who it is who cares, as well as what it is that counts as knowledge.

If locations help identify senses in expanded philosophical notions of perception and its knowing, notions of performance and practice help identify the enacted life of locations. Michel de Certeau distinguishes place as the stable and inert co-existence of things from place relations or space as "the intersections of mobile elements," which is dependent on numerous variables that in effect produce it (de Certeau 1984, 117). Place becomes alive and active through spatial relations and so becomes ambiguous and indeterminate. It is not clear what de Certeau would do with the possibility suggested by Abram that what appear to be inert places have life in their own animating variables, including those of withdrawal and absence. But de Certeau's notion of places as performed spaces destabilizes the quasi-Platonist phenomenology that guides Abram's orientation of an original fit between individual and place. Instead, de Certeau's approach indicates the rhetorical and thus indeterminate character of sense-knowing as speakers and audiences and places engage each other. His perspective provides ways to consider how such engagements happen as a way of doing ethics that articulates interactions and infusions of locating-responding-listening, so that medical ethics is not something that appears to come from nowhere, nor is it the transparent, positivist result of somewhere. Instead, we can consider the place relations of medical ethics, including the rhetorical spatial relations of bodies, particularly the extensions and alterations of bodies in touch.

BODIES AS SITES OF TOUCH

Whether or not touch, as Diane Ackerman claims, is the oldest sense, touch not only extends the world (including coming up against limits), but also makes us aware that the world is three-dimensional in arrangement and variegated in texture (Ackerman 1990, 80, 94). Because many in the hospital are wary of touching people with AIDS, Verghese's ease and sometimes aggressive willingness to touch his patients when all others have distanced themselves (Verghese 1994, 180) indicate that touch articulates multiple place relations of presence and absence. Percussing the body of any patient is Verghese's first, most trusted practice as his hand reaches out to extend both bodies, his and the patient's, to sense and be sensed (Verghese 1994, 416–17). Percussing, the process of feeling what is going on in the body through drumming the fingers across its surfaces, could be identified philosophically as "haptic." In discourse theory, haptic refers to culturally variant uses of body contact to communicate (Kinneavy 1971, 23), a referent that helps loosen and also relies on the Platonic lineage of haptic as the knowledge given and received through awareness of movement within the body and of the body through space, in the interstices of its habitation (Walter 1988, 134).

Verghese's calculated risks in touching would put doctors less trained more at risk (Levine 1991, 208); surgeons sometimes accept his offer to accompany them when operating on AIDS patients. His wife Rajani cautions him to wash his hands, feeling a continuous fear for him, herself, and their young children, which Verghese later realizes he intentionally and insensitively ignored as he enacted the doctor-hero and suppressed his own fears of infection. For associating with his patients, he is shunned by many of his colleagues. The continuous presence of death makes the sexual advances of a female secretary more tempting. These performances of touch take place not with a generalized body but with specific, felt bodies, what Adrienne Rich calls "the geography closest in" (Rich 1986, 212). Even in their separations and tensions, medicine and ethics share in the production of a deracinated approach to which Verghese's experiences of bodies are irrelevant or irrational: his need to touch his patients' bodies to find out what is going on, the dangers of infection, the pleasure of touch to sense and to explore, the capacities of touch to evoke and to account for, the pariah status of his patients, the pariah status he often feels from his colleagues and his wife, the denial of touch in resisting a weekend fling.

Any placement of bodies is some kind of touching. Maurice Drury takes to heart his former teacher Wittgenstein's recommendation to sit down by the patient's bed as a practicing physician instead of assuming the authoritarian pose of standing over it (Drury 1996, 154). Daniel Baxter, writing of his AIDS patients at the Spellman Center for HIV Related Disease in New York City, speaks of the need for physicians to know when touch better takes over from verbal language (Baxter 1997, 235). Even with sensitive doctors, there are places where people may recoil from contact invasive to their manner of bodily habitation. John Sassal notes a patient's discomfort where he pushes a needle into his chest at a spot that should have been relatively painless. The man responds: " 'That's where I live, where you're putting that needle in.' 'I know,' Sassal said, 'I know what it feels like. I can't bear anything done near my eyes. . . . I think that's where I live, just under and behind my eyes' " (Berger 1967, 50). Yet we also smooth our hands or clasp ourselves in search of comfort, or may even go to the doctor "to be patted, stroked, listened to, inspected, handled" (Ackerman 1990, 119–20), a part of healing unavailable when a doctor refuses to touch or touches inappropriately.

As a mode of persuasion, touching is rhetorical and the touching of one body to another need not include the "literal," which may prevent healing. In the Hmong community, the shaman discerns without direct touch, his own body mediating as he works with the ill person's body fully clothed, in contrast to the undressing and the touching of United States hospital examinations and treatment procedures that so offend the Hmong people who live here (Fadiman 1997). This is also the case with the Maori, whose attention to dreams prompts notions of bicultural medical ethics among doctors in New Zealand (Campbell, Gillett, and Jones 1992, 166–67). When illness and healing are understood in terms of balance, direct attention to the soul or spirit is necessary, with or without Western medicine.

All of these registers articulate knowledge and experience that indicate the mixture and mobility of sense, emotion, intellect, physicality, and spirit in the body. The consequent unraveling of the material and immaterial duality of the mind-body opposition contests the notion that the mind is the locus of productive knowledge that can be applied to a physical site such as the body, which is itself unable to produce knowledge—though the body may thwart the mind. Postmodern reversals in which bodily desire is the locus of all knowing assume the same dualism as modern associations of bodies with feelings considered private, mute, and antithetical to the public, discursive intellect (Cooey 1994, 44–47). Feminists have argued that the dualism of knowing and feeling, intellect and body, are attained in and posited by the reified gaze of theory that is imbued with the authority to grant productivity to its object only when the object is completely subsumed by the theory's power; the gaze of law grants recognition to its object only when it is fully compliant with technical regulation.

De Certeau argues that all law is inscribed on bodies, and he observes a current shifting from legal notions of individuals to medical notions of well-being (de Certeau 1984, 139–42). This problem is what Michel Foucault has in mind when he argues that, in post-Enlightenment medical-moral practices, bodies are sites of control and obedience, their "docility" part of the micropower of the institutional life of the healthy and the good (Foucault 1979, 136–37). In Foucault's analysis, feminism and homosexuality are among the resistances that disrupt these institutions (Foucault 1977, 216). But the life and death of any one body resists Foucault's own tendency to portray bodies as transparent objects of knowledge that divide the overseeing consciousness from the institutional-bodily struggle for power and control (see de Certeau 1984, 62–64). Still, Foucault makes clear that post-Enlightenment disciplinary knowledge entails rhetorical-spatial categories that do not leave out the body, as is sometimes argued, but order bodies and suppress those that resist regimes of moral, legal, and medical control (Foucault 1973).

Infused with other senses, touching extends and is extended by language, becoming what Abram, following Merleau-Ponty, calls "the flesh of language" (Abram 1996, 73). These gestures join others in the micro-ordering of bodies that Foucault has in mind. They also meet each other in momentary co-extensions of the participation that Abram has in mind. Abram describes iterating in bodily senses the experience of learning to ride a bike while watching another and so feeling not just what his body remembers, but what the other person is feeling, a process that can be refined as we get to know another person or place (Abram 1996, 126–27). For Abram such experiences seem to entail some kind of inherent moral quality regarding how we relate to living beings. This quality is more specified in the idea of co-extension present in Diana Fritz Cates's account of her own body lurching out to join her young daughter Hannah's as the child falls (Cates 1997, 140–41). Cates is arguing for a less remote notion of compassion that includes a more expansive sense of self coming forward in particular attention to *"this* (God-related) person's" suffering (226). The experience with Hannah pushes the notion of compassion into murkier terrain with the displacement and re-placement of boundaries of self and the desires and perceptions of this "mess of feelings in immediate complacency" (150), which participate in what Cates calls "well-empassioned thinking" (196).

It is, by Abram's account, not only in humans with other humans that co-extension can take place; nothing is without the possibility of participation. "Every phenomenon, in other words, is potentially expressive" (Abram 1996, 81). Everything is potentially touching-speaking-listening to everything else. Abram, again drawing on Merleau-Ponty, speaks of the spontaneity of sensory events, which may collaborate in various ways, but he also speaks as if there is only one way for events to combine, only one way for participation to take place, bringing aspects of Foucault again to mind. Abram acknowledges that language carries the experience both directions— expressing place and reworking the sense of place—but there is no debate about the character of these moments of joining that appear to be composed of univocal claims of what is true for that moment. In this space of unity and totality, no alternative or error appears to be possible, except that of not participating; or perhaps error and alternative are irrelevant. Foucault and Abram intensify and codify senses of place with their respective considerations of humans as part of an ancient life-world and a modern institutional one; each has a tendency to assign social and moral symmetry to the rhetorical activity of place, so that people are, in different valences, either participating or alienated (Abram), obedient or resistant (Foucault). Yet places are rough and unfinished, and the registers of natural co-extensions and institutional environments are multiple and embedded in each other in the particular ways of any one moment of touching. The hotel staff watches with disapproval as writer Fenton Johnson assists his weakened partner Larry from the dining room during their last few days together before Larry's death of AIDS in Paris (Johnson 1996, 182). When Gordon Vines dies at home, their family funeral director balks at preparing his body for burial; an indignant Essie finds someone else (Verghese 1994, 149).

VICKIE AND CLYDE McCRAY'S FRONT PORCH

One day, Verghese drives on up the highway to visit Vickie and Clyde McCray in Tester Hollow. Tester Hollow is north of Johnson City, off state route 11-E. This whole area is lower in elevation than the Blue Ridge, but higher than the valley and ridge province that gradually flattens out into the Appalachian Plateau. From Verghese's account of Vickie's directions, I imagine that the McCrays lived in the foothills of Holston Mountain, between the Holston and Watauga Rivers, a drive that on that fall afternoon would have been shockingly beautiful.

Clyde McCray is seriously ill with AIDS; his symptoms include a dementia of childhood regression. Vickie, diagnosed as HIV-positive, has taken charge of his care while raising their two children and holding a full-time job at Pet Dairy. As a result of Clyde's illness a new family arrangement has emerged: Clyde in his deterioration becomes the baby, his young son becomes his brother, Vickie assumes the position of head of household, and her daughter becomes the mother (Verghese 1994, 139). When Verghese arrives, Clyde is asleep. After the tour she volunteers to give of their modest trailer, Vickie McCray and Abe Verghese sit on the front porch talking about and letting go of her anger about Clyde's infidelities and infection with AIDS, her subsequent infection, and their difficult life in the small community of the hollow. Vickie's forthright speech carries the strength of her body, personality, and the local manner, and Verghese is a good listener. In addition, one senses the camaraderie that can develop as patient and doctor support each other in a demanding situation. Sitting on the porch is peaceful, and Verghese takes in the play of light and shadow on its wooded surroundings, as he and Vickie smoke and talk (208–13).

Many aspects comprise this moment that are not conventionally part of medical ethics and that a spatial-rhetorical perspective helps locate. Everyone knows that doctors do not make house calls, much less sit on makeshift porches, except in old movies. As a specialist, Verghese has little to offer as he responds to Vickie's keen analytic description of Clyde's changing condition and decline. The conversation is outside the place-and-time relations of an office appointment, a procedure, or a decision, lacking the more generally agreed upon means of rhetorical exchange between doctor and patient, ethicist and doctor, patient and ethicist. The conversation slowly gives itself shape, starting in easy quiet, and then stumbling into temporary awkwardness that feeds the momentum of Vickie's story of her and Clyde's relationship, the person who infected Clyde, and relationships with neighbors and family whose homophobia and fear of infection have left her with almost no help. On the porch, Vickie McCray and Abe Verghese are involved in a conversation that sticks to the bone and places neither in an exclusive role, confusing ready associations of rational knowledge with the masculine and nurture with the feminine: Vickie is an analyst of Clyde's illness, a breadwinner, a patient, and care taker; Verghese is an analyst of disease and patterns of infection, concerned about his patients and about how they, with cooperation and antagonism of family and friends, manage from day to day (Verghese 1994, 214–18). The domestic context is nonbourgeois; Vickie and Clyde have struggled to support life in a trailer that would only express transience by middle-class standards and whose porch evades bourgeois divisions of public and private. As extension and juncture, the porch's edge reaches out from the house to the hollow and the hills that encompass it. The Appalachians are the oldest mountain range on this continent. In looking at them, one feels the comfort and mystery of their relative stability—how well they protect and isolate their inhabitants, how well they are known among the different groups that have long traversed them, and how well they keep their secrets to themselves.

The moral uptake of this situation could be accounted for with a rhetoric of care often characterized as attention to relationship. Perspectives about care have been a primary way feminists have argued against the orientations of an individualistic autonomy, claiming that both medicine and ethics need healing in their isolated, alienated stances toward life and in their oppressive power relations (Holmes 1989, 3–4). Care presents a context that begins with the assumption of connections to be met with appropriate responses, instead of radical individuality that must be adjudicated in terms of the rights of separation and authority. Feminists have also argued that in its segmentation of the doctor-patient relationship, medical ethics has isolated itself from its own politics. The rhetoric of autonomy and choice masks the larger problem of offering women an unacceptable range of choices in the first place—for example, with reproductive technologies—and of overriding or negating women's presence in medical situations with the rhetoric of scientific and moral authority (Sherwin 1989, 62–63).

The lack of critical attention to the political claims of moral claims also pertains to feminist articulations inasmuch as they present care as unproblematic and complete. Vickie McCray and Abraham Verghese would supply one more confirming example of something already understood and spoken for, except that neither of them fits the gender, class, and racial figures of these categories. The question is not only one of a political-moral critique, however, but also one of how that moment is morally performed, which involves rhetorical-spatial relations more heterogenous than any single, controlling noun such as care.

The modern moral rhetoric of care emerges in oppositional and complementary figures with nineteenth-century notions of judgment, reason, and justice. Together they constitute the dominant cultural referents of moral performance across various distinctions and divisions, such as charity and philanthropy, missions and welfare, domesticity and marketplace (Smith 1988), by which care is located and relocated. The relations of care are complicated and its moral authority destabilized in a number of current studies that analyze difficulties of care as a moral referent, some of which are part of the misfit of care with Vickie McCray and Abe Verghese. Emily Townes looks to a wider range of discourses from African American institutions in tension with the neglect of African Americans in white institutions of medical care (see also Schulman 1999) and the legacies of care in relations of slavery and servitude (Townes 1997). Joan Tronto argues that care must be placed critically in its moral and political power relations (1994), though she continues to give care the authority "to account for all need" (Tronto 1995, 144). Paul Lauritzen criticizes the association of moral care with child bearing and raising that continues a romantic and narrow basis for an ethic, inasmuch as it identifies agency and goodness exclusively with biological motherhood (Lauritzen 1989, 39). From another perspective, the narrowness and romanticism are part of the capitalist regulation of the erotic, as Jane Gallop argues; care is a demand for order and obedience, a depletion of pleasure that never runs rapid, or spills over, or surprises (Gallop 1988, 117).

These difficulties expand and reconfigure moral spaces regarding the who, what, and how of moral activity, identifying the impulse to tidy things up too quickly from either a homogenous, unreflective view of experience, what Lauritzen calls "experiential foundationalism" (Lauritzen 1997, 97), or the pressure to reach a smooth conclusion, as if the place relations of care have never been established or were made stable and predictable by being assigned domestic locations. Life in places, however, is never completely certain, and even the predictable qualities of places often take us by surprise. The upper-middle-class, divorced woman who asks Verghese if he will care for her ill son, whom she wants to bring home from California, comes to the doctor's office in secrecy because of her longtime friends' derogatory comments about gay men (Verghese 1994, 324). Even home ownership and class status do not protect her position in the face of illness, nondominant sexuality, and death. In his "concrete metaphysics" of household spaces, Bachelard locates the unsettled qualities of place in the imagination that is forever restless and in the mobility of identity in memory, dream, association, and the gestures through which one moves about a house: "But is he who opens a door and he who closes it the same being?" (Bachelard 1994, 224). The indeterminate qualities of what might be considered most certain—family and home—are antithetical to a notion of ethics as the stable point beyond the fray, but we cannot perform morally without the fray and the questions it raises about who we are and what we are doing.

Wittgenstein derides philosophers for retreating to the "icy surface" of removed generalities, away from the "rough ground" of experience whose friction challenges idealizations about what something is and how to respond to it (Wittgenstein 1968, 107). The locus of "rough ground" is an argument against naive empiricism, with its narrow view of particulars, and naive rationalism, with its universal view of overarching rules. Human activity, from Wittgenstein's perspective, is neither transparent nor unavailable by some prior philosophical commitment. Instead, we poke around, look at things, pay attention, exercise curiosity, try something out, discard it, walk around the next corner. We bring dispositions, habits, and other experiences that may or may not work; we have to find out. Wittgenstein would commit none of this to ethics per se, but I would, along with the outlook that the difficulties of finding one's way may result in a variety of moral rhetorics that take shape as they are performed.

One could understand medical ethics as an activity that brings order to the fragmentation and intensity of experiences by leaving the rough ground, but this view assumes the moral-epistemological unproductivity of places and contexts as impediments to the medical and the ethical. In the hospital, the institutions of science, medicine, and ethics come together, not as one voice, but in a rhetoric of opposition that is itself part of an agreement about the negotiations of expertise and the performances of authority. Science, medicine, and ethics define the rhetorical situation in a jostling of shared and cross-referential signs indicating conditions of placelessness and designating the moral and the material. I am not arguing for a resolved medical ethic, nor am I arguing that the current approach is without effectiveness. Medical ethics by definition will always entail tension, a factor that contributes to people's fascination with medical-moral dilemmas portrayed on television.

My point is that many tensions in current articulations of medicine, science, and ethics also articulate consensus about the spatial and rhetorical terms by which medical ethics and its arguments are produced, terms that may work to the detriment of patients, as part of the "good" being done. Medical ethics can benefit everyone involved; its articulations may be crucial. But it can also contribute to the regulation of patients and those close to them within the place relations of health care institutions for which ethics can be one more way to extend their control, even in the altruism of volunteers who carry out narrow regulations of state HIV/AIDS programs (Patton 1989, 123) or the image of comforters who cannot face the physical, bodily placed experience of death (Bronski 1989, 226).

Consider further the exchange between Vickie McCray and Abe Verghese on Vickie's porch as the production of medical ethics. One could parse the situation as a fulfillment of responsibilities and obligations or the precursor to a series of principled decisions or an attempt to invoke a greater good. One could parse the situation as an expression of responsiveness, attention, mutuality, and support. One could argue for the applicability of narrative, of a story within a story, as Vickie relates her own story to Verghese, who at the end encourages her and Clyde to join the local support group (eventually they do). But this would assign the performance of ethical activity to the evocation of a group of nouns, instead of a rhetorical situation of strangeness and friendliness, Vickie's bravado amidst her fears, Verghese's anxiety about the limits of what he as a doctor can do, the pleasure of sitting on the porch, the comfort and alienation of the hollow. Consider that whatever we would call medical ethics in this moment comes as these different registers of place in their specific intersections. Registers of place are not an accompaniment to the moral but help constitute it.

Sitting on the porch in the hollow challenges codes of ordering here, sidesteps them there. In going to see Vickie and Clyde, Verghese leaves the institutional place relations of modern professional activity and its complementary site of middle-class domesticity. As a formulation of their activity, the idea of care giver and care taker could be combined in Vickie, and the idea of autonomy and care in Verghese, but the ordering functions of these are displaced by their attribution of moral disorder to the nonwhite and nonbourgeois. What emerges is a rhetorical sorting and sifting in which the exigency of the moment gains language and sensation, falters, and moves on, or just hangs there, as Verghese "hears Vickie to speech," in the words of Nelle Morton, whose family home in Holston Mountain would have been not too far away (Morton 1985, 54–55). Vickie also hears Verghese in his need for information, his desire to help, and his desire to feel at home. There is no summary to this moment of sorting out life, living with death, and pondering how to go on. Light, dark, and shadow are not suppressed or condensed as is so often the case in the hospital, but participate more freely as a topistic diet. The rhetorical-topistic moment articulates whatever "there" refers to, to produce its moral geography.

THE CONNECTION

Periodically, Verghese works with local Red Cross director and activist Olivia Sells to present information about AIDS in public venues. Early in Verghese's years in Johnson City, where Sells grew up, they arrange to hold a program at The Connection, the one public place in the region for gay men to hang out, drink, and dance. The evening of the talk, Verghese is nervous about being seen anywhere near The Connection, much less going into the bar, located near the university and adjacent to a popular middle- and upper-middle-class neighborhood; he stops circling the block only when he sees Olivia arrive. About twenty people come into the back room, while others linger at the doorway for the information video, the talk, and the question period. A number later come to the Medical Center for testing, all with negative results. After the program, Verghese remains for a while and observes the flirtation and anxiety that mark the crowded outer room (Verghese 1994, 63–68). The bar scene intimidates him, and his initial nervousness returns after he leaves the rhetorical space of expertise that the presentation creates. Looking on from a corner table, Verghese senses the negotiation of identity going on among these men, and also among his own registers of professional, familial, migrant, and sexual situatedness.

Again, Verghese is not in the customary spaces in which medical ethics is produced, though in joining Olivia Sells in public health work, he iterates earlier, turn of the century approaches to illness that preceded scientific medicine (Starr 1982). Those approaches more often assumed the doctor-patient relation as one of doctor-patient-community, which Grant Gillett identifies as the trio at issue in medical ethics. Gillett argues that AIDS in particular confronts doctors with the need to get over their upper-middle-class sexual prejudices and enlist the help of their patients in extending health care into the community (Gillett 1989, 31). Even as Verghese does this, he recalls during the evening at The Connection his homophobic fears of his first HIV/AIDS work in Boston, and he will wonder later if his now more opened egalitarianism merely hides a deeper prejudice regarding his patients' self-worth and fear of losing his own self-worth in his associations with this community (Verghese 1994, 253). Verghese is drawn to borders, as if re-enacting his own migrations provides the most familiar orientation, yet this border—the turf of gay men—disorients him, and he is relieved to return home.

The Connection is well advertised, and men travel from some distance to get to the place, which later changed its name and moved to a larger building closer to a nexus of regional roads and major highways connecting

Tennessee, North Carolina, Kentucky, West Virginia, and Virginia. Patterns of travel and migration are important in tracing the coming of AIDS to the Appalachian highlands, and in his research Verghese finds the paths cut by talented, young men who leave the region in order to live their lives more freely, only to return as they become ill with a fatal infection from life in the cities on which they had staked their hopes (Verghese 1994, 400–3). For some men the migration went only as far as the partner who had been out of the region and returned; for some as far as a regional truck stop on the interstate highway; some returned ill after a period of liberation in a large city only to barely make it home; some returned to cruel isolation; some returned grateful to leave city life behind and reclaim the region as home with their families who may have gulped hard, but welcomed them; and some returned with no regrets and a keen sense of the ironies of migration that had provided many gay men with what they saw as far more sophisticated notions of beauty and of human behavior than those heterosexual men whose performance of masculinity left them unable to create any aesthetic of life and, above all, left them dependent on their hatred of gay men (Verghese 1994, 252).

Such migrations belie simple claims about the moral goodness of home and community (Sandoval 1993). And, as with other modern and older migrations, adventure and the moral, educational, and aesthetic gifts of travel are neither discounted nor disconnected, even in the face of death. In Walter's consideration of sickness and "placeways," he observes that for human beings since the agricultural revolution, plague has been an illness of one place to another, involving transit routes within and between towns, tiny organisms, and human bodies (Walter 1988, 45–47). Migration is existentially familiar to Verghese, who came to the United States for advanced medical education and sits in The Connection with his green card marked "foreign alien" (Verghese 1994, 58). As an Indian who grew up and first trained medically in Addis Ababa, Ethiopia, he is aware of the distance of his parents' Indian and Syrian Christian household from the local culture he observed as a child on daily bicycle travels (Verghese 1998, 23–28). In the United States, he worked for a year as an orderly before finding through Greyhound Bus travels an acceptable intern placement. He knows he figures in the ethnic hierarchy feeding hospitals in the United States, which attracts the most ambitious from other countries and then hires them on the low ends of the American health care system (Verghese 1994, 279; 1997, 70–88).

Verghese is a configuration of many situations that identify him with transactions at once large scale and small in the migratory life of his patients and himself, with their stable and unstable points of fixity and motion: the persistence of homophobia, the thrill of sexual encounter, the need to hide, the desire to love, the lure of freer bodies and cities, the burdens of economic survival, the push for education, the trip home, the search for home, the infection that has no cure, the fears and experiences of death. Easy distinctions between local and global fall away in the transit patterns of gay men and transnational doctors. There is a strong Indian community in Johnson City, and a number of Indian doctors work in the area around the hospital where Verghese met Essie Vines. Verghese stops short from time to time, recognizing that just as he is finding himself at home in East Tennessee, he is also set apart by his brown skin, his origins in former colonies, and his work as an internist to which the Indian community, like others, assigns less status than other specialties. Yet the region he has come to call home lives with national judgments that its inhabitants are ignorant and that many suffer from a kind of poverty sometimes called "third world." Fenton Johnson finds himself the object of ridicule for his Kentucky dialect and small-town ways when he goes to Stanford University as a young man to find freedom from sexual prejudice (Johnson 1996, 61). Simultaneously considered depraved and exotic, people from this part of the country negotiate a range of tropes not unlike those associated with inhabitants of a former colony. The placelessness of moral discourse itself is part of colonial relations of disassociation and reassociation by which cultural-geographic referents appear not to exist at all (Ross 1993) or to circulate in naturalistic relations of how cultural production does and does not occur in figures of novelty, entertainment, stupidity, intelligence, creativity, isolation, and refuge.

In moral theory, when notions of how moral activity happens are articulated as the application of moral principle or example onto the situation, each aspect—application, moral, and situation—is decontextualized, suppressing the contexts by which they are already enmeshed in each other. De-contextualization is the kind of place and rhetorical performance that has been identified as the abstraction necessary for systematically thinking about morality and establishing other kinds of knowledge, taken so habitually to be the rhetorical situation of theorizing that even a committed theory, such as that of care, easily loses its rough and contested grounds. Verghese, Olivia Sells, and the patrons in the bar are in an unexpected space in the existence of the bar at all and in its medical performance. The point is not only that spaces considered outside medical institutions are morally significant for medicine and ethics, but that spaces actively reconfigure in varying ways moral notions of self, knowledge, action, and place entailed in any one instance of things that do and do not take place. To pay attention to what has been designated as the unrefined world of appearances involves everything from the speakers'-audiences' exigencies of the back room public health presentation to where to sit in a bar in which the doctor is out of place, to the kinds of moral musings that are prompted about Verghese's relations with his patients, issues that potentially connect ethical studies with ritual studies (J. Smith 1987; Sullivan 1986). This approach is not to dismiss the moral question of Verghese's willingness to go, though it is to recognize that Verghese's willingness is not a simple, segmented moral quality, but a complex, social-moral one embedded with fear and reluctance, and finally pulled forward by Olivia's ease and his own curiosity at an event both medical and exotic. What I want to emphasize even more is the improvisational quality of the evening and the moral images and questions that appear when a site and a particular imagination engage each other.

In modern accounts, moral rhetoric and its place relations not only articulate willing, knowing, and judging, but also articulate rules and orders regarding what is withheld, as if everything that really mattered about ethics were already known and decided. With the emergence of people with HIV/AIDS in Johnson City, Verghese is in a new situation. He comes to it with his cultural histories and memories, his family, and his medical education. Even how to be a good doctor is not clear in this context, nor is it always clear how to be a good patient or family member, partner, or friend. The situation is not one of rhetorical place relations that are out of control; rhetorical habits and place relations are highly patterned, though they must continuously be re-invented and elaborated. Yet sometimes they fail us or falter because we are in a situation we have never been before. Many medical situations are just that; they leave us feeling that we have to recover our ground and that this ground is not ours anymore because something startling has happened. That is why the term "improvisation" in two senses suits so much of what Verghese, his patients, and those associated with them do in the immediacy of events, which are not "put on hold momentarily" to achieve distance (Cates 1997, 196), but are engaged in the moment.

Improvisation in one sense comes with practices so highly developed that one can play off of them, sometimes into virtually another practice. Because one is good at something, one has the flexibility to take it someplace strange, unexpected, and independent. In another sense, improvisation emphasizes working with the stuff of the moment, which may or may not relate to established practices, to the people usually there and what they usually would do. Medical ethics is not the scene of the application of thought; medical ethics is an activity. Medical ethics cannot be identified with one kind of person, one kind of speech, and one kind of space. It is the participation and rhetorical performance of places and people confronted with an event that has to be figured out and lived and possibly died with. What makes the participation specifically moral may be difficult and even unnecessary to define. One of the interesting things about improvisation is that what makes someone good at it may include attributes and practices not officially considered moral. Part of Verghese's effectiveness comes from his curiosity, his impulsiveness, his clinical discipline, and the confluent geographies of migration and work that are at play in his medical-moral practice. With their own improvisations, his patients, their partners, and families engage events they had neither imagined nor prepared for. The Connection may seem like a simple opposite to the Johnson City Medical Center, but the back room of the HIV/AIDS talk and the front room of the dancing play on each other as sites of uncertainty and invention for the doctor and the group of men who happened to be there that night.

RE-SITUATING MEDICAL ETHICS

The concerns that Wittgenstein expresses regarding experience are well-taken regarding place relations: to consider terrain without reaching for naive empiricism with its narrow view of particulars or for naive rationalism with its universal view of overarching rules (Wittgenstein 1968, 402). To consider *My Own Country* as a performance of medical ethics is not to recommend it as a statement of universal practice or as a group of variables in predictable relations of causality. Spatial-rhetorical orientations evade these kinds of determinism, the complete freedom from place that is considered productive on metaphysically ultimate terms and the complete boundedness to place that is considered unproductive on metaphysically inert terms. What one finds instead is not a serial list of features that modify the nouns of place or agency, but fields of activity including the still activities of waiting, silence, introspection, and reception, the suppression of activity, and resistance activity, and including figures of self-transforming and self-diminishing activity. This seems perhaps not to be ethics but to be something else; yet place relations have that quality of suggesting something else— the thought out of nowhere, the loose tendrils of situations, the expected and unexpected qualities that spaces and people produce.

Amidst their argument that the emergence of the primary care physician entails rejecting older practices of medical authority, Harmon Smith and Larry Churchill stop to inject that they are not making the case for a physician who is simply easy to get along with, but without expertise; the doctor sitting beside your bed can be pleasant and incompetent (Smith and Churchill 1986, 44). But patients still cannot count on the most minimal of human civilities from doctors, and more to the point of my argument, we do not have adequate ways of accounting for what goes on morally when doctors and patients attend well to such relations. In Verghese's practice we are able to see how rhetorical-spatial relations of illness and medicine are active in and beyond the hospital, not because he gives guidelines for what to do, but because he goes out to have a look around, nudged by his commitment to bedside doctoring, to AIDS as a community issue, to his own interest and research, and to his search for home and for the next place.

Several things shift in medical ethics. The most obvious is the site. As a patient, Gordon Vines challenges the site assumptions of modern hospitals because HIV/AIDS has no cure and its infectious qualities are not well understood. He also challenges the site of modern ethics because he is not a regular candidate for autonomy in society at large. Interestingly, he may also experience autonomy in its senses of respect, dignity, and exchange of information to a greater degree in the hospital than outside it, given the right doctor, X-ray technician, or nurse. Verghese's office becomes a context of social service efforts, as when he and his nurse try to find a desperate patient a job; and of resistance, as when he begins to read the radical medical journals of his most activist patient. It is a site of secrecy as parents, partners, and patients begin to put together medical histories fragmented by lives lived covertly and often far from home. The places of kitchen table, front porch, and bar are thus not the only participating spaces in re-situating medical ethics; any place involved with HIV/AIDS is recontextualized.

With shifting sites, the rhetorical activity shifts. The ownership arrangements of language change by default, opposition, and living where one has not been before. Fresh moral discourse emerges in new rhetorical situations. Decisions are not always the orienting rhetorical frame of moral activity, which can instead address how to get through the day, the feeling of getting to speak and of being heard, the sorting of self in pondering one's relationships, the willingness to sit and spend time, to do things that "waste time" and that may happen in nonprofessional spaces or can radically change the character of professional space. Agencies and places shift as they mediate each other. Loci for the production of medical ethics are diffuse, not only because of their infusion with all kinds of personal-economic-political relations, but also because the events to which they speak are among the most far-reaching of human experiences.

In recent years my two sisters and I spent time at the Johnson City Medical Center with one or the other of our parents. In trying to care properly for our parents, we used every resource we could find, including my medical ethicist colleague, Thomas Shannon, but also including doctors, nurses, ward staff, social workers, ministers, extended family, and the steadfast friends from my parents' fifty years in that one town. Sometimes we were making decisions, sometimes we were figuring things out, sometimes we were waiting, sometimes we were being there; always, my sisters, brother-in-law, parents, and myself were groping. Certainly there were moments when explicit decisions had to be made—the most identifiable situation in the dominant rhetorical practices of medical ethics. At those moments we needed good information and people with whom to mull things over. We also needed a sense of the medical and moral language used in hospitals these days—though even as an ethicist I found myself translating that language not just into the situation, but into something more flexible and capacious to be able to sense our parents' wishes about extraordinary care, their thoughts and feelings about how they wish to die, their dismay and disorientation at their dependency, their changing relations with their sensory-reasoning selves, their house, their neighbors, the Medical Center.

Even the moment of decision never stands alone; it is invaded by all others that brought you there and that immediately take you to the next place. The nodal points of moral performance shift and turn, flatten and re-form somewhere else, as you find your way, and then are immediately moved along to where you have never been before, to a place that was not even a "where" before. The question is not only one of ordering versus resistance, but also of how to work with what is going on, the question that haunts every day of any extended illness and raises every kind of question of living and dying—a territory much too large and rough to be limited to the rhetorical-spatial practices that have dominated much of medical ethics and ethics itself.

Lucy Lippard reconfigures the deep ecologists' term "bioregionalism" to convey the combination of shifting human populations and land and water masses with their life forms, and the ways in which a region's inhabitants identify it, not as a subject of study, but as a dwelling (Lippard 1997, 35). For her, the term indicates the presence of multicenters to express many contemporary individuals' significant connections with multiple places, and I would add, with the many places of any one place. Bioregional seems one way to imagine reconstituting ethics as an activity that always goes on somewhere, even as that "somewhere" diffuses and mingles with the "where" around the curve and the "where" at the corner on the left-hand side. The vectors are not the above and below of theory and matter, which themselves come with bioregions being staked out and having the stakes pulled out from under them. This figure is not a solution or a resolution, but it is an approach to medical ethics that does not start with a priori connections or disconnections, with answers only to be applied or applications only to be reproduced. The production of medical ethics happens every day as doctors and other health care workers, patients, friends, partners, and families make, find, and find themselves in places, ask questions, receive fine to acceptable to awful answers, tolerate a great deal of uncertainty and sometimes of certainty, and compose gestures both subtle and bold.

References

Abram, David. 1996. *The Spell of the Sensuous*. New York: Vintage Books.

Ackerman, Diane. 1990. *A Natural History of the Senses*. New York: Random House.

Bachelard, Gaston. 1994. *The Poetics of Space*. Boston: Beacon.

Baxter, Daniel. 1997. *The Least of These My Brethren: A Doctor's Story of Hope and Miracles on an Inner-City AIDS Ward*. New York: Harmony Books.

Berger, John. 1967. *A Fortunate Man: The Story of a Country Doctor*. New York: Vintage Books.

Bronski, Michael. 1989. Death and the Erotic Imagination. In *Taking Liberties: AIDS and Cultural Politics*, ed. Erica Carter and Simon Watney, 119–228. London: Serpent's Tail.

Campbell, Alastair, Grant Gillett, and Gareth Jones. 1992. *Practical Medical Ethics*. Auckland: Oxford University Press.

Cates, Diana Fritz. 1997. *Choosing to Feel*. Notre Dame, Ind.: University of Notre Dame Press.

de Certeau, Michel. 1984. *The Practice of Everyday Life,* trans. Steven Rendall. Berkeley: University of California Press.

Code, Lorraine. 1995. *Rhetorical Spaces: Essays on Gendered Locations*. New York: Routledge.

Cooey, Paula. 1994. *Religious Imagination and the Body: A Feminist Analysis*. New York: Oxford University Press.

Drury, M. O'C. 1996. *The Danger of Words and Writings on Wittgenstein*. Bristol, England: Thoemmes.

Elliot, Carl. 1992. Where Ethics Comes from and What to Do About It. *Hastings Center Report* 22 (July-August): 28–35.

Fadiman, Anne. 1997. *The Spirit Catches You and You Fall Down: A Hmong Child, Her American Doctors, and the Collision of Two Cultures.* New York: Farrar, Straus, and Giroux.

Foucault, Michel. 1973. *The Birth of the Clinic,* trans. Alan Sheridan. New York: Pantheon.

———. 1977. *Language, Counter-Memory, Practice: Selected Essays and Interviews,* trans. Donald F. Bouchard and Sherry Simon. Ithaca, N.Y.: Cornell University Press.

———. 1979. *Discipline and Punish: The Birth of the Prison,* trans. Alan Sheridan. New York: Vintage Books.

Gallop, Jane. 1988. *Thinking Through the Body.* New York: Columbia University Press.

Gillett, Grant. 1989. *Reasonable Care.* New York: St. Martins.

Grant, Jacquelyn. 1993. The Sin of Servanthood. In *A Troubling in my Soul,* ed. Emily Townes, 199–218. Maryknoll: Orbis.

Holmes, Helen Bequaert. 1989. A Call to Heal Medicine. *Hypatia* 4 (summer): 1–8.

Johnson, Fenton. 1996. *Geography of the Heart: A Memoir.* New York: Scribner.

Kinneavy, James. 1971. *A Theory of Discourse.* New York: Norton.

Lauritzen, Paul. 1989. A Feminist Ethic and the New Romanticism—Mothering as a Model of Moral Relations. *Hypatia* 4 (summer): 29–44.

———. 1997. Hear No Evil, See No Evil, Think No Evil: Ethics and the Appeal to Experience. *Hypatia* 12 (spring): 83–104.

Levine, Robert J. 1991. AIDS and the Physician-Patient Relationship. In *AIDS and Ethics,* ed. Frederic G. Reamer, 188–211. New York: Columbia University Press.

Lippard, Lucy. 1983. *Overlay.* New York: Pantheon

———. 1997. *The Lure of the Local: Senses of Place in a Multicentered Society.* New York: The New Press.

Morton, Nelle. 1985. *The Journey Is Home.* Boston: Beacon.

Patton, Cindy. 1989. The AIDS Industry: Construction of "Victims," "Volunteers" and "Experts." In *Taking Liberties: AIDS and Cultural Politics,* ed. Erica Carter and Simon Watney, 113–25. London: Serpent's Tail.

Rich, Adrienne. 1986. Notes Toward a Politics of Location. In *Blood, Break, and Poetry: Selected Prose 1979–1985,* 210–31. New York: Norton.

Ross, Kristin. 1993. Rimbaud and Spatial History. In *Space and Place: Theories of Identity and Location,* ed. Erica Carter, James Donald, and Judith Squires, 357–77. London: Lawrence and Wishart.

Sandoval, Alberto. 1993. Dios bendiga nuestro hogar. *Un Piso Trece Gay* 2 (September/December): 13.

Schama, Simon. 1995. *Landscape and Memory.* New York: Vintage Books.

Schulman, Kevin A. et al. 1999. The Effect of Race and Sex on Physicians' Recommendations for Cardiac Catheterization. *New England Journal of Medicine* 340 (February 25): 618–26.

Sherwin, Susan. 1989. Feminist and Medical Ethics: Two Different Approaches to Contextual Ethics. *Hypatia* 4 (summer): 57–72.

Smith, Harmon L., and Larry Churchill. 1986. *Professional Ethics and Primary Care Medicine: Beyond Dilemmas and Decorum.* Durham: Duke University Press.

Smith, Jonathan Z. 1987. *To Take Place: Toward Theory in Ritual.* Chicago: University of Chicago Press.

Smith, Ruth. 1988. Moral Transcendence and Moral Space. *Journal of Feminist Studies in Religion* 4 (fall): 21–37.

————. 1997–1998. Negotiating Homes: Morality as a Scarce Good. *Cultural Critique* 38 (winter): 177–95.

Sontag, Susan. 1990. *Illness as Metaphor and AIDS and its Metaphors.* New York: Doubleday.

Spretnak, Charlene. 1991. *States of Grace: The Recovery of Meaning in the Postmodern Age.* San Francisco: Harper.

Starr, Paul. 1982. *The Social Transformation of American Medicine.* New York: Basic Books.

Sullivan, Lawrence E. 1986. Sound and Senses: Toward a Hermeneutics of Performance. *History of Religions* 26 (August): 1–33.

Townes, Emily M. 1997. "The Doctor Ain't Taking No Sticks": Race and Medicine in the African American Community. *Embracing the Spirit: Womanist Perspectives on Hope, Salvation and Transformation,* ed. Emily M. Townes, 179–94. Maryknoll, NY: Orbis.

Tronto, Joan C. 1994. *Moral Boundaries: A Political Argument for an Ethic of Care.* New York: Routledge.

————. 1995. Care as a Basis for Radical Political Judgments. *Hypatia* 10 (spring): 141–49.

Verghese, Abraham. 1994. *My Own Country: A Doctor's Story.* New York: Vintage Books.

————. 1997. The Cowpath to America. *New Yorker* 73 (June 23 and 30): 70–88.

————. 1998. *The Tennis Partner: A Doctor's Story of Friendship and Loss.* New York: HarperCollins.

Walker, Margaret Urban. 1993. Keeping Moral Space Open: New Images of Ethics Consulting. *Hastings Center Report* 23 (March-April): 33–40.

Walter, E.V. 1988. *Placeways: A Theory of the Human Environment.* Chapel Hill: University of North Carolina Press.

Wittgenstein, Ludwig. 1968. *Philosophical Investigations,* trans. G.E.M. Anscombe. New York: Macmillan.

INDEX